PINNA

Surgery
for the Physician Assistant

Roberto E. Kusminsky, MD
Robert M. Blumm, MA, PA-C

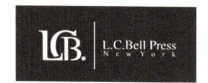

Executive Editor: Laura Kusminsky
Book Design: DesignForBooks.com

Copyright © 2014 by L.C. Bell Press, Ltd.
www.lcbellpress.com
Published by L.C. Bell Press, Ltd.

First Edition

All rights reserved. This book is protected by copyright. No part of this book may be reproduced, stored in a retrieval system, or transmitted in any form or by any means, electronic, mechanical, photocopying, recording, or otherwise, without prior written permission of the publisher. To make inquiries visit www.lcbellpress.com.

ISBN: 978-0-9913169-0-8 (paperback)
ISBN: 978-0-9913169-2-2 (ePub)
ISBN: 978-0-9913169-3-9 (Mobi/Kindle)

Get the right digital edition for your favorite eReader: Get the ePub for iPads and Nook, and Mobi for Kindle and the Sony eReader.

DISCLAIMER

Care has been taken to confirm the accuracy of the information presented and to describe generally accepted practices. However, the authors, editors and publisher are not responsible for errors or omissions or for any consequences from application of the information in this book and make no warranty, expressed or implied, with respect to the currency, completeness, or accuracy of the contents of the publication. Application of this information in a particular situation remains the professional responsibility of the practitioner. The clinical treatments described and recommended may not be considered absolute and universal recommendations.

The authors, editors, and publisher have exerted every effort to ensure that drug selection and dosage set forth in this text are in accordance with the current recommendations and practice at the time of publication. However, in view of ongoing research, changes in government regulations, and the constant flow of information relating to drug therapy and drug reactions, the reader is urged to check the package insert for each drug for any change in indications and dosage and for added warnings and precautions. This is particularly important when the recommended agent is a new or infrequently employed drug.

Some drugs and medical devices presented in this publication have Food and Drug Administration (FDA) clearance for limited use in restricted research settings. It is the responsibility of the health care provider to ascertain the FDA status of each drug or device planned for use in their clinical practice.

To purchase additional copies of this book, visit L.C. Bell Press at www.lcbellpress.com.

1 2 3 4 5 6 7 8 9 10

Contents

Preface   vii

About the Authors   ix

Contributors   xi

Online Access   xv

Topic I: Basic Principles   1

1. Perioperative Care   3
2. Wound Healing and Care   17
3. Common Postoperative Complications   31

Topic II: Endocrine   45

4. Thyroid and Parathyroid   47
   Clinical Keys: Questions and Answers   63
5. Adrenals and Multiple Endocrine Neoplasias   65
   Clinical Keys: Questions and Answers   76

Topic III: Thoracic   79

6. Esophagus   81
   Clinical Keys: Questions and Answers   92
7. Lung   95
   Clinical Keys: Questions and Answers   108

Topic IV: Breast, Skin, and Soft Tissue   111

8. Breast   113
   Clinical Keys: Questions and Answers   126
9. Melanoma, Soft Tissue Infection, and Skin Cancer   127
   Clinical Keys: Questions and Answers   135

Topic V: Cardiac and Vascular   137

10. Heart   139
    Clinical Keys: Questions and Answers   155
11. Vascular Surgery   157
    Clinical Keys: Questions and Answers   175

Topic VI: Abdomen   179

12. Stomach and Duodenum   181
    Clinical Keys: Questions and Answers   191
13. Small Intestine   193
    Clinical Keys: Questions and Answers   202
14. Colon, Rectum, and Anus   203
    Clinical Keys: Questions and Answers   235
15. Liver and Portal System   237
    Clinical Keys: Questions and Answers   248
16. Biliary System   251
    Clinical Keys: Questions and Answers   262
17. Pancreas   265
    Clinical Keys: Questions and Answers   278
18. Spleen   281
    Clinical Keys: Questions and Answers   288
19. Abdominal Wall Hernias   289
    Clinical Keys: Questions and Answers   296

Topic VII: Urology   299

20. Common Urologic Problems   301
    Clinical Keys: Questions and Answers   312

Interpreting Common Presentations   315

Algorithm 1: Managing Jaundice   316

Algorithm 2: Managing Acute Abdominal Pain   320

Algorithm 3: Managing Acute GI Bleeding   324

Algorithm 4: Managing Acute Limb Ischemia   327

Algorithm 5: Managing Acute Mesenteric Ischemia   331

Appendix   337

Surgical Signs and Syndromes by Chapter   339

Case Study Questions   349

Answers and Rationales   369

Index   387

Preface

The Pinnacle series is a new concept. Until the publication of this book, PA students have not had a series of textbooks designed specifically for their needs. Traditionally, PA students have been using textbooks designed for medical students. Yet these texts fail to focus the information to best prepare PAs for their specific end-of-rotation examinations and boards. Furthermore, PA training is condensed into a much shorter time frame than that allotted to medical students, so PAs were in need of a resource that could provide just the information they needed—no more, no less—in a streamlined fashion.

With this in mind, L.C. Bell Press set out to design a series of concise, manageable references for PAs to use while in the academic portion of their studies, on their rotations, or in preparation for their boards. To that end, we reached out to the top specialists in the fields of medicine and surgery to help author a new series of books especially designed for this population of students. Combining our expertise in medical pedagogy with our authors' backgrounds in teaching budding clinicians, we have developed the Pinnacle series specifically geared toward the PA student.

In content, format, and focus, each book in the series addresses the immediate educational needs of the PA student during every stage of his or her studies. The books support students' clinical experience through a clear, systematic approach that mirrors the thought process of arriving at a diagnosis and treatment. The Pinnacle series can be used to study disease processes, learn how to organize your thoughts with a clinical approach, augment classroom training, and prepare for the PANCE with the included case study questions and answer rationales.

We are always eager to hear your feedback. Please send your comments or thoughts about any book in the Pinnacle series to info@lcbellpress.com, or go to www.lcbellpress.com to contact us.

We wish you much success in your training and beyond.

The Publisher, L.C. Bell Press, Ltd.

About the Authors

Roberto Kusminsky, MD, MPH, FACS, is a Professor and Chair of the Department of Surgery at the Charleston Division of West Virginia University. He is a Fellow of the American College of Surgeons and has been involved in medical education for over 35 years, with a dedication to advancing the learning experience of his students. He trained at the Medical College of Pennsylvania and Baylor University Medical Center, and has served in a myriad of roles through the years. He has taken on a leadership role in surgical quality improvement for years, and until recently he was the Clinical Director for Quality Improvement of Surgical Services at Charleston Area Medical Center, a 900-bed tertiary care facility. His primary interests are in surgical oncology in general and breast surgery in particular, and he currently serves as the Medical Director of the Breast Center in Charleston, West Virginia. He also maintains a keen interest in advancements in genetics and pharmacogenomics, and for years he has been interested in the future of surgery and the changing roles of surgeons. All of these issues have been at the core of many of the lectures he has delivered to a variety of professional audiences. He is a noted researcher, and many of his contributions continue to be published in peer-reviewed journals. His cumulative experience and that of this book's contributors has made the material presented here well suited to the needs of its intended audience. He is most enthusiastic about the unique design of this book, which he feels is grounded in the practical reality and needs of the student's experience in the clinical arena.

Robert M. Blumm, MA, PA-C, DFAAPA, received his early training as a combat medic in the Republic of Vietnam from 1965 to 1968. He has been a PA for the past forty years and received the first AAPA Paragon Award for the Physician/PA Team along with his Supervising Physician Gerald Acker, MD. Mr. Blumm is the fifteenth recipient of the John W. Kirklin, MD Award for Excellence in Surgery. He has served as an administrator, clinician, and mentor. He was Instructor of Surgery and Emergency Medicine at Hofstra University PA Program for five years and is a Distinguished Fellow of the AAPA and a member of AFPPA, AASPA, APSPA, AAPA, NYSSPA, and PAs for Tomorrow, where he currently serves as vice president. He chaired the Surgical Congress of the AAPA for four years and served as the AAPA Liaison to the American College of Surgeons for five years. He is a past president of the New York State Society of Physician Assistants, American Association of Surgical Physician Assistants, American College of Clinicians, and Physician Assistants in Plastic and Reconstructive Surgery. Mr. Blumm is the co-author and co-editor of the textbook *Skin and Soft Tissue Injuries and Infections, a Practical Evidence Based Guide.* He is a contributing author to two additional textbooks and has authored in excess of three hundred articles. He is a national conference speaker for PAs, NPs, and physicians and is on the Editorial Board of *Advance for NPs and PAs*. He is Chairman of the PA Advisory Board for clinician1.com. In addition, Mr. Blumm is on the faculty of Fitzgerald Health Education Associates (FHEA) and has delivered lectures at their conferences as well as past conferences of the Nurse Practitioner Association (NPA), the Nurse Practitioner Associates for Continuing Education (NPACE), Vermont Association for Naturopathic Physicians (VANP), and the National Conference for Nurse Practitioners (NCNP). He has served as a faculty trainer for NP programs. He is on the staff of two Urgent Care Clinics and has worked closely with the same surgeon for forty-two years. Currently, he is a course director in the professional education department of Ethicon Wound Closure Academies for surgical residents. He is presently engaged in a new endeavor as Manager of Business Development for Quality Surgical Services of New York State to place surgical First Assistants in operating rooms throughout the state.

Contributors

Nicholas Baker, MD
Resident
Department of Cardiothoracic Surgery
University of Pittsburgh Medical Center, Presbyterian

Genevieve M. Boland, MD, PhD
Fellow, Surgical Oncology
The University of Texas
MD Anderson Cancer Center

John E. Campbell, MD
Assistant Professor of Surgery and Medicine
Division of Vascular/Endovascular Surgery and Medicine
Department of Surgery
West Virginia University, Charleston Division

Patrick Chan, MD
Resident
Department of Cardiothoracic Surgery
University of Pittsburgh Medical Center, Presbyterian

Chris C. Cook, MD
Assistant Professor of Surgery
Chief of Cardiac Surgery
Division of Adult Cardiac Surgery
Department of Cardiothoracic Surgery
University of Pittsburgh Medical Center, Passavant

John A. DeLuca, MD, FACS
Associate Professor of Surgery
Section of Trauma and Critical Care
Department of Surgery
West Virginia University, Charleston Division

Benjamin W. Dyer, MD
Assistant Professor of Surgery
Section of General Surgery
Department of Surgery
West Virginia University, Charleston Division

Michael Elmore, MD
Assistant Professor of Surgery
Section of Surgical Oncology
Department of Surgery
West Virginia University, Charleston Division

Michael D. Hall, MD, FACS
Assistant Professor of Surgery
Section of Trauma and Critical Care
Department of Surgery
West Virginia University, Charleston Division

Richard S. Mangus, MD, MS, FACS
Associate Professor of Surgery
Director, Adult/Pediatric Intestine and Multivisceral Transplantation
Transplant Division, Department of Surgery
Indiana University, School of Medicine

Albeir Y. Mousa, MD, MPH, RPVI
Associate Professor of Surgery
Division of Vascular/Endovascular Surgery and Medicine
Department of Surgery
West Virginia University, Charleston Division

Bryan K. Richmond, MD, MBA, FACS
Professor of Surgery
Section Chief, General Surgery
Department of Surgery
West Virginia University, Charleston Division

Lara Schaheen, MD
Resident
Department of Cardiothoracic Surgery
University of Pittsburgh Medical Center, Presbyterian

Gerald T. Simons, MPAS, CRT, PA-C
Lecturer in Surgery
Physician Assistant Program
Weill Cornell Graduate School of Medical Sciences
Physician Assistant, East Hampton Urgent Care
East Hampton, NY

Patrick Stone, MD, FACS
Associate Professor of Surgery
Division of Vascular/Endovascular Surgery and Medicine
Department of Surgery
West Virginia University, Charleston Division

Richard K. Umstot, Jr., MD, FACS
Assistant Professor of Surgery
Section of Trauma and Critical Care
Department of Surgery
West Virginia University, Charleston Division

Jonathan R. Van Horn, PA-C
Senior Physician Assistant
Legacy Emanuel Trauma Services
Adjunct Faculty
Pacific University School of Physician Assistant Studies
Portland, OR

Lawrence M. Wyner, MD
Associate Professor of Surgery
Section of Urology
Joan C. Edwards School of Medicine
Marshall University

Online Access

Find more interactive PANCE-style questions online at www.lcbellpress.com. Simply create a username and enter the password below:

35!LK@Bk

Topic I

Basic Principles

Perioperative Care

PREOPERATIVE CARE

The goals of **preoperative evaluation** of a patient are to (1) **detect and correct** any comorbidity that might increase operative risk, (2) assess the **risk of the operation** (high, intermediate, or low risk), (3) assess the **severity of the illness,** and (4) determine whether the surgical procedure is **elective or emergent.** Examples of the relative risks of surgical procedures and their relationships to the likelihood of cardiac complications are presented in Table 1-1.

Table 1-1. Types of Procedures and Associated Risks of Cardiac Complications

Type of Operation	Percent Cardiac Complication
High-Risk Procedures 　Aortic 　Major vascular 　Peripheral vascular 　Esophageal 　Emergent surgery in elderly patients	>5%
Intermediate-Risk Procedures 　Abdominal 　Head and neck 　Carotid 　Hysterectomy	<5%
Low-Risk Procedures 　Hernia 　Breast 　Cataract 　Endoscopic 　Surgical procedures outside major body cavities	<1%

History and physical examination. The first step in assessing surgical patients is to perform a complete **history and physical examination.** Some institutions use a questionnaire (Table 1-2) that enables the clinician to detect potential causes of increased risk of complications. This helps to determine which, if any, preventive or therapeutic interventions may be needed. Such a system has the advantage of creating a standardized methodology.

Table 1-2. Preoperative Questionnaire

Question	Y	N
Have you experienced chest pain or discomfort?		
Do you get short of breath when walking, going uphill, or sleeping?		
Have you ever had a heart attack?		
Have you ever had a stroke?		
Have you ever had complications from an anesthetic?		
Do you have kidney or liver disease?		
Have you been told you snore, choke, or gasp while sleeping?		
Do you have asthma?		
Do you have diabetes?		
Do you take aspirin or blood thinners?		
Do you have seizures?		
Do you have frequent respiratory infections?		

In addition to identifying preexisting medical conditions, allergies and a surgical history and related complications should be noted. Use of prescription and over-the-counter medications, herbal remedies, tobacco, alcohol, and illicit drugs should also be documented.

Specific risk factors. The importance of using a systems approach (eg, cerebrovascular system, cardiovascular system, pulmonary system, renal system, and endocrine system) to discover a patient's risk factors promotes a more accurate prediction of specific perioperative complications. For example, risk factors for **perioperative stroke** (an uncommon operative complication) include a history of stroke, hypertension, and coronary artery disease.

Of note, one-third to one-half of perioperative deaths are due to **cardiac events.** Therefore, evaluation of **cardiac risk factors** is exceedingly important. A common method is to use the Goldman criteria, developed in the 1970s and later modified to improve the precision of the scale. These criteria assign a point value to a number of variables that increase risk, such as (1) a history of **myocardial infarction** within the past 6 months, (2) **arrhythmias or conduction** defects, (3) **valvular disease,** (4) the **type of surgical procedure** (see Table 1-1), (5) **age over 70 years,** (6) **creatinine value,** (7) **unstable angina,** and other factors. The total points are used to categorize patients into 1 of 4 classes, each with a cardiac predicted mortality that increases from 0.2% for class 1 to 56% for class 4 patients. In some cases, evaluation of cardiac risk requires a preoperative stress test.

After cardiac events, **pulmonary complications** are the most common source of postoperative morbidity and mortality, and preexisting lung disease significantly increases this risk. Chronic obstructive pulmonary disease (COPD) is the most important risk factor for pulmonary complications. Every effort should be made to reduce the risk of pulmonary complications; smoking cessation prior to surgery is one of the most important elements of prevention.

Other systematic diseases, such as renal disease and diabetes mellitus increase operative risk. In fact, patients with diabetes have an approximately 50% increase in risk of perioperative mortality and morbidity compared to nondiabetic patients.

Exercise capacity is an important determinant of overall risk—patients who exercise regularly can withstand intensive operative procedures better than those with a poor functional capacity.

Age is considered a relatively minor indicator of preoperative risk. However, mortality increases linearly with age for most surgical procedures, and it is twice as high for patients older than 80 years than it is for those aged 65 to 69 years. Much of the risk associated with age is linked to the number of associated comorbidities.

Other factors that influence risk must be assessed, such as **nutritional status,** and risk factors for the development of **deep vein thrombosis** and **pulmonary embolization** (eg, lack of mobility, coagulation disorders). A history of weight loss equal to 10% or more over 6 months must be investigated.

The **risk of anesthesia-related complications** is determined using the American Society of Anesthesiologists (ASA) physical status classification system (Table 1-3), which remains one of the most widely employed scales because of its predictive accuracy and simplicity of use.

Preoperative diagnostic testing and preparation. **Laboratory testing** does not need to be done routinely. Instead, it should be performed for specific reasons and for patients with clear indications for doing so. For instance, obtaining a creatinine level is indicated in patients who (1) are older than 50 years and undergoing intermediate- or high-risk surgery; (2) have a history of renal disease, diabetes, or hypertension; or (3) will be receiving nephrotoxic medications. An ECG is appropriate for patients who are scheduled for a vascular procedure, have a history of cardiovascular disease, or are over 50 years old. A history suggesting a bleeding tendency should trigger appropriate testing and consultations. A pregnancy test is indicated when the pregnancy status is in question. The most common laboratory abnormality found in the preoperative patient is **anemia,** and a workup and treatment is appropriate.

In general, patients must not eat or drink for an appropriate period before surgery to decrease the volume and acidity of the gastric contents and minimize the chances of aspiration.

Table 1-3. ASA Physical Status Classification

ASA Class	Preoperative Physical Condition	Example
1	Healthy	No organic, physiologic, or psychiatric disturbance; good exercise tolerance
2	Mild/moderate systemic disease under control	Patient has 1 body system with well-controlled disease, such as medically managed diabetes, hypertension, or asthma; mild obesity
3	Severe systemic disease	Patient has more than 1 body system with well-controlled disease; poorly controlled hypertension, morbid obesity, history of angina or myocardial infarction in previous 6 months, COPD with intermittent symptoms
4	Severe systemic disease as constant life threat	Patient has a minimum of 1 poorly controlled or severe disease; severe heart failure, symptomatic COPD, uncontrolled diabetes or hypertension; advanced renal disease
5	Moribund patient not expected to survive without surgery	Ruptured abdominal aortic aneurysm, head trauma with increased intracranial pressure, multiorgan failure, sepsis
6	A brain-dead patient whose organs are to be harvested	
E	Suffix attached to emergency surgery	

Abbreviations: ASA, American Society of Anesthesiologists; COPD, chronic obstructive pulmonary disease.

INTRAOPERATIVE CARE

Anesthesia. The type of anesthesia administered may be general, regional, or local. **General anesthesia** produces a controlled and reversible state of unconsciousness. It is obtained using intravenous and inhaled agents and allows for muscle relaxation. It can be adapted to operations of different duration and complexity. It is frequently associated with airway control, which requires tracheal intubation. Evaluation of the airway prior to surgery is therefore an essential step. Possible predictors of a difficult intubation include a short neck, a small or receding jaw, poor dentition, orofacial trauma, poor neck extension (eg, a patient with severe cervical arthritis), or cervical traction. A widely used scoring system is the Mallampati scale, which is used to determine the **ease of intubation.** The airway is assigned a class from 1 to 4 depending on the ability to visualize the pharynx through the open mouth.

Patients arrive to the operating room (OR) usually after receiving premedication, which is most commonly a **benzodiazepine** such as midazolam. Next, they undergo the stage of **induction,** a critical phase in which an intravenous agent is administered in combination with a strong opioid such as fentanyl. At this point, the airway is secured with an endotracheal tube, which is connected to a respirator. **Maintenance** is the final phase of general anesthesia, and its depth varies with the type and duration of the procedure.

Regional or **local anesthesia** affects a specific larger or smaller area according to need. This type of anesthesia is induced with local anesthetics, which have different durations of action. When used for regional effect, the anesthetic agent can be injected peripherally, as is the case with a **nerve block** (eg, brachial plexus block) or delivered centrally via an **epidural** or **spinal** route. Typically, epidural anesthesia is administered by entering the epidural space and placing a catheter that allows for continuous infusion. Spinal anesthesia is administered by piercing the dura mater (the outermost layer of meningeal coverings) and entering the subarachnoid space into which the anesthetic is then delivered.

Propagation of nerve impulses occurs through a modification of the ionic gradient of sodium and potassium, and this mechanism of **depolarization** is inhibited by local anesthetics. All local anesthetics have a degree of **lipophilia.** This characteristic is directly related to their **potency** because lipid solubility enables diffusion through the highly lipophilic nerve cell membrane. The **duration of action** is determined by the protein-binding capability of the local anesthetic, because the anesthetic receptors in the nerve cell membrane are proteins. Local anesthetics belong to the ester group or the amide group. **Esters** are metabolized by the enzyme **pseudocholinesterase,** which in rare cases is genetically defective. When this is the case, there is an increased risk for important toxic effects from this type of anesthetic. This genetic abnormality is particularly significant when a patient is under general anesthesia, because some agents used to induce muscular paralysis, like succinylcholine, are also metabolized by pseudocholinestarase. Therefore, a patient with this genetic defect will require ventilator support for a long period until the effect of the drug dissipates.

The **amide group** of local anesthetics is metabolized by enzymes in the liver. The clinician should be aware that a fair number of drugs inhibit these enzymes, including some antiarrhythmics, antibiotics, and antidepressants. Excessive administration of a local anesthetic produces central nervous system (CNS) manifestations. Cardiovascular-related toxicity is also possible, but most often this is due to the addition of epinephrine to the anesthetic.

Some genetic defects are associated with a biochemical chain reaction called **malignant hyperthermia,** triggered by amide local anesthetics, certain volatile general anesthetics, and succinylcholine. Malignant hyperthermia results in high fever, muscle rigidity, and dark brown urine, and it can be fatal if unrecognized and untreated.

Physiologic monitoring. Physiologic parameters are monitored intraoperatively and postoperatively to allow for early and rapid corrective intervention should any problems arise.

Hemodynamic parameters like blood pressure and heart rate are a basic evaluation carried out continuously during a procedure. Occasionally, it may be necessary to monitor these through a direct invasive method, usually achieved by inserting a catheter into an artery, most commonly the radial artery.

Electrocardiographic monitoring of heart function is done continuously and is displayed on a monitor.

Cardiac output and other measures of cardiac function are frequently monitored through a catheter inserted into the central venous system that is threaded into the pulmonary artery. This allows the anesthesiologist to measure ventricular function, mixed venous oxygen concentration, and ejection fraction. This type of monitoring, however, is now being used less frequently because it is associated with a higher risk of complications and mortality, and its effectiveness is in question. Assessment of right and left ventricular function and ejection fraction is done accurately with **transesophageal echocardiography,** which is now used in the immediate postoperative period as well.

Respiratory monitoring is performed by routine measuring of airway pressures in mechanically ventilated patients, and by obtaining arterial blood gas levels as needed. This is complemented by the use of pulse oximetry, a noninvasive way of assessing arterial oxygen saturation, and capnometry, which measures Pco_2 in the airway throughout the respiratory cycle.

Renal function is assessed by monitoring urine output with a bladder catheter. Normal renal function in an adult produces a urinary output of 0.5 mL/kg/h. Measuring bladder pressure allows for oliguria and elevated intra-abdominal pressure to be detected. These 2 findings in combination with high peak airway pressures define **abdominal compartment syndrome,** which is associated with edema and hypoperfusion of intra-abdominal organs.

Prevention of complications. Maintaining **normothermia,** defined as a core temperature between 36°C and 38°C, decreases the risk of adverse outcomes. Keeping body temperature stable sometimes requires warming the anesthetic gases and the IV fluids that are administered during the surgical procedure. Normothermia should be maintained during the immediate postoperative period. **Prophylactic antibiotics** are chosen according to the pathogens that are most likely to be encountered during the procedure (Table 1-4). The antibiotic must be administered within 1 hour of the incision time. Prophylactic antibiotics should be discontinued 24 hours postoperatively.

Glucose control should be maintained throughout the procedure, usually with an average glucose level of 150 mg/dL. **Hair removal** must be done immediately prior to the preparation of the surgical field, using clippers instead of shavers. **Skin antiseptics** should be applied and allowed to air-dry. Chlorhexidine-containing solutions have been declared the agents of choice, but whether they are superior to iodine-containing agents is still questioned. **Oxygenation** during surgery should be maintained at approximately 80% of the inspired air. Prophylaxis of **venous thromboembolism** includes the use of mechanical methods, such as pneumatic compression of the calves, and systemic anticoagulant therapy, most often initiated postoperatively.

Table 1-4. Common Organisms in Surgical Procedures

Organism Type	Organism Name
Aerobic, gram-positive cocci	*Staphylococcus aureus* *Staphylococcus epidermidis* *Streptococcus pneumoniae*
Aerobic, gram-negative bacilli	*Escherichia coli* *Haemophilus influenzae* *Klebsiella pneumoniae* *Proteus mirabilis* *Pseudomonas aeruginosa* *Serratia marcescens*
Anaerobic, gram-positive	*Clostridium perfringens* *Clostridium tetani* *Clostridium difficile*
Anaerobic, gram-negative	*Bacteroides fragilis*
Fungi	*Candida albicans* *Cryptococcus neoformans*
Viruses	Hepatitis B and C *Cytomegalovirus* Epstein-Barr Herpes simplex HIV

POSTOPERATIVE CARE

Fluids, electrolytes, and acid-base disorders. Balancing fluids and electrolytes is an essential element of managing surgical patients, and it requires a clear understanding of the basic mechanisms of homeostasis. The clinician is primarily concerned with the fluctuations of water volume and the concentration of sodium and potassium.

Total body water (TBW) represents approximately 60% of adult body weight (Fig. 1-1), but the relationship between TBW and weight varies according to the amount of fat and muscle in the body. A greater amount of body fat results in lower TBW, and a greater amount of muscle results in higher TBW in relation to body weight. Infants have a higher proportion of TBW than adults, and older individuals have less muscle mass, which results in lower TBW. **Intracellular water** (ICW) is the largest fluid compartment, and water diffuses freely across the semipermeable membrane of the cell through the process of osmosis. It moves from a compartment with less solute to a compartment with more solute until equilibrium is achieved. The main **intracellular cation** is potassium (K^+), and the main cation in **extracellular water** (ECW) is sodium (Na^+). The volume and composition of body fluids is regulated by the kidneys through filtration and reabsorption of sodium and regulation of water excretion in response to **antidiuretic hormone** (ADH) secretion. These mechanisms are essential to maintain equal **osmolality** (a measure of solute concentration) within all body compartments.

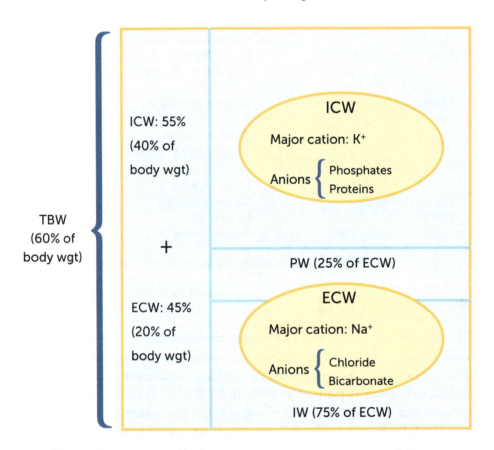

Fig. 1-1. Water Compartments in the Adult Patient

Abbreviations: ECW, extracellular water; ICW, intracellular water; IW, interstitial water; PW, plasma water; TBW, total body water; wgt, weight

In the surgical patient, losses of fluids and electrolytes are common. These losses can occur with vomiting, diarrhea, obstruction, nasogastric (NG) tubes or drains, bleeding, and so on. Other losses can be related to the use of diuretics, sweating, burns, trauma, adrenal insufficiency, and fluid sequestration and edema following surgery. As a result, adequate replacement of fluid and electrolytes is necessary. This requires understanding the effects that the specific surgical procedure has on the composition of body fluids (Table 1-5).

Table 1-5. Average Daily Volume and Electrolyte Concentration of Body Fluids[a]

Fluid	Volume	Sodium	Potassium	Chloride	Bicarbonate
Saliva	400	50	20	40	30
Gastric contents	1500	70	15	100	0
Bile	700	140	5	100	50
Pancreatic fluids	700	140	5	80	100
Small intestine contents	2000	140	5	100	40
Colon contents	150	60	40	25	10
Urine[b]	1200	NA	NA	NA	NA

Abbreviation: NA, not applicable.
[a]Volume is measured in mL, and electrolyte concentrations are measured in mEq/L.
[b]Electrolyte concentrations in urine only determined from 24-hour collection.

Clinically, estimates of volume depletion can be made by measuring intake and output, changes in body weight, vital signs and physical signs, blood urea nitrogen (BUN) level, creatinine level, and others.

Hyponatremia is common in the postoperative patient, usually caused by excessive administration of sodium-free fluid coupled with the water retention caused by stimulation of ADH secretion. Severe hyponatremia may cause nausea, lethargy, and even coma. **Hypernatremia** leads to weakness, altered mentation, and thirst.

Hypokalemia produces myalgias, weakness, ileus, and an inverted T wave and widened QRS complexes on ECG. **Hyperkalemia** may cause paralysis, metabolic acidosis, peaked T waves on ECG, and even ventricular fibrillation or asystole.

Other electrolytes can produce symptomatic alterations that must be recognized and corrected. **Hypocalcemia** may induce laryngospasm, perioral paresthesia, a prolonged QT interval on ECG, and tetany. The latter may manifest as Chvostek's sign or Trousseau's sign. **Chvostek's sign** is typically observed as spasms in the facial muscles, usually a twitch in the nose or lips, when the facial nerve is tapped near the parotid gland, at the angle of the jaw. **Trousseau's sign** is seen when blood flow to the forearm and hand is cut off, such as with a tourniquet or blood pressure cuff. Ischemia and low blood calcium level induces spasms in muscles of the hand and forearm. **Hypercalcemia** causes weakness, depression, lethargy, and if severe, coma and death. A serum calcium concentration greater than 12 mg/dL must be considered an emergency. **Hypomagnesemia** can develop in acute pancreatitis, diabetic acidosis, and burns. The symptoms are similar to those of hypocalcemia, with tetany, tremors, and sometimes convulsions. **Hypermagnesemia** is rare in surgical patients, and it is mostly associated with renal disease. It causes CNS symptoms like lethargy and ECG changes similar to those seen in hyperkalemia.

Respiratory and metabolic disturbances leading to **acid-base disorders** are a common problem affecting the surgical patient. An arterial blood gas (ABG) analysis provides the clinician with the pH, $Paco_2$, and bicarbonate (HCO_3^-) level, which are used in combination with physical signs to identify and correct the acid-base abnormality (Table 1-6).

Table 1-6. Characteristic Findings of Primary Acid-Base Abnormalities

Acid-Base Abnormality	pH	Paco$_2$	Bicarbonate	Causes	Treatment
Respiratory acidosis[a]	↓	↑		Aspiration, atelectasis, abdominal distention	Spirometry, deep breathing, pain control, ventilation
Respiratory alkalosis[b]	↑	↓		Hyperventilation, sepsis	Pain control, CO$_2$ rebreathing
Metabolic acidosis[c]	↓		↓	Shock, renal failure, ischemic bowel	Volume resuscitation, correct underlying cause
Metabolic alkalosis[d]	↑		↑	Volume loss, potassium loss	Volume replacement (NaCl solution) and K$^+$ replacement

[a]Bicarbonate level may increase to compensate.
[b]Bicarbonate level may decrease to compensate.
[c]Paco$_2$ decreases to compensate.
[d]Paco$_2$ increases to compensate.

Metabolic alkalosis is the most common acid-base abnormality in surgical patients, likely because of conditions that produce a combination of decreased volume and reduced levels of hydrogen and potassium ions, which are seen with vomiting and/or nasogastric aspiration and lack of oral intake. Replacement therapy is based on a calculated estimate of the fluid deficits and serum electrolyte measurements. In situations that cause acute volume loss, approximately half of the calculated deficit should be replaced within 24 hours, and at that point the patient's fluid requirements must be recalculated. Daily and obligatory losses must be accounted for in the fluid administration plan, taking into consideration the information derived from Table 1-5. Most of the time it is possible to administer isotonic solutions and modify the therapy according to the patient's response, which is measured by urine output and serum electrolyte levels.

The nutritional needs of the surgical patient must be considered, with the goal of optimizing all elements of care until oral intake can be resumed. Some basic caloric requirements can be partly satisfied by providing dextrose in the administered fluid. Solutions with 5% dextrose contain 50 g/L dextrose and provide 200 kcal/L. Dextrose contributes to the maintenance of osmolality if the solution infused contains less than 0.45% sodium. If the period of anticipated starvation is long, appropriate nutritional replacement therapy must provide calories via enteral (if possible) or parenteral routes.

Typical fluids given to surgical patients include normal saline (0.90% sodium chloride; composed of 154 mEq/L Na^+ and 154 mEq/L Cl^-) or half-normal saline (0.45% sodium chloride), and lactated Ringer's solution, which contains sodium, chloride, potassium, calcium, and lactate. Lactated Ringer's and normal saline are isotonic and may be used to replace GI extracellular volume losses. Sodium chloride solutions are well suited for replacement in cases with volume deficits associated with hyponatremia, hypochloremia, and metabolic alkalosis. Half-normal saline solutions are commonly used for replacement of GI losses and postoperative maintenance.

BIBLIOGRAPHY

Dumville JC, McFarlane E, Edwards P, Lipp A, Holmes A. Preoperative skin antiseptics for preventing surgical wound infections after clean surgery. *Cochrane Database Syst Rev.* 2013 Mar 28;3:CD003949.

O'Doherty AF, West M, Jack S, Grocott MP. Preoperative aerobic exercise training in elective intra-cavity surgery: a systematic review. *Br J Anaesth.* 2013;110(5):679-689.

Wound Healing and Care

WOUND HEALING PHASES

The process of wound healing follows a pattern that is artificially divided into 3 overlapping phases, each with characteristic biochemical and cellular events leading ultimately to the restoration of tissue integrity (Table 2-1, Fig. 2-1). The phases, in order, are inflammation, proliferation, and maturation, also referred to as *remodeling*.

Inflammatory Phase (Few Seconds to 5 Days)

Vascular Stage As soon as an injury occurs, **hemostasis**, a process that arrests bleeding in roughly 3 overlapping steps, is initiated. First, the injured vessels **vasoconstrict** to limit the amount of blood flow. In the second step, the **platelet phase,** the endothelial cells of the vessels retract, exposing subendothelial collagen, to which incoming platelets adhere. The platelets that adhere to the vessel walls release chemical messengers that cause aggregation (the "sticking together") of nearby free platelets. This results in the formation of a platelet plug. These activated platelets release chemotactic and growth factors, which initiate the third step, the **coagulation phase.** This last phase involves an intricate series of steps that ultimately result in the formation of an insoluble **fibrin clot.** The clot material both promotes hemostasis and acts as a scaffold for the inflammatory cells that will migrate to the wound. The fibrin matrix is essential to wound healing, which would be impaired without it. The clot is confined to the injured site because the normal cells away from the injury produce prostacyclin, an inhibitor of platelet aggregation. This chain of events includes the release of vasoactive substances, like histamine and serotonin. In response to these substances, the vessels dilate, vascular permeability increases, and cells (eg, neutrophils) migrate easily by **diapedesis** (the passage of cells through intact vessel walls). Increased vascular permeability and vasodilatation are responsible for the **clinical findings of inflammation: rubor** (erythema), **tumor** (swelling), **calor** (heat), and **dolor** (pain).

Cellular Stage This stage occurs almost simultaneously with the hemostatic response and is characterized by different types of cells arriving at the wound to mount an **inflammatory response.** The first cells to enter the injured area are **neutrophils** (polymorphonuclear leukocytes, or *PMNs*), which are the predominant cell type during the first 24 to 48 hours postinjury. Neutrophils cleanse the wound by hunting for and phagocytizing debris, foreign material, and bacteria and survive only for approximately 24 hours. They are a major source of cytokines, which are mostly glycoproteins with intercellular communication functions. The number of neutrophils declines once contamination is under control. The next cells to arrive at the wound are **macrophages** (or tissue phagocytes), which derive from circulating monocytes and are crucial to wound healing. They appear when PMNs decline, and their number peaks between 48 and 96 hours postinjury. They remain until wound healing is complete. Macrophages have multiple functions, acting as phagocytes, regulating matrix synthesis, and recruiting and activating various types of cells through the production of more than 30 cytokines and growth factors. They also produce nitric oxide, which has antibacterial properties. T lymphocytes migrate to the wound around the fifth postinjury day and peak at 1 week, bridging the transition between the inflammatory and proliferative phases. Their role in wound healing is not completely understood.

Proliferative Phase (4 Days to 3 Weeks)

During this phase, characterized by the formation of granulation tissue, wound continuity is restored. It can be thought of as the **fibroblastic phase,** divided loosely into 3 stages: **angiogenesis, fibroplasia,** and **epithelialization.**

Angiogenesis This is the process of new blood vessel formation, which begins 2 or 3 days after injury. It is stimulated by coagulation first and then by the hypoxic and acidic wound microenvironment, which induces secretion of potent angiogenic factors, first from platelets and then macrophages. Angiogenesis is a required component of wound healing, which in this phase results in the formation of **granulation tissue,** the typical beef-red layer seen in a healing open wound and often referred to as "proud flesh."

Fibroplasia If the wound is clean, **fibroblasts** are recruited and become the predominant cell type 3 to 5 days after injury. Fibroblasts develop from mesenchymal cells that are resting in connective tissue. The time it takes for these cells to differentiate into fibroblasts is called the *lag phase* of wound healing, usually lasting 4 to 5 days. A wound that is reopened 4 or 5 days after closure returns to the healing phase it was in when the process was interrupted, because the fibroblasts are already in place.

The main function of fibroblasts is to **synthesize collagen,** which is essential for wound repair and integrity. There are at least 27 types of collagen; type I is the most common and the principal collagen of skin and bone. In the fibroblastic phase, however, the more immature type III collagen becomes most prominent and acquires a significant role in the repair process until it is replaced by type I collagen.

During the proliferative phase, the initial matrix of fibrin and platelets is broken down, and fibroblasts synthesize the replacement extracellular matrix (ECM). The ECM is a provisional scaffold of complex structure and behavior, and it is different from the ECM in normal tissue. It regulates cells that come in contact with it. The structural components of ECM are mostly secreted by fibroblasts and include the proteins collagen, fibronectin, and elastin. Fibroblasts also synthesize polysaccharide chains of glycosaminoglycans (GAGs), which form proteoglycans by linking to the proteins in the ECM. Proteoglycans weld the wound edges together and constitute a major portion of the ground substance, the nonfibrous portion of ECM that is a component of granulation tissue.

Another element of granulation tissue is the *basal lamina,* a flexible, thin layer of specialized ECM that separates cells and epithelial surfaces from the surrounding connective tissue. Among its many functions, it acts as a molecular filter and also as a selective cellular barrier. The basal lamina, for instance, prevents fibroblasts from entering the injured area and inducing contraction of the epithelial layer, but it allows the passage of macrophages and lymphocytes. The basal lamina and collagen combine to form the basement membrane.

Epithelialization This is a proliferative stage that overlaps with the initial period of healing. The process of replacing the epithelial covering begins within hours of injury, so that, for example, a clean surgical wound is resurfaced and sealed within 24 to 48 hours. In this manner, protection from water losses and bacterial invasion is provided rapidly. Epithelial cells first detach from their connections to other cells, then migrate across the wound surface under the overlying eschar. Once continuity is reestablished, the cells proliferate and restore epithelial thickness. The basal lamina must be present for epithelialization to occur.

Maturation or Remodeling Phase (3 Weeks to 2 Years)

Contraction This stage usually starts 7 to 8 days after injury, after fibroblasts have had time to differentiate into myofibroblasts. They are attracted to the wound by fibronectin and growth factors. The myofibroblasts are thought to be the main cells generating contractile forces. The contraction process is a centripetal movement of the skin surrounding the injury, which significantly decreases the size of the wound and therefore the amount of new tissue required. This process does not occur in closed surgical incisions. It must not be confused with a contracture, a clinical situation in which scar formation leads to restricted function.

Remodeling During this period, the number of fibroblasts decreases, and so does the crowded capillary network. Collagen synthesis diminishes after 4 weeks, and at this point there is a state of equilibrium between collagen synthesis and collagen degradation by the action of collagenases. As type III collagen is replaced by a larger proportion of type I collagen over an average of 6 to 8 weeks, the tensile strength increases to approximately 80% of the preinjury values. However, a scar never recovers the same strength of unwounded tissue. The increase in strength during this period is due mainly to the cross-linking of the deposited collagen. Scars have no hair or epidermal appendages, and early in their development they are red because of the dense capillary network present. Once they reach maturity they become hypopigmented.

Table 2-1. Phases of Wound Healing

Phase	Stages	Cellular Activity	Timing
Inflammatory	a. Vascular b. Cellular	First: platelets Second: neutrophils Third: macrophages	Few seconds to 5 days
Proliferative	a. Angiogenesis b. Fibroplasia c. Epithelialization	Macrophages Fibroblasts Epithelial cells	4 days to 3 weeks
Maturation/ Remodeling	a. Contraction b. Remodeling	Myofibroblasts Fibroblasts	3 weeks to 2 years

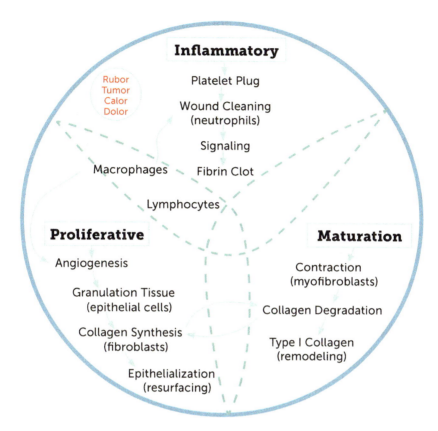

Fig. 2-1. Overlapping Phases of Wound Healing

FACTORS AFFECTING WOUND HEALING

The elements that influence wound healing can be divided into local and systemic factors. Local factors include those that directly affect the wound, whereas systemic ones refer to the health of the individual as a whole.

Local Factors

Wound Oxygen Pressure Although a local factor, wound oxygen pressure is also a reflection of the host's general status, because it demonstrates the adequacy of the inspired oxygen, the availability of hemoglobin for transport, and the condition of the vessels perfusing the wound. Appropriate oxygen levels are essential for normal function of neutrophils and fibroblasts. If the partial pressure of oxygen falls to less than 40 mm Hg, collagen synthesis is not possible. Hypoxia leads to capillary vasodilatation, leakage, and edema, which increases tissue pressure and further compromises perfusion.

Bacteria Infection leads to hypoxia, increased collagenase activity, and impaired angiogenesis and epithelialization.

Hydration/Desiccation The rate of epithelialization is faster in a well-hydrated wound than in a dry one. Dryness slows down all phases of wound healing. A moist wound environment allows appropriate cell function and migration and diffusion of chemical factors. Using wet-to-dry dressings, a common technique of wound débridement, is sometimes counterproductive because pulling off adherent dry gauze also removes new tissue. Occlusive dressings hasten epithelial repair.

Temperature A cold wound temperature (below 12°C) reduces tensile strength. The opposite is true when the temperature is greater than 30°C.

Foreign Material Contaminants increase susceptibility to infection and prolong the inflammatory phase.

Pressure Increased pressure on a wound leads to ischemia. This is the typical mechanism by which a decubitus ulcer forms.

Host Factors

Age A variety of changes seen with advanced age influence healing, such as a reduction in and increased fragility of small blood vessels, reduction in collagen levels, and slower inflammatory and immune responses.

Nutrition Protein depletion, indicated by low albumin levels, adversely affects wound healing. The presence of the essential amino acid methionine is critical for wound healing, because it serves as part of the bonds needed for collagen synthesis. In addition to providing the general increase in energy required for repair, carbohydrates are an energy source for white blood cells, which are critical for removal of bacteria and necrotic materials from the wound. Carbohydrates, in the form of glycoproteins, proteoglycans, glycolipids, and carbohydrate polymers, are key components in the cells and connective tissue of structures that were damaged and need to be replaced. Cell adhesion and migration, processes that are critical for all stages of wound healing, are mediated by proteins and lipids that are all, to some degree, glycosylated.

Vitamin A appears to have an effect against the inhibitory action of steroids on wound healing. Vitamin C is important to maintain normal capillary stability, which is important during angiogenesis, but vitamin E appears to have an inhibitory effect on wound healing. Nutritional supplements containing glutamine, glycine, and zinc improve wound healing. Copper and magnesium are needed as well for normal healing.

Drugs Steroids inhibit all phases of wound healing. Antineoplastic agents do as well, but it appears their effect wears off 14 days after discontinuation. Nonsteroidal anti-inflammatory drugs (NSAIDs) decrease collagen synthesis.

Radiation Production of growth factors that are necessary in all stages of wound healing is inhibited by radiation exposure. Radiation impairs collagen synthesis and also induces fibrosis of the vascular bed, which interferes with healing by preventing circulation of nutrients, growth factors, and oxygen. A healthy wound bed is crucial for epithelialization.

Comorbidities Diabetes and cancer affect healing through a variety of mechanisms. Some diseases are associated with impaired healing. Osteogenesis imperfecta, Ehlers-Danlos, and Marfan's syndromes are associated with defective collagen disorders.

Smoking Collagen synthesis associated with wound healing is inhibited in smokers. Nicotine adversely affects wound healing by its actions as a vasoconstrictor, which reduces oxygen levels in the wound. It also inhibits generation of macrophages and fibroblasts, two cell types that are crucial for normal wound healing.

ACUTE WOUND CARE

Types of Wounds

The most common types of wounds are listed in Table 2-2. Wounds may be acute or chronic, and they may have associated tissue loss. Burns are a category of wounds with specific local and systemic effects. Knife and bullet wounds are commonly associated with significant organ or system injuries. Complex wounds such as crush injuries, severe avulsions, and degloving trauma, often need care in the operating room under regional or general anesthesia.

Table 2-2. Types of Wounds

Wound Type	Wound Name		Wound Characteristics
Open	Incision		Clean, sharp edges
	Laceration		Linear or stellate, usually caused by blunt trauma; most common type
	Abrasion		Superficial, involves epidermis (scrapes)
	Puncture		Includes stings and insect bites
	Complex	Avulsion	Loss of tissue
		Degloving	Skin and fat separate from muscle
		Mutilation	Traumatic amputation
Closed	Contusion		Subcutaneous tissue damage
	Complex crush injury		Extensive tissue damage under intact skin with possible laceration

Classification of Surgical Wounds

There are clear differences between the care rendered to an accidental wound and one created under controlled circumstances, as is the case with surgical wounds. However, the principles of wound healing are universal, so the clinician must be aware of the steps involved in wound care regardless of the wound type. Surgical wounds might be created electively in the clean environment encountered during an operation such as a hernia repair, or emergently in an infected field, such as during the débridement of a soft tissue infection. The more contaminated the operative field, the greater the chances of a postoperative infection. Operative wounds are categorized into 4 classes (Table 2-3).

Table 2-3. Classification of Surgical Wounds

Class	Wound Type
I. Clean	Clean, operative field; nontraumatic, uninfected wound; no break in technique; respiratory, gastrointestinal, and genitourinary tracts not entered
II. Clean-contaminated	Nontraumatic wound; minor break in technique; gastrointestinal, genitourinary, or respiratory tracts entered without major spillage
III. Contaminated	Traumatic, contaminated wound; major break in technique; entrance into the genitourinary or biliary tracts; gross spillage
IV. Dirty-infected	Traumatic, infected wound (eg, abscess drainage)

Types of Wound Healing

Wounds may heal by **primary, secondary,** or **tertiary intention.** Healing by primary intention refers to wounds that are closed by approximation of wound margins at the appropriate time. A typical example is a surgical incision that is closed under aseptic conditions. Wounds that are closed by primary intention heal the fastest and provide the best cosmetic results. Healing by secondary intention describes a wound that has been left open and is allowed to close by contraction and epithelialization. This technique is commonly used in the management of contaminated or infected wounds. Healing by tertiary intention (also called *delayed primary closure*) means that a wound has been left open for 3 to 4 days to minimize the chances of infection and is then closed. Even with the delay, this type of wound heals as if it had been closed soon after the injury. This method is commonly used with certain incisions in cases where the disease process had been associated with an obvious infection or contamination. For instance, a patient might require surgery because of a diverticular abscess, and the wound contamination under these circumstances justifies delayed wound closure. Delayed closure results in the same rate of tensile strength gains as would have been achieved if the wound had been closed primarily.

Wound Management

History and Examination The ultimate goal of wound care is to achieve a closed wound, so that the best functional and cosmetic outcome may be accomplished. The first step of wound care is to obtain a rapid but comprehensive history, and this should be followed by careful inspection and examination of the wound. The clinician should be exceedingly attentive to the possible functional deficits that might be present prior to attempting any repair. For instance, a finger laceration should be assessed for the possibility of an associated nerve, vascular, or bone injury.

Irrigation and Hemostasis If the wound can be managed without requiring general anesthesia, a local or regional anesthetic is injected next. It is possible to first use a topical anesthetic such as benzocaine to minimize the discomfort associated with an injection. Benzocaine is sometimes used in spray form, and if used on an open wound, it is absorbed systemically. Rarely, a high dose of benzocaine may lead to methemoglobinemia, a severe and life-threatening complication in which oxygen is not released appropriately to the tissues. This condition requires immediate treatment.

The wound must next be rid of foreign material and necrotic and nonviable tissue. This is accomplished by thorough irrigation with normal saline solution, exposing all surfaces of the wound to the irrigant. It is not necessary to add antibiotics to the fluid. Next, hemostasis must be achieved, usually by applying compression and ligating bleeders. The wound is then ready for closure.

Timing of Closure The clinician must decide if it is best to close the wound or allow it to heal by secondary intention. In general, two factors will influence this decision: the type of wound and the time elapsed since the injury occurred.

Abrasions are seldom closed. In some cases, such as abrasions resulting from motorcycle accidents, foreign material is difficult to remove entirely. Puncture wounds are best left to heal by secondary intention.

Lacerations should be closed within 6 to 8 hours postinjury, but in certain body locations, the margin of time is greater and a wound can be closed even after 24 hours. An example of this is a wound on the face, because the area has a rich vascular supply and the desired outcome includes the best possible cosmetic results. If necrotic tissue or foreign material cannot be removed, however, the wound should not be closed primarily. Other typical situations where a wound should be left open include high velocity injuries and bites.

Infection Human bites are considered infected from the moment they take place, so they should not be closed and must be treated with antibiotics. Commonly identified aerobes in human bites include *Eikenella corrodens* and *Staphylococcus* species, and anaerobes include *Bacteroides* and *Peptostreptococcus* species. Cat bites are associated with a high risk of infection, usually caused by *Pasteurella multocida*.

Additional Treatments Some wounds require incision and débridement and afterward are left open for healing by secondary intention. Injection, extravasation, and high velocity injuries sometimes require this approach. Occasionally, wounds (other than burns) are so large that a skin graft is required to close them.

Closure Techniques Wounds must be closed without tension, and the edges must coapt with neither overlap nor inversion. Sutures must be taut enough to just approximate the tissue gently (Fig. 2-2).

Materials used for closure include adhesives, staples, and sutures. In general, it is best to use the finest material that will bring tissues together. In some cases, staples work best. For instance, scalp lacerations that are closed with staples appear to have a lower infection rate than those closed with sutures.

Suture material may be absorbable or nonabsorbable. Absorbable material degrades over variable periods, which range from 50 to 120 days. Suture material can also be made of monofilament or multifilament strands (braided or twisted), which are more likely to harbor microorganisms.

Summary Understanding the process of wound healing and the factors affecting it allows the clinician to optimize care. Treating the wound means treating the patient, so an effort to control all systemic factors must be done in conjunction with local wound care. Nutrition, systemic cardiopulmonary issues, local perfusion, and oxygenation must be addressed. The wound must be cleansed and débrided, and a moist and clean environment must be provided, commonly through the use of an occlusive dressing. Desiccation and pressure on the wound must be prevented. These principles apply to the intraoperative handling of surgical wounds as well. Antibacterials must be applied to the skin before making an incision. During a long procedure, it is best to cover exposed surfaces with warm saline moistened sponges, and tissue must be handled with minimal trauma to reduce the amount of cellular debris. Fluids and blood should be removed by gentle blotting, not rubbing. Wounds must be closed without tension, and all instruments and materials must be used in ways that do not cause additional trauma.

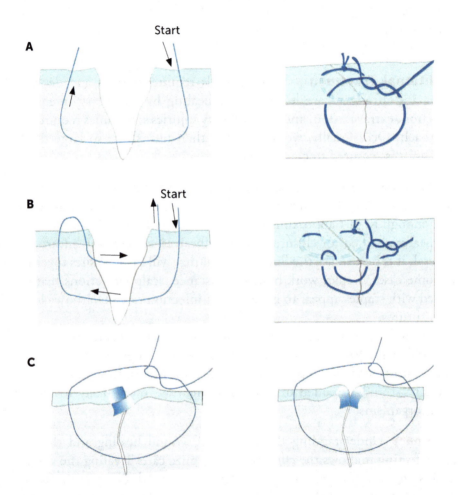

Fig. 2-2. Common Types of Stitches **A.** Simple stitch. **B.** Mattress stitch **C. Left panel:** Incorrectly completed stitch with skin overlap. **Right panel:** Incorrectly completed stitch with skin inversion.

BIBLIOGRAPHY

Greer N, Foman NA, MacDonald R, et al. Advanced wound care therapies for nonhealing diabetic, venous, and arterial ulcers: a systematic review. *Ann Intern Med.* 2013;159(8):532-542.

O'Meara S, Al-Kurdi D, Ologun Y, Ovington LG, Martyn-St James M, Richardson R.

Antibiotics and antiseptics for venous leg ulcers. *Cochrane Database Syst Rev.* 2013 Dec 23;(12):CD003557.

Common Postoperative Complications

Postoperative complications may be classified as systemic, wound-related, or procedure specific. Each of these categories can be further divided into infectious and noninfectious events.

Postoperative fever higher than 38°C is common and is usually the result of the inflammatory response provoked by surgery. It frequently resolves spontaneously. However, when other clinical manifestations are noted, it is necessary to investigate the cause of the fever, which is aided by the time of its onset. **Fever** is the most common postoperative sign suggesting a complication.

A mnemonic commonly cited to remember common causes of postoperative fever that tend to occur on specific postoperative days is the **5 Ws:** wind, water, walking, wound, and what. "Wind" refers to pulmonary complications, such as atelectasis; "water" refers to urinary tract infections (UTIs); "walking" refers to venous complications such as thromboses; and "what" is a reminder to consider the procedure(s) performed, including the use of intravenous lines, urinary catheters, or medications.

Another way to remember the postoperative days as they correlate to complications is the mnemonic **P-Ur-Vie-W–1-3-5-7.** "P" stands for pulmonary; "Ur" stands for urinary; "V" stands for venous; and "W" stands for wound. So, for example, on postoperative day 1, a common complication is atelectasis; on day 3, a urinary tract infection; on day 5, a deep vein thrombosis (DVT); and on day 7 or later, a wound infection or other wound complication (see Table 3-1). These are, of course, clinical approximations because many of these complications may develop earlier or later. Devices such as IV lines, catheters, drains, and implants (eg, a vascular graft) in many cases are the source of or contribute to the development of infections, so they should be cultured during the workup of postoperative fever or infection. Medications are the most common noninfectious cause of fever, with antimicrobials and heparin at the top of the list.

Table 3-1. Postoperative Fever, Complications and Timing of Their Appearance

Complication	Postoperative Day[a]						
	1	2	3	4	5	6	7
Pulmonary Atelectasis Pneumonia		→→→→	→→→→	→→→→	→→→→	→→→→	→→→→
Urinary tract infection			→→→→	→→→→	→→→→	→→→→	→→→→
Deep vein thrombosis			→→→→	→→→→	→→→→	→→→→	→→→→
Wound[b]		→→→→	→→→→	→→→→	→→→→	→→→→	→→→→

[a]Color emphasis indicates the most common time a complication develops.
[b]Rarely, a wound might be infected in the first 24–48 hours by *Clostridium* species or group A beta-hemolytic streptococcus, both capable of causing necrotizing infections.

ORGAN-SYSTEM COMPLICATIONS

Pulmonary Complications

ATELECTASIS

Definition Atelectasis refers to a collapse of pulmonary alveoli (mostly located peripherally).

Etiology Factors that contribute to the development of atelectasis include the effects of anesthesia, pain that causes shallow breathing, and the use of narcotics.

Epidemiology Atelectasis is the most common pulmonary complication that develops after an abdominal procedure, occurring in 25% to 30% of patients. Virtually all patients who undergo a thoracic or abdominal operation have an altered breathing pattern, which predisposes to atelectasis. The degree of atelectasis is influenced by existing patient risk factors, with smoking the most significant. Additionally, pulmonary and cardiac disease, and malnutrition increase the risk.

Symptoms and Signs These are typically noted within the first 24 postoperative hours. Clinically, they typically manifest as tachypnea, tachycardia, and fever. However, currently there is controversy relating to whether there is indeed a direct relationship between atelectasis and a febrile response. On auscultation, rales and decreased breath sounds may be noted, and commonly the rest of the physical exam is normal.

Diagnosis The diagnosis is made with the clinical presentation and a chest radiograph. The radiographs may show only a wedge-like density or a larger area of airless consolidation.

Prevention Prior to an operative procedure, smoking cessation should be encouraged. Postoperatively, early mobilization/ambulation, frequent position changes, encouragement to cough, and incentive spirometry are recommended.

Treatment Coughing, therapeutic chest percussion, nasotracheal aspiration, administering nebulizers with bronchodilators and mucolytic agents, and bronchoscopy are treatment modalities. If untreated, secretions accumulate and may cultivate infection, and pneumonia almost certainly follows.

PNEUMONIA

Definition Pneumonia is an inflammation with a consolidation of part or the entire lung, most commonly due to an infection. Consolidation means that the alveoli fill with exudate (fluid), usually composed of inflammatory cells and fibrin. Occasionally pneumonia may be caused by inhalation of irritants, as can occur with the aspiration of gastric contents.

Etiology Atelectasis, increased and stagnant bronchial secretions, and weak cough efforts are common causes of pneumonia. Endotracheal intubation may cause a deficiency of the mucociliary transport mechanism, which can contribute to the development of pneumonia. Patients with infections and those requiring postoperative ventilator support are at the highest risk for pneumonia. Ventilator-associated pneumonia, or VAP, is usually caused by *Streptococcus pneumoniae*,

Haemophilus influenzae, or *Staphylococcus aureus.* Late-occuring VAP (developing after 4 days of ventilation) is typically caused by antibiotic-resistant nosocomial organisms such as *Pseudomonas aeruginosa, Enterobacter,* and methicillin-resistant *Staphylococcus aureus* (MRSA). Grossly apparent aspiration is a cause of pneumonia (known as aspiration pneumonia) associated with high mortality, in the range of 50%.

Epidemiology One-quarter of postoperative deaths are due to pulmonary complications, and more than half of these deaths are due to pneumonia. Over 50% of the postoperative pulmonary infections are due to gram-negative organisms. The greatest mortality rate is associated with VAP, reported to be as high as 46%. VAP represents approximately 15% of hospital-acquired infections.

Symptoms and Signs Usually these are noted on the third postoperative day, although the timing can fluctuate as depicted in Table 3-1. Tachypnea, fever, rales on auscultation, and signs of consolidation such as **dullness to percussion** and **decreased or absent breath sounds** may be noted.

Diagnosis Chest radiographs are used to diagnose pneumonia. Induced sputum is used for bacterial culture and antibiotic sensitivity testing.

Prevention Measures to prevent pneumonia are the same as those used to prevent atelectasis. For patients on a ventilator, the "ventilator bundle," which is a combination of prophylactic measures, should be employed. This includes elevation of the head of the bed to at least 30 degrees, a daily "sedation vacation," a daily assessment of the need to continue intubation, and prophylaxis for deep vein thrombosis and peptic ulcer disease. Aspiration pneumonia prevention is accomplished by protecting the airway to reduce the chances of aspirating gastric contents and by implementing a nothing-by-mouth (NPO) status before anesthesia.

Treatment Aggressive pulmonary toilet facilitates removal of bronchial secretions. Broad-spectrum antibiotics may be administered until culture results become available, at which point antibiotic coverage is tailored to the organisms identified. Aspiration must be addressed immediately with oxygen therapy and suctioning of the bronchial tree. Routine use of steroids to treat aspiration pneumonia is no longer recommended.

Cardiac Complications

Myocardial Infarction

Definition A myocardial infarction (MI) is the **irreversible necrosis of heart muscle,** and it is more accurately considered as 1 condition within a constellation of clinical presentations known as acute coronary syndromes. These include unstable angina, ST segment elevation MI (STEMI), and non–ST segment elevation MI.

Etiology Ischemia, almost always a result of **coronary artery disease** (CAD), is the main cause of perioperative MI. It may also be precipitated by hypotension, hypoxia, or severe anemia.

Epidemiology It is estimated that 30% of patients who undergo surgery have a certain degree of CAD. The risk of ischemia and a subsequent MI is greatest in the first 48 postoperative hours. The incidence of postoperative MI increases when patients undergo an operation for manifestations of atherosclerosis (eg, vascular operations). Approximately 10% of postoperative deaths are a result of cardiac complications.

Symptoms and Signs In the postoperative period, the classically described symptoms of an acute MI (eg, chest pain with radiation to the jaw or arm) are infrequent. Patients instead may manifest shortness of breath, mental status alterations, changes in vital signs and cardiac rate, or respiratory symptoms. In patients with diabetes, a significant elevation of glycemia levels may be noted.

Diagnosis ECG and elevated troponin levels guide diagnosis.

Prevention Beta-blockers should be considered and administered starting preoperatively in eligible patients. Postoperative shortness of breath and dysrhythmias warrant aggressive investigation. Patients with increased risk factors must be managed appropriately.

Treatment ICU admission, high-flow oxygen administration, IV nitroglycerin administration, and anticoagulation must be initiated if there is no contraindication for doing so. Pain management is commonly implemented.

Arrhythmias

Definition An arrhythmia is an alteration in cardiac rhythm.

Etiology A host of factors may induce intraoperative or postoperative arrhythmias. Stress, electrolyte imbalances, hypoxemia, hypercarbia, and medications are common causes.

Epidemiology Dysrhythmias are divided into **tachyarrhythmias** (of supraventricular or ventricular origin), **bradyarrhythmias,** and **heart block.** Intraoperative arrhythmias occur in approximately 20% of patients. One-third of these occur during anesthesia induction. The most common postoperative tachyarrhythmia is atrial fibrillation (AF), which usually develops around the third postoperative day, coinciding with the mobilization of interstitial fluid. One-third of patients develop ventricular ectopy in the postoperative period, most commonly premature ventricular contractions (PVCs).

Symptoms and Signs Most arrhythmias are transient and unassociated with symptoms. When they do produce physiologic changes, the spectrum of symptoms and signs can include palpitations, chest pain, shortness of breath, and hypotension.

Diagnosis ECG guides diagnosis.

Prevention This includes control of comorbidities such as hypertension and diabetes, smoking cessation, preventing hypotension and hypoxemia, and continuous electrocardiographic monitoring in appropriate cases.

Treatment In hemodynamically stable postoperative patients with a supraventricular arrhythmia, control of heart rate and blood pressure are the most important steps. In the unusual event of AF causing hemodynamic instability, cardioversion might become necessary. Initiating anticoagulation therapy must be considered if persistent AF develops. Ventricular dysrhythmias have a more significant effect on cardiac performance compared to supraventricular alterations in rhythm. They should be treated with oxygen administration, correction of fluid and electrolyte imbalances, and sedation and analgesia as appropriate. If a sustained run of ventricular arrhythmia occurs, immediate therapy with intravenous lidocaine is indicated.

Urinary Complications

Retention

Definition Urinary retention is the inability to empty a full bladder.

Etiology This complication results from interference or discoordination of the neural mechanisms involved in urination, most commonly seen after pelvic and perineal operations. Urinary retention occasionally develops after spinal anesthesia.

Epidemiology This complication most commonly develops in the elderly. Benign prostatic hypertrophy contributes to the development of urinary retention.

Symptoms and Signs Discomfort in the hypogastrium increases to frank pain and urgency as retention worsens.

Diagnosis Symptoms in addition to a lack of urine output for several hours guides diagnosis.

Prevention Methods include the insertion of a urinary catheter when the operative procedure is extensive or performed for pelvic disease (eg, a low anterior resection of the rectum). Early ambulation after surgery, pain control, and judicious administration of IV fluids are other preventative steps.

Treatment Insertion of a Foley catheter is the mainstay of treatment.

Urinary Tract Infection

Definition A urinary tract infection (UTI) is an infection of the lower urinary tract.

Etiology Eighty percent of hospital-acquired UTIs are caused by the presence of a urinary catheter. Urinary retention and instrumentation are significant risk factors.

Epidemiology UTIs are the most frequent hospital-acquired infection. They are more common in females because they have a shorter urethra than males. Hospital-acquired UTIs are frequently associated with antibiotic resistant organisms because of extended lengths of stay and exposure to antibiotics. Common causative organisms include

Escherichia coli, Proteus mirabilis, Klebsiella pneumoniae, Pseudomonas aeruginosa, and enterococci. After 30 days of use, the presence of a Foley catheter is associated with bacteriuria in 100% of patients.

Symptoms and Signs The typical symptoms of urgency, burning with urination, and frequency in association with fever are not present in catheterized patients. Patients instead may experience pelvic pressure and lower abdominal discomfort. Fever should be worked up with the intention of ruling out or confirming a UTI.

Diagnosis Bacteriuria with more than 100,000 CFU/mL and growth of a predominant pathogen in culture confirms the diagnosis.

Prevention A clear indication for urinary catheter use is imperative. Following proper infection control protocols (eg, standard sterile Foley insertion, careful disposal of urine and urinary catheter systems, hand washing after handling a urinary catheter system) is an important step in minimizing the incidence of UTIs. Other measures include prompt removal of a catheter when it is no longer needed and using condom catheters for short-term needs when feasible.

Treatment Antibiotic(s) tailored to the causative organism and adequate hydration are the main steps. Bacteriuria without symptoms may not require treatment. Removal of the urinary catheter is essential.

VENOUS THROMBOEMBOLISM (VTE)

Deep Vein Thrombosis

Definition A deep vein thrombosis (DVT) is the formation of thrombi in the deep veins of the legs or arms.

Etiology **Virchow's triad,** 3 factors that predispose to the development of thrombosis, includes **venous stasis, endothelial injury,** and a **hypercoagulable state** as the primary mechanisms of DVT development.

Epidemiology Without appropriate prophylaxis, the incidence of postoperative DVT following abdominal procedures is close to 30%. This incidence in association with orthopedic procedures is in the range of 50% or greater. It is highest in patients who suffer spinal cord injury, where the incidence is 60% to 80%. Ten percent of patients placed on bed rest for a week will develop DVT, and for those with pulmonary disease on bed rest for 3 days, the incidence is 25%. The incidence for patients in a medical ICU and for those in a critical unit following an MI is 30%.

Symptoms and Signs It is common for early DVT to be unassociated with clinical symptoms. When the more proximal veins are involved, patients might develop recognizable clinical signs. Pain along the course of venous trunks might be reported, but it is an unreliable sign. **Homan's sign,** or pain elicited in the calf with dorsiflexion of the foot, is also an unreliable clinical indicator. However, when it is positive, a workup to confirm or rule out the diagnosis is required.

In cases of massive DVT where the iliofemoral venous system is affected, the patient may develop a condition known as **phlegmasia alba dolens** (painful white edema), which presents with pitting edema and pain and blanching without cyanosis. It is a common condition in the third trimester of pregnancy, when the uterus can compress the left common iliac vein against the pelvic rim. Unlike phlegmasia alba dolens, in which the thrombosis involves only the deep major veins of the extremity, in **phlegmasia cerulea dolens** (painful blue edema), the thrombosis extends to collateral venous channels, resulting in massive venous congestion. Clinically, this manifests with significant **edema** and **pain,** and **cyanosis.** The condition may lead to venous gangrene and amputation if untreated.

Diagnosis The test of choice is a **duplex ultrasound,** combining Doppler analysis with color-flow imaging. The **D-dimer** test measures the **degradation of fibrin,** and its negative predictive value is greater than 99%. However, in the postoperative period, fibrin degradation is increased; therefore the D-dimer test has limited value.

Prevention Early postoperative ambulation is encouraged. Other prophylactic measures include the use of compression devices, elastic stockings, or low-dose heparin administered every 8 hours. The use of low-molecular-weight heparin (LMWH) is the optimal approach for the patient with a moderate to high risk for DVT.

Treatment DVT is treated first with IV anticoagulation therapy until the transition can be made to an oral agent. The duration of treatment continues to be a point of controversy, although a minimum of 3 months is currently accepted. If the patient has a known hypercoagulable state (eg, malignancy), anticoagulation must be continued for life. An untreated DVT leads to propagation of the thrombus, postthrombotic syndrome (leg pain, edema, skin discoloration), and recurrent DVT in 30% of cases.

Pulmonary Embolism

Definition A pulmonary embolism (PE) develops when an embolus lodges in the pulmonary circulation, resulting in hypoxia, hemodynamic compromise, pulmonary hypertension, and increased right ventricular afterload, which may lead to right ventricular failure.

Etiology Emboli usually arise from a DVT of the lower extremities. They can, however, originate in the pelvis, arms, and even in the heart chambers.

Epidemiology PE is estimated to occur in as many as 80% of patients with DVT. More than 50% of these cases are asymptomatic. Approximately 10% of patients with PE die within an hour, and if the first episode is untreated, 30% die from a subsequent occurrence. Massive PE with hemodynamic consequences and death occurs in 5% to 10% of patients. Major trauma victims experience fatal PE in 1% to 2% of cases. The incidence of PE in patients with subclavian or axillary vein thrombosis is 9%. Most PEs are multiple.

Symptom and Signs The most common symptoms include dyspnea, pleuritic chest pain, cough, and hemoptysis. However, most patients with PE have no symptoms. Atypical symptoms include mental status alterations, wheezing, fever, and cardiac dysrhythmias. Pulmonary infarction is unusual because of the presence of collateral bronchial arterial circulation. The most commons exam findings are tachypnea and rales. A fourth heart sound is present in 25% of patients with PE.

Diagnosis The test of choice is a CT angiogram (CTA). This imaging study is particularly accurate for a centrally-located PE and helps to rule out other causes of pulmonary complications. If CTA is not available, a V/Q (ventilation-perfusion) lung scan is an acceptable test, although CTA has rendered it practically obsolete.

Prevention It is based on DVT prophylaxis (see earlier section, "Deep Vein Thrombosis").

Treatment Anticoagulation is the mainstay of treatment. If the patient has a contraindication to anticoagulation (eg, bleeding, hemorrhagic stroke), or has recurrent VTE despite adequate anticoagulation, placing an inferior vena cava (IVC) filter should be considered.

OTHER COMPLICATIONS

The clinician must be aware of other fairly common postoperative complications, including postoperative bleeding, renal failure, alterations of mental status (eg, "ICU syndrome" of the elderly), adrenal insufficiency, and *Clostridium difficile* colitis.

WOUND COMPLICATIONS

Surgical Site Infections

Definition A surgical site infection (SSI) may be superficial incisional (involving the skin and subcutaneous tissue only), deep incisional (involving the fascia and muscle), or organ space (involving the organs operated on).

Etiology SSIs are caused by bacterial invasion of the surgical site, which may originate from skin flora, bowel contents, a break in sterile technique, and so on. All surgical wounds are contaminated with bacteria, but host defenses are usually sufficient to prevent infection. The most common organism responsible for surgical infections is *Staphylococcus aureus*. A variety of risk factors influence the development of an SSI: the type of surgery, the length of hospital stay, history of smoking, diabetes, cardiovascular disease, obesity, malnutrition, immunosuppression, and radiation exposure at the site.

Epidemiology SSIs usually develop between the fifth and eighth postoperative days, but they can develop earlier or later. Eighty-five percent of SSIs occur within the first 30 postoperative days, and approximately 40% develop after the patient has been discharged from the hospital.

Symptoms and Signs Erythema, tenderness, edema, and occasionally drainage are present.

Diagnosis Presence of an SSI is determined by clinical exam. An ultrasound can help determine if a collection requiring drainage is present.

Prevention This includes meticulous surgical technique, prevention of tissue trauma or ischemia, antibiotic prophylaxis, appropriate skin preparation with an antiseptic agent, control of glycemia, and maintenance of normothermia. Hypothermia leads to vasoconstriction and decreased oxygen tension in tissues. Hair should be clipped, not shaved, immediately before surgery.

Treatment An infected wound must be opened, drained, and sometimes débrided. It is then left open to heal by secondary intention. The presence of crepitus suggests necrotizing fasciitis (caused by *Clostridium perfringens,* a rod-shaped bacteria), and in these cases the wound must be opened emergently. Significant associated cellulitis in an infected wound requires antibiotic therapy.

Dehiscence

Definition Postoperative disruption and separation of the fascial layer.

Etiology Multiple factors contribute to the development of this complication. It is most commonly the result of a surgical error, usually because of sutures that are placed under excessive tension or placed too close to the edge of the wound. Other contributing factors include obesity, infection, increased intra-abdominal pressure, malnutrition, and comorbidities.

Epidemiology Dehiscence occurs in 1% to 3% of abdominal operations, most commonly between the fifth and the eighth postoperative days.

Symptom and Signs Commonly, salmon-colored fluid drains from the wound. Opening the incision may reveal evisceration, in which abdominal organs protrude through the wound.

Diagnosis This is based on clinical findings and is usually accomplished by probing the wound or opening the incision if confirming the presumptive diagnosis is necessary.

Prevention Careful attention to wound closure is essential. Preferably, a running suture should be used, four times as long as the length of the incision.

Treatment The degree of fascial disruption dictates the method to be used for repair. The relevance of this is that the fascia should not be closed under tension. If the fascia is intact, a primary closure is acceptable. Otherwise, the fascia might require débridement, and closure should be performed by any method that assures no tension. This can be accomplished using a synthetic mesh or the recently developed bioprostheses (eg, human cadaveric or porcine dermis derivatives).

PROCEDURE-SPECIFIC COMPLICATIONS

Certain procedures are associated with specific complications, and awareness of their clinical manifestations dictates the course of the workup and leads to appropriate therapy. Examples include anastomotic leaks after bowel surgery, bile duct injury after hepatobiliary procedures, stroke after carotid artery surgery, recurrent laryngeal nerve injury after thyroid surgery, and others.

Topic II

Endocrine

Thyroid And Parathyroid

4

The thyroid (Fig. 4-1) is a bilobed gland that lies anterior to the trachea, just below the cricoid cartilage. The right and left lobes are connected by an isthmus at the midline.

The thyroid receives a rich blood supply from the superior and inferior thyroid arteries.

The thyroid gland produces thyroxine (T_4), which regulates many metabolic functions. Elemental iodine is an essential cofactor in this process.

The release of T_4 is controlled by thyroid-stimulating hormone (TSH) released from the pituitary gland. Once released from the thyroid, T_4 is converted to triiodothyronine (T_3), which is physiologically more active.

The parathyroid glands produce parathyroid hormone (PTH), which regulates serum calcium levels. PTH release is stimulated when serum calcium levels are low and is inhibited when serum calcium levels are above the normal range.

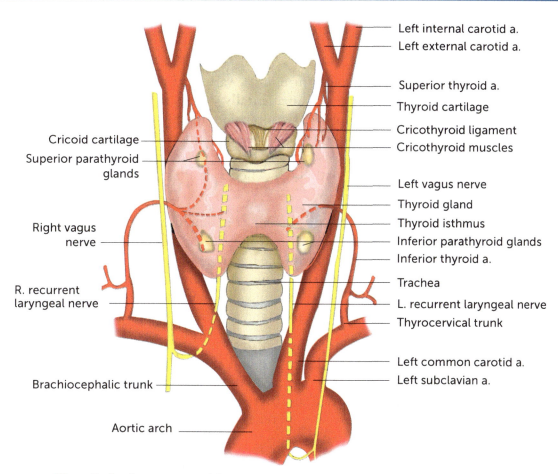

Fig. 4-1. Anatomy of Thyroid and Parathyroid Glands and Major Arteries

Solitary Thyroid Nodule

Definition A solitary thyroid nodule is a **single solid mass** within the thyroid parenchyma. This nodule contrasts with a cyst, which is a fluid-filled structure, and a complex cyst, which has both solid and cystic components.

Etiology Thyroid nodules may be malignant or benign, and their causes are not always identified. However, nodules are more common in patients with a history of radiation exposure, persons with a family history of thyroid disease, and individuals living in iodine-deficient areas of the world.

Epidemiology It is estimated that 50% of Americans over 50 years of age have thyroid nodules, and 4% of the general population have nodules large enough to palpate. Thyroid nodules are 4 times more common in females than in males. A vast majority (90%–95%) are benign.

Symptoms Thyroid nodules manifest a variety of symptoms. Many thyroid nodules are found **incidentally** during unrelated imaging studies or on routine physical examination. If symptoms are present, the patient may describe a sensation of fullness in the neck, changes in the voice, frank hoarseness, or dysphagia. Metabolic symptoms of hyperthyroidism may also be noted if the nodule is "toxic" (hyperfunctioning).

Physical Exam and Signs If palpable, a nodule may be evaluated by retracting the sternocleidomastoid muscle laterally with one hand and palpating the thyroid with the fingers of the other hand. A solitary nodule moves with swallowing. Attention should be given to degree of firmness, size of the thyroid gland and the nodule, any fixation to surrounding tissues, pain, and associated lymphadenopathy.

Differential Lymphadenopathy: Enlarged lymph nodes may be confused with thyroid nodules on physical exam or could coexist with them. **Goiter:** Diffuse enlargement of the thyroid gland, with or without a thyroid nodule(s). **Thyroglossal duct cyst:** Congenital abnormality suggested by a midline mass at the level of the hyoid bone; moves during swallowing.

Diagnosis Fine-needle aspiration (FNA) is the cornerstone of the evaluation of thyroid nodules and is generally recommended for all

solid thyroid nodules greater than 1 cm. FNA is performed under ultrasound guidance with a 22- to 25-gauge needle, and the material obtained is submitted to a cytopathologist. Examples of the diagnostic categories and recommendations for each category are displayed in Table 4-1.

Labs. Serum TSH is the only recommended initial laboratory study; ↑TSH signifies hypothyroidism; ↓TSH signifies hyperthyroidism; normal TSH signifies a euthyroid state.

Imaging. The initial imaging is an **ultrasound** of the thyroid (Fig. 4-2), which may **show a hypoechoic, solid nodule.** If the cause is a hyperfunctioning nodule, this is best imaged with a nuclear thyroid scan.

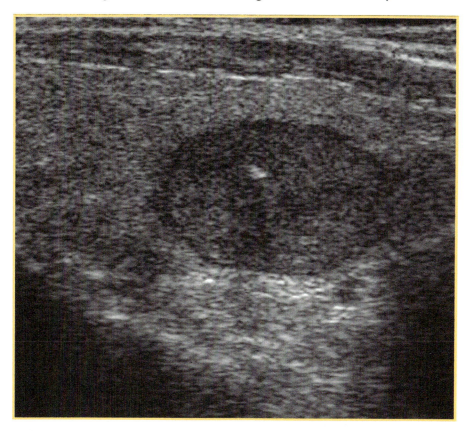

Fig. 4-2. Ultrasound of Thyroid Nodule

Table 4-1. The Bethesda System for Reporting Thyroid Cytopathology

FNA Category	Risk of Malignancy	Recommendation
Benign	0%–3%	Observation, follow-up
Unsatisfactory	Undefined	Repeat biopsy[a]
Atypia/follicular lesion of uncertain significance (AUS/FLUS)	5%–15%	Repeat biopsy[b]
Suspicious for follicular neoplasm	15%–30%	Thyroidectomy (lobectomy)[c]
Suspicious for malignancy	50%–75%	Thyroidectomy
Malignant	97%–99%	Thyroidectomy

[a]Repeated under ultrasound guidance. If still unsatisfactory, surgery is recommended.
[b]Typically, 50% will be reclassified as benign.
[c]Follicular neoplasms (benign or malignant) are indistinguishable on FNA biopsy.

Complication(s) Development of thyroid cancer. Problems may arise from the local compressive effects of a large nodule on adjacent structures, resulting in hoarseness or dysphagia.

Treatment Symptomatic nodules are evaluated for surgical treatment, as are those with FNA results that elicit concern. The typical operation is **thyroid lobectomy/isthmectomy,** in which the entire lobe containing the nodule and the isthmus of the gland is removed. A **total thyroidectomy** may be appropriate when malignancy is suspected or is diagnosed preoperatively by FNA. Simple removal of the nodule itself is not an acceptable procedure.

Hyperthyroidism

Definition This term refers to **overproduction of thyroid hormone** by the thyroid gland, resulting in a **hypermetabolic state.** The disease is also referred to as *thyrotoxicosis*.

Etiology Hyperthyroidism may result from **Graves' disease** (an autoimmune disorder caused by immunoglobulins targeted against TSH receptors), a **toxic adenoma** (hyperfunctioning nodule), or **toxic nodular goiter** (multiple hyperfunctioning nodules).

Epidemiology The overall prevalence of hyperthyroidism is 1.3%. Women are affected 5 times more frequently than men. **Graves' disease** is the most common cause of hyperthyroidism.

Symptoms Hyperthyroidism may be characterized by anxiety, weight loss, palpitations, insomnia, increased appetite, heat intolerance, weakness, and psychiatric disturbances.

Physical Exam and Signs Hyperthyroid patients may appear **anxious** or **irritable.** Other signs of hyperthyroidism may include an enlarged, palpable thyroid, hyperreflexia, hair loss, and muscle wasting. Patients often exhibit tachycardia and may develop a cardiac arrhythmia such as atrial fibrillation. Nonpitting edema of the pretibial areas may be evident, described as *pretibial myxedema*. Patients with Graves' disease may exhibit an anterior bulging of the eyes, or *exophthalmos*.

Differential The differential includes the causes of hyperthyroidism mentioned under "Etiology."

Diagnosis The diagnosis of hyperthyroidism is made with a combination of lab findings and ultrasonography.

Labs. ↓TSH, ↑T_3, and ↑T_4.

Imaging. An ultrasound may show a hypoechoic, solid thyroid nodule. ^{123}I nuclear medicine thyroid scanning is useful for diagnosis of a toxic adenoma.

Complication(s) If untreated, patients may have continued muscle wasting, life-threatening arrhythmias, psychosis, or visual impairment, or they may develop **thyroid storm.**

THYROID STORM, a potentially deadly complication of hyperthyroidism, is characterized by a severe hypermetabolic state caused by excessive release of thyroid hormones in patients with hyperthyroidism. The mortality rate ranges from 10% to 30%.

Symptoms. The symptoms are an exaggeration of the symptoms of hyperthyroidism. Agitation, delirium, psychosis, and stupor may be noted. Nausea, vomiting, diarrhea, and abdominal pain may occur.

Physical Exam and Signs. Tachycardia is often present and may exceed 140 bpm. A fatal arrhythmia may occur, as can hypotension and cardiovascular collapse. Fever may exceed 105°F. Jaundice may be present, indicating hepatic failure.

Diagnosis. The diagnosis is based on clinical findings and lab results.

Labs. ↑T_4, ↑T_3, and ↓TSH; degree of thyroid hormone elevation does not correlate with the severity of the syndrome.

Imaging. No specific findings.

Treatment

Hyperthyroidism: **Radioactive iodine therapy** (RAI) in the form of ^{131}I is the treatment of choice for most cases of Graves' disease, although a **total thyroidectomy** is indicated in some cases. RAI has no long-term side effects, but sometimes several treatments are required. A toxic adenoma requires a lobectomy of the affected side only. For a toxic nodular goiter, a total thyroidectomy is preferred. Patients undergoing surgical therapy are first rendered **euthyroid** with antithyroid medications such as **propylthiouracil (PTU)** or **methimazole**, both of which inhibit the production and release of thyroid hormone. These are administered concurrently with a **beta-blocker** to treat the tachycardia associated with high circulating thyroid hormone levels.

Thyroid storm: Early recognition and treatment are essential in preventing death. **Beta-blockers** should be administered to control tachycardia and arrhythmias. **Antithyroid medications** should be administered to counteract hormone overproduction. **Glucocorticoids** (hydrocortisone) should be given intravenously to promote vasomotor stability and to limit the conversion of T_4 to the more active T_3. Administration of potassium iodide solution (Lugol's solution) is helpful in inhibiting further release of thyroid hormone from the gland. After recovery, patients should be offered definitive treatment for their hyperthyroidism such as RAI or thyroidectomy.

THYROID CANCER

Definition A malignancy of the thyroid gland.

Etiology Unknown. Risk factors include radiation exposure and a family history of thyroid cancer. Some thyroid cancers are inherited.

Epidemiology The most common type of thyroid cancer is **papillary carcinoma** (70%–80%), followed by **follicular carcinoma** (10%–15%). These 2 types arise from the thyroid follicle and are well differentiated. Next is **medullary carcinoma** (2%–4%), which is followed by **anaplastic (undifferentiated) carcinoma** (1%). Medullary carcinoma may be sporadic or inherited (see Chapter 5: Adrenals, Pituitary, and Multiple Endocrine Neoplasias). The thyroid rarely harbors metastases. Papillary and follicular carcinomas exhibit 10-year survival rates of 95% and 85%, respectively. The 10-year survival rate of medullary carcinoma is approximately 65%. Anaplastic carcinoma of the thyroid is uniformly fatal.

Symptoms When symptoms are present, they often occur in the setting of more advanced disease. Patients may exhibit pain, hoarseness, dysphagia, or odynophagia.

Physical Exam and Signs A nodule or a diffusely enlarged thyroid may be noted. Fixation of a mass suggests local invasion of adjacent structures. Associated lymphadenopathy may indicate metastases to regional lymph nodes. Hoarseness may indicate tumor involvement of the RLN.

Differential The differential centers around all of the benign and malignant thyroid conditions.

Diagnosis **FNA** is the test of choice to diagnose thyroid cancer. The false-negative rate is less than 5%. The diagnosis is confirmed afterward from the surgical specimen. **Papillary carcinoma** has classic histologic features such as nuclear grooves/cytoplasmic clearing (**"Orphan Annie eye nuclei"**) and areas of calcification (**psammoma bodies**). Follicular neoplasms may be malignant (follicular carcinoma) or benign (follicular adenoma). The distinction between the 2 is based on the presence or absence of capsular or vascular invasion by cells within the nodule. **Medullary carcinomas** can be diagnosed with special stains that detect the presence of calcitonin. **Anaplastic carcinoma** is characterized by wildly pleomorphic nuclei, necrosis, and no identifiable normal follicular tissue.

Labs. Laboratory findings are nonspecific for diagnosing malignancy. Calcitonin is elevated in medullary cancer. Thyroglobulin and calcitonin levels are useful as tumor markers after treatment.

Imaging. **Ultrasound** is the initial test of choice for working up suspicious clinical findings. Features that suggest **malignancy** within a nodule include **irregularity, hypervascularity,** and the presence of **microcalcifications** within the area of concern. The regional lymph nodes should be assessed preoperatively by ultrasound and clinically at the time of surgery.

Complication(s) Local complications include tumor involvement of the RLN and resultant vocal cord paralysis. The trachea and the esophagus may be invaded. Thyroid cancer may metastasize to regional lymph nodes and to distant sites.

Treatment The mainstay of thyroid cancer treatment is **thyroidectomy,** but the extent of surgery varies by histologic type. **Papillary carcinoma** is treated with total thyroidectomy for tumors greater than 1 cm; a lobectomy may be considered for smaller tumors. A selective neck dissection is performed to remove any clinically enlarged lymph nodes. **Follicular carcinoma** is treated by total thyroidectomy. **Medullary carcinoma** is treated with total thyroidectomy and at least central compartment lymph node removal because this type of cancer is associated with early spread to regional lymph nodes. **Anaplastic thyroid carcinoma** is an aggressive and uniformly lethal form of cancer; surgery is not curative and often is not technically possible because of local invasion of adjacent structures. Often, patients require a tracheostomy to prevent airway obstruction. Chemotherapy and radiation serve only a palliative role, and survival rarely exceeds 1 year, even with multimodality treatment. Postoperatively, patients with papillary and follicular carcinomas may receive adjunctive therapy with **RAI** to ablate small remnants of thyroid tissue and to eliminate metastatic disease. After surgery and RAI, patients are treated with **oral levothyroxine** at higher than normal doses to achieve suppression of TSH levels to less than 0.1 mIU/L, thereby inhibiting stimulation of any residual tumor cells. Thyroglobulin, which is produced by the normal thyroid and by these types of well-differentiated tumors, should be undetectable after treatment; therefore, a postoperative thyroglobulin elevation suggests a recurrence. Periodic assessment of the neck with ultrasound is recommended. If a recurrence of a follicular or papillary carcinoma is suspected, a whole body iodine nuclear scan may be useful for visualizing metastases. Medullary carcinoma is not treated with RAI postoperatively because the malignancy arises from the C cells of the thyroid, and iodine does not bind to them. Follow-up consists of periodic ultrasound of the neck and measurement of calcitonin levels, which decrease with successful treatment and rise with a recurrence.

INFLAMMATORY THYROID DISEASE

Definition Inflammatory thyroid disease, or *thyroiditis*, is a **group of disorders** characterized by thyroid inflammation. Thyroiditis may be acute, subacute, or chronic.

Etiology Thyroiditis may be caused by infectious or autoimmune processes. **Chronic lymphocytic thyroiditis (Hashimoto's thyroiditis)** is a chronic autoimmune thyroid inflammation caused by the formation of antithyroid antibodies. Patients with Hashimoto's thyroiditis develop hypothyroidism at a rate of 5% per year. **Subacute granulomatous thyroiditis (de Quervain's thyroiditis)** is the most common cause of a painful thyroid gland. It is most likely caused by a viral upper respiratory tract infection. Mumps, coxsackievirus, adenovirus, influenza, and Epstein-Barr virus are some of the infectious agents implicated. Symptoms of hyperthyroidism develop in as many as 70% of patients, and normal function returns in 4 to 6 months. Permanent hypothyroidism resulting from destruction of thyroid tissue may be seen in 5% of patients. **Acute suppurative thyroiditis** is a rare form of thyroiditis caused by a bacterial infection with *Streptococcus* or *Staphylococcus*. Patients may develop pain, fever, dysphagia, and dysphonia. A fluctuant mass indicates an abscess. **Invasive fibrous thyroiditis** (*Riedel's struma*), the rarest form of thyroiditis, is characterized by progressive fibrosis of the thyroid gland and fibrosis of other sites—sclerosing cholangitis and retroperitoneal fibrosis may develop. Goiter may be present, as can symptoms of airway, esophageal, or RLN compression. In some cases, the cause remains unknown.

Epidemiology The incidence of thyroiditis is estimated at 12.1 in 100,000 individuals. Ninety-five percent of cases occur in women, and most cases are seen in individuals between 30 and 50 years of age.

Symptoms Thyroiditis may be asymptomatic. Some patients present with painful enlargement of the thyroid gland caused by a goiter or, rarely, an abscess. Fullness or "tightness" in the neck, sore throat, or fever may be reported.

Physical Exam and Signs The thyroid may be enlarged and tender. Patients may present with pharyngitis and fever, which is more likely if an abscess is developing. In this case, a fluctuant area of localized pain may be palpated over the affected area. Symptoms of hyperthyroidism or hypothyroidism may be present.

Differential The differential includes the causes of thyroiditis mentioned under "Etiology."

Diagnosis The clinical presentation and lab results direct the diagnosis.

> *Labs.* Measurement of T_3, T_4, and TSH is indicated because many patients with thyroiditis develop hyperthyroidism or hypothyroidism, which may require pharmacologic treatment. An increased erythrocyte sedimentation rate (ESR) is common but not specific. Anti-thyroid peroxidase and antithyroglobulin antibody levels should be obtained to exclude chronic lymphocytic thyroiditis. If an abscess is drained, cultures should be taken.
>
> *Imaging.* Ultrasound is useful for demonstrating thyroid enlargement and any dominant nodules. Patients with a dominant nodule should undergo FNA, as chronic thyroiditis may increase the risk of thyroid carcinoma.

Complication(s) Thyroiditis may result in hyperthyroidism, which is usually transient, or hypothyroidism, which is frequently permanent. Thyroid carcinoma may develop in patients with chronic thyroiditis, particularly in those with chronic lymphocytic thyroiditis. In acute suppurative thyroiditis with abscess formation, local edema may lead to life-threatening airway compromise. Invasive fibrous thyroiditis may result in progressive airway compromise, esophageal compression, and hoarseness caused by damage to the RLNs.

Treatment Surgical treatment is rarely required. **Hyperthyroidism** is treated with antithyroid medications and beta-blockers. **Hypothyroidism** is treated with oral levothyroxine supplementation. **Chronic lymphocytic thyroiditis** treatment is supportive. Any suspicious nodules seen on thyroid ultrasound should undergo FNA. Thyroidectomy is performed for suspicious FNA results or for symptoms resulting from progressive enlargement of the thyroid, such as hoarseness or dysphagia. Occasionally, a short course of treatment with oral corticosteroids (methylprednisolone) may be required. In acute suppurative thyroiditis, prompt recognition and drainage of an abscess are essential, as is appropriate anti-infective therapy guided by culture results. Invasive fibrous thyroiditis may be self-limited. Corticosteroids may be useful in some patients. Thyroidectomy is indicated for symptoms of airway, esophageal, or recurrent laryngeal nerve compression.

GOITER

Definition Goiter (benign nontoxic goiter) is an abnormal enlargement of the thyroid gland (Fig. 4-3). It may be nodular or diffuse and may involve one or both lobes of the thyroid. Patients with goiter may be hypothyroid, euthyroid, or hyperthyroid.

Etiology Goiter may develop as a result of **chronic dietary iodine deficiency** (now rare in industrialized nations because of the iodination of table salt), which is the most common cause of goiter worldwide. In hypothyroid patients, goiter may result from chronically elevated TSH levels. Goiter associated with hyperthyroidism can be seen in patients with Graves' disease or toxic adenoma. In many cases, an exact cause is not identified.

Epidemiology Goiter may be present in as many as 10% of adults in the United States. Females are affected more often than men.

Symptoms Goiter may be asymptomatic or may present with tenderness. Symptoms of hypothyroidism or hyperthyroidism may occur. Fullness or "tightness" of the neck and symptoms of local compromise such as hoarseness, dysphagia, or odynophagia may be noted.

Physical Exam and Signs The thyroid may be visibly enlarged, and this is confirmed by palpation. The enlargement may be diffuse or limited to a single lobe. A dominant nodule may be present, suggesting a coexisting carcinoma. With a substernal goiter, a portion of the thyroid descends into the mediastinum. This type of thyroid can be large and symptomatic, often resulting in displacement of the trachea.

Differential Thyroid carcinoma: Enlargement of the gland. **Graves' disease:** Diffusely enlarged gland; hyperthyroidism. **Toxic nodular goiter:** Associated with hyperthyroidism.

Diagnosis Clinical exam, lab analyses, and imaging guide diagnosis.

Labs. T_3, T_4, and TSH typically reflect a euthyroid or hypothyroid state in benign nontoxic goiter.

Imaging. Ultrasound should be obtained in all patients, with attention to any suspicious nodules. Dominant or suspicious nodules should undergo FNA. Chest X-ray may demonstrate tracheal deviation or substernal extension of the goiter. CT scan of the neck and chest is useful for delineating the gland precisely and for determining its relationship to other structures and the degree of substernal extension, if present.

Complication(s) Malignant degeneration of a benign goiter may occur in 5% to 10% of cases.

Treatment Benign nontoxic goiter management is based on the presence of symptoms. Thyroidectomy may be offered for relief of significant dysphagia, dyspnea, hoarseness, and tracheal deviation, and for those with suspicious FNA results. Total thyroidectomy is the operation of choice; lobectomy is appropriate if the goiter involves a single lobe.

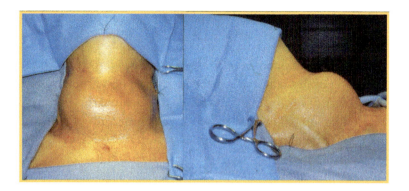

Fig. 4-3. Goiter

Hyperparathyroidism

Definition Hyperparathyroidism (HPT) refers to overproduction of PTH by 1 or more abnormal parathyroid glands, often resulting in **hypercalcemia**.

Etiology Three types of HPT have been identified. In **primary HPT,** the most common type, overproduction of PTH is caused most often by a benign parathyroid adenoma. **Secondary HPT** often occurs in patients with end-stage renal disease (ESRD) and is the result of enlargement, or *hyperplasia,* of all 4 parathyroid glands. Overproduction of PTH is due to the chronic hypocalcemia characteristic of ESRD. **Tertiary HPT** is triggered by the development of autonomous function of the hyperplastic glands in a patient with secondary HPT. For example, this may occur in a patient who has undergone a kidney transplant, which has resulted in restoration of normal renal calcium and vitamin D metabolism; however, hyperplastic parathyroid glands continue to overproduce PTH.

Epidemiology The incidence of primary HPT is approximately 1 in 1000 individuals (0.1%). Eighty percent of cases of HPT are caused by a single adenoma, 10% by a double adenoma, and 10% by hyperplasia of all 4 parathyroid glands.

Symptoms Mild HPT may be asymptomatic. However, patients may present with kidney stones, bone pain, abdominal pain, and psychiatric symptoms ("stones, bones, groans, and moans"). Other symptoms include weakness, lack of energy, reflux, and irritability.

Physical Exam and Signs No specific physical findings have been reported. The exception is the rare case of a hypercalcemic crisis.

Differential **Hypercalcemia of malignancy:** May occur as the result of a coexisting malignancy, as can be seen with bone metastases or with paraneoplastic syndrome. **Familial hypocalciuric hypercalcemia (FHH):** Hereditary condition with ↑calcium and ↑PTH in asymptomatic patients; history of relatives with hypercalcemia.

Diagnosis The diagnosis is made largely on the basis of lab results.

Labs. **In primary HPT,** ↑serum calcium (>10.5 mg/dL) and ↑PTH, normal/↓vitamin D levels, ↑24-hour urinary calcium level. **Secondary HPT** does not cause ↑serum calcium.

Imaging. Imaging studies are helpful in determining the operative approach. The test of choice is a technetium Tc 99m sestamibi nuclear scan, which will detect a parathyroid adenoma approximately 80% of the time (Fig. 4-4). **Ultrasound** is an effective localization method, with reported sensitivity and specificity similar to those of nuclear medicine scanning.

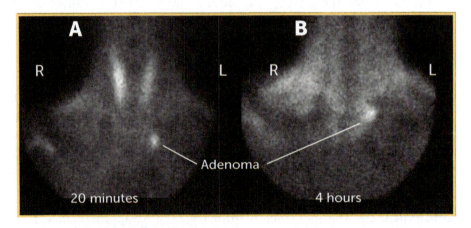

Fig. 4-4. Parathyroid Adenoma (Sestamibi Scan). **A.** At 20 minutes. **B.** At 4 hours.

Complication(s) Untreated HPT can cause nephrolithiasis, osteoporosis, or osteopenia. **Hypercalcemic crisis,** in which the serum calcium rises to above 15 mg/dL, is characterized by weakness, lethargy, confusion, and arrhythmia. This serious, potentially life-threatening condition requires immediate intervention.

Treatment **Surgery** is the treatment of choice for primary and tertiary HPT. **Secondary HPT** is treated medically with **cinacalcet,** which acts directly on the parathyroid gland to inhibit release of PTH. In **primary HPT,** identification and excision of the adenoma(s) require removal of the diseased gland(s). In the rare case of 4-gland hyperplasia, a subtotal parathyroidectomy is performed, in which 3.5 glands are removed. This leaves enough functional tissue to prevent hypoparathyroidism. An alternative approach in cases of 4-gland hyperplasia is total parathyroidectomy with autotransplantation, in which a portion of 1 gland is transplanted into the sternocleidomastoid muscle or the muscles of the forearm. Some of the tissue is preserved by freezing in case the grafted parathyroid tissue fails to remain viable. **Tertiary HPT** is treated with a subtotal or total parathyroidectomy with autotransplantation. During surgery, a 50% drop in the PTH level revealed by a rapid assay determines whether the source has been removed. Failure of the intraoperative PTH level to drop indicates that the offending gland(s) has not been excised, and exploration continues. The success of surgery for HPT is approximately 95% or higher. Hypercalcemic crisis requires initial vigorous hydration with normal saline, followed by administration of furosemide. **Bisphosphonates** such as pamidronate or zoledronic acid may maintain the serum calcium level within an acceptable range until an urgent parathyroidectomy can be performed.

Table 4-2. Hyperparathyroidism: Causes and Treatment

Type	Cause(s)	Laboratory Findings	Treatment
Primary	Adenoma (80%), double adenoma (10%), hyperplasia (10%)	Hypercalcemia, ↑PTH	Surgical
Secondary	ESRD with 4-gland hyperplasia	Hypocalcemia or normocalcemia, ↑PTH	Medical (cinacalcet)
Tertiary	Autonomous function of hyperplastic glands in patients with secondary HPT	Hypercalcemia, ↑PTH	Surgical (subtotal or total parathyroidectomy with autotransplantation)

BIBLIOGRAPHY

Bahn R, Burch H, Cooper D, et al. Hyperthyroidism and other causes of thyrotoxicosis: management guidelines of the American Thyroid Association and American Association of Clinical Endocrinologists. *Endocr Pract.* 2011;17(3):456-520.

Cooper D, Doherty G, Haugen B, et al. Revised American Thyroid Association guidelines for patients with thyroid nodules and differentiated thyroid cancer. *Thyroid.* 2009;19(11):1167-1214.

Clinical Keys: Questions And Answers

Question	Answer
What initial imaging is used to assess a solitary thyroid nodule?	Thyroid ultrasound
What percentage of thyroid nodules are benign?	90% to 95%
What is the most common cause of hyperthyroidism?	Graves' disease
What are the 2 most common types of thyroid cancer?	Papillary carcinoma (70%–80%), followed by follicular carcinoma (10%–15%)
What are classic histologic features of papillary carcinoma?	Nuclear grooves/cytoplasmic clearing ("Orphan Annie eye nuclei") and areas of calcification (psammoma bodies)
What features on ultrasound suggest malignancy?	Irregularity, hypervascularity, and the presence of microcalcifications
Which medications are used to treat hyperthyroidism before surgery?	Propylthiouracil (PTU) or methimazole and a beta-blocker
What are the signs and symptoms of hyperthyroidism?	Anxiety, weight loss, palpitations, insomnia, increased appetite, heat intolerance, weakness, psychiatric disturbances, enlarged thyroid, hyperreflexia, hair loss, and muscle wasting
What is goiter?	Abnormal enlargement of the thyroid gland
What is the most common type of hyperparathyroidism?	Primary HPT (caused by a parathyroid adenoma)

Adrenals, Pituitary, and Multiple Endocrine Neoplasias

The adrenal, or *suprarenal*, glands (Fig. 5-1) are a paired set of glands that rest on top of the kidneys.

The adrenals are highly vascularized and receive their arterial blood supply from the phrenic arteries, the aorta, and the renal arteries.

The largest portion of the adrenal glands **is the outer adrenal cortex**, which has 3 distinct zones that produce steroid hormones: (1) **the outer zona glomerulosa**, which produces mineralocorticoids (mainly aldosterone); (2) **the middle zona fasciculata**, which produces the glucocorticoids cortisol, corticosterone, and cortisone; and (3) **the inner zona reticularis**, which produces androgens.

The **adrenal medulla** is centrally located and produces the catecholamine hormones epinephrine, norepinephrine, and dopamine (only small amounts of the latter).

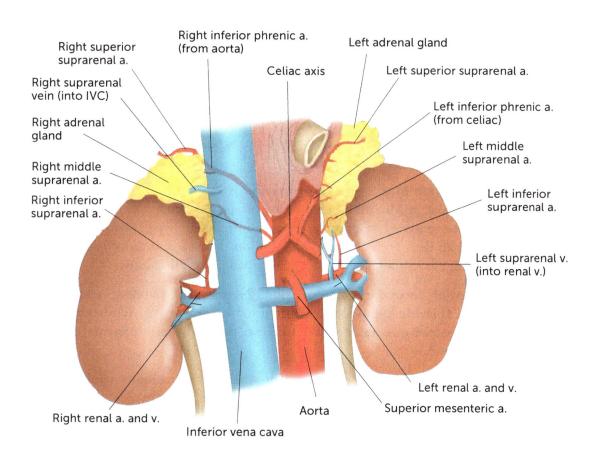

Fig. 5-1. Anatomy and Blood Supply of the Adrenal Glands

Primary Aldosteronism

Definition Primary aldosteronism (PA) is the presence of nonsuppressible hypersecretion of aldosterone, manifesting as resistant hypertension and hypokalemia.

Etiology Traditionally, the most common causes of PA have been cited as **aldosterone-producing adrenal adenomas** (APAs) (60%–75%), but more recent studies reveal that **idiopathic bilateral adrenal hyperplasia** (IHA) may be responsible for as many as 75% of cases. Adrenal adenomas most often arise from the zona fasciculata. Adrenal carcinoma is a distant third and rare cause of the syndrome. Secondary aldosteronism is caused by conditions that trigger the renin-angiotensin-aldosterone system in response to renovascular hypertension, cirrhosis, and other causes.

Epidemiology It is estimated that 7% to 15% of hypertension cases are due to aldosteronism, but this varies according to different sources. PA is more common in women than in men.

Symptoms Weakness may occur secondary to hypokalemia—which occurs as sodium is preferentially reabsorbed in the distal tubules of the kidneys—but this is not a significant symptom unless the potassium falls to below 2.5 mEq/L.

Physical Exam and Signs **Hypertension** is the most common finding, and signs due to its complications such as bruits, proteinuria, and congestive heart failure may be present. Severe hypokalemia may cause an ileus with abdominal distention. Edema is an uncommon finding, so its presence should raise suspicion for other causes.

Differential Secondary hypertension: Normal aldosterone-to-renin ratio. **Thiazide hypokalemia:** History of thiazide intake. **Syndrome of apparent mineralocorticoid excess:** Family history; presents in childhood.

Diagnosis The diagnosis of PA is made with a combination of clinical findings (moderate diastolic hypertension) and lab values.

Labs. Hypokalemia (<3.5 mEq/L), inappropriate kaliuresis (>30 mEq/dL), ↑plasma aldosterone (>15 ng/dL), ±hypernatremia, and ±metabolic alkalosis. A ratio of plasma aldosterone to plasma renin of >20 to >25 (↑aldosterone, ↓renin) suggests PA.

Nonsuppressibility of aldosterone (>14 μg/24 h) after salt and volume loading confirms the diagnosis. An aldosterone-to-plasma renin ratio <10 suggests secondary aldosteronism.

Imaging. **Thin-cut (2 mm) CT scanning with contrast** may localize an adrenal tumor if a unilateral mass at least 1 cm in diameter is present. If CT scan does not localize the tumor, selective venous sampling of cortisol and aldosterone levels from the right and left adrenal veins may be performed and levels compared with those of hormones in the peripheral circulation. NP-59 iodocholesterol I 131 nuclear scanning is almost 90% accurate in discriminating between an aldosteronoma and adrenal hyperplasia. However, the scan is not sensitive for small tumors.

Complication(s) The complications of PA are related to hypertension and the biochemical manifestations.

Treatment Aldosteronomas are removed **surgically**, with a greater than 90% success rate. Idiopathic bilateral adrenal hyperplasia is treated **medically** with 200 to 400 mg daily of spironolactone.

ACUTE ADRENAL INSUFFICIENCY

Definition Acute adrenal insufficiency (AI) refers to **insufficient adrenal production of the glucocorticoid cortisol** from the **adrenal cortex**. (Addison's disease is a chronic form of adrenal insufficiency that should not be confused with an adrenal crisis, which is an acute presentation.)

Etiology AI can be **primary** (Addison's disease), which means the adrenals do not produce enough hormones despite adequate adrenocorticotropic hormone (ACTH), or **secondary,** which is the result of ACTH deficiency. The surgeon is concerned with **secondary AI,** a presentation that is most commonly caused by **abrupt withdrawal of exogenous corticosteroid therapy.** When this occurs, the adrenal cortex is unable to secrete glucocorticoids and mineralocorticoids appropriately. Other causes of secondary AI include sepsis and the systemic inflammatory response syndrome seen in critically ill patients. Less common causes of secondary AI include fungal infection, adrenal bleeding induced by metastatic tumors (eg, carcinoma of the lung), amyloidosis, and others.

Epidemiology Thirty percent of critically ill patients may manifest acute AI.

Symptoms Common symptoms include nausea, vomiting, diarrhea, and fatigue.

Physical Exam and Signs **Severe hypotension** is a significant sign; other signs of acute AI may include dehydration and altered mental status. Fever can be quite high.

Differential Septic shock is a presentation requiring discrimination from acute AI in the critically ill patient.

Diagnosis Patients with acute AI are more likely to be in the ICU or to be trauma victims. Commonly these patients have a history of steroid dependency.

  Labs. Hyperkalemia, hyponatremia, ↓cortisol, azotemia, and hypoglycemia. A rapid ACTH stimulation test is used to test for AI by measuring plasma cortisol levels at timed intervals after administration of synthetic corticotropin.

  Imaging. CT scanning may assist in determining some of the causes of secondary AI (eg, adrenal parenchymal bleeding due to metastatic disease).

Complication(s) If untreated, acute AI can be fatal.

Treatment Acute AI should be treated immediately with **large-volume resuscitation** with isotonic or hypertonic saline and dextrose, along with administration of an **IV glucocorticoid,** such as 4 mg dexamethasone. Afterward, 100 mg hydrocortisone is administered every 6 to 8 hours until the patient's condition stabilizes and steroids may be tapered.

PHEOCHROMOCYTOMA

Definition Pheochromocytoma is a **catecholamine-producing tumor** that may induce life-threatening hypertension. Most pheochromocytomas secrete predominantly **norepinephrine** and lesser amounts of **epinephrine.**

Etiology Unknown, although several genetic mutations have been identified. Pheochromocytomas are derived from the chromaffin cells of the sympathoadrenal system.

Epidemiology Pheochromocytoma is known as the disease with **"the rule of 10s"**: Approximately 10% are malignant, 10% are discovered incidentally, 10% occur in children, 10% are bilateral, and 10% are extra-adrenal. The vast majority of pheochromocytomas (85%–90%) develop in the **adrenal medulla.** The most common extra-adrenal location is the organ of Zuckerkandl in the retroperitoneum. Pheochromocytoma may be associated with multiple endocrine neoplasia (MEN) II.

Symptoms Headaches, palpitations, diaphoresis, flushing, or anxiety. Nausea and weakness may occur. Symptoms become more frequent over time.

Physical Exam and Signs **Paroxysmal or sustained severe hypertension** is the most common sign. Tremor, fever, and arrhythmias are possible. Anesthesia, opiates, beta-blockers, or metoclopramide may precipitate a hypertensive crisis.

Differential Several conditions associated with hypertension or its complications, such as labile hypertension, stroke, renovascular hypertension, and cardiogenic pulmonary edema.

Diagnosis **Twenty-four–hour urine collection** for catecholamines and metanephrines is almost 100% specific.

Labs. Increased urinary epinephrine and norepinephrine and their metabolites (metanephrine, normetanephrine, and vanillylmandelic acid); ±hyperglycemia; plasma levels of chromogranin A can assist in the identification of a pheochromocytoma or its recurrence.

Imaging. **CT** is the imaging test of choice and is approximately 85% to 95% accurate. MRI is best for imaging pheochromocytomas in children. A scintigraphy scan after administration of metaiodobenzylguanidine I 131 (MIBG) is reserved for cases in which a pheochromocytoma is confirmed biochemically but does not appear on CT or MRI.

Complication(s) Cardiac arrhythmias, myocarditis. A crisis may precipitate hypertensive encephalopathy or stroke.

Treatment Surgical resection is the treatment of choice—via a laparoscopic approach when feasible—but it must be preceded by careful preoperative management. An alpha-blocker should be started first to control hypertension, followed by a beta-blocker if tachycardia or arrhythmias develop. Volume correction should be achieved via liberal salt intake and administration of isotonic sodium chloride solution.

INCIDENTAL ADRENAL MASS

Definition An incidental adrenal mass (incidentaloma) is an adrenal tumor(s) larger than 1 cm discovered as an incidental finding.

Etiology Most incidentalomas are benign adenomas. They can, however, occur as metastatic masses, pheochromocytomas, hemorrhage, hyperplasia, or others.

Epidemiology High-resolution CT scanning reveals incidentalomas with a frequency of 4%, which rises with age. The prevalence is higher in patients with diabetes and hypertension. Incidentalomas are bilateral in 10% to 15% of cases, and in some cases one side might be functional while the other is not. Approximately 85% to 90% of incidentalomas are nonfunctional. The remaining 10% to 15% most commonly produce **cortisol.** An adrenal mass larger than 4 cm is highly likely to be malignant.

Symptoms None, unless the mass is functional. If subclinical Cushing's syndrome is present, patients may exhibit hypertension and diabetes.

Physical Exam and Signs None.

Differential The differential focuses on whether the mass is benign or malignant and is functional.

Diagnosis Lab values and findings on imaging vary with the hormone produced and the etiology of the mass, respectively.

Labs. The most common abnormality is a ↓**cortisol level,** inducing **subclinical Cushing's syndrome.** Patients should undergo a 1-mg dexamethasone suppression test, a 24-hour measurement of urinary cortisol, measurement of serum sodium and potassium, and measurement of metanephrines and their metabolites to rule out pheochromocytoma.

Imaging. **Noncontrast CT** is helpful in discriminating between a benign adenoma and a malignant mass. If the images reveal the density of adipose tissue, the likelihood of the finding corresponding to a benign adenoma is almost 100%, although not all adenomas contain large amounts of fat. A pheochromocytoma may have increased vascularity, as well as cystic and hemorrhagic changes. A carcinoma may be large and may have an irregular shape and calcifications.

Complication(s) Related to the etiology of the mass.

Treatment If clinically significant secretory activity is noted, or if the mass is proven to be carcinoma, surgery should be performed. A pheochromocytoma should be resected, and the same is true for most incidentalomas larger than 4 cm. Incidentalomas smaller than 4 cm may be followed clinically.

PROLACTINOMA

Definition Prolactinoma is a **prolactin-producing tumor** of the **anterior pituitary**.

Etiology Unknown. Prolactinoma is caused by neoplastic transformation of the lactotrophs (prolactin-producing cells) in the anterior pituitary.

Epidemiology Prolactinomas represent 30% of all pituitary adenomas. In young patients (up to age 20 years), they represent 75% of all pituitary adenomas. Sixty percent of males present with macroadenomas (>1 cm), and 90% of females present with microadenomas (<1 cm).

Symptoms Females present with oligomenorrhea or amenorrhea, or with galactorrhea. Men may exhibit galactorrhea and signs of hypogonadism, such as decreased libido and erectile dysfunction. Large adenomas may be associated with headaches or visual disturbances.

Physical Exam and Signs Patients should be assessed for the presence of galactorrhea. Some patients may exhibit compromised extraocular movements.

Differential **Polycystic ovarian disease:** Abnormal menses. **Hypothyroidism:** ±Menstrual irregularities and ↑prolactin levels. **Cirrhosis and chronic renal failure:** ±↑Prolactin levels.

Diagnosis The diagnosis of prolactinoma is made on the basis of lab findings and imaging tests.

  Labs. Prolactin level >200 ng/mL (normal level in a nonpregnant female is 2–30 ng/mL) is almost certainly the result of a prolactinoma. Serum TSH should be drawn to determine that prolactin elevation is not due to ↑TRH (seen in hypothyroidism). If amenorrhea is reported, a pregnancy test must be performed.

  Imaging. MRI is better for small lesions. CT is more helpful if bone alterations have occurred.

Complication(s) Large adenomas may produce visual or other local compressive problems.

Treatment Asymptomatic microadenomas can simply be observed. If symptomatic, medical treatment with **bromocriptine** or **cabergoline**—dopamine agonists that inhibit the synthesis of prolactin—should be initiated. If medical therapy fails, or if a macroadenoma is identified, **surgical excision** is performed by a **transsphenoidal approach**.

MULTIPLE ENDOCRINE NEOPLASIAS I AND II

Definition MEN I and MEN II are rare familial syndromes that result in an inherited predisposition to develop various types of benign or malignant tumors originating from endocrine or neuroendocrine tissues. Both are inherited in an **autosomal dominant** fashion. They manifest as overproduction of hormones and/or tumor growth.

  MEN I is called the syndrome of the "3 *P*s," as it is characterized by tumors of the **parathyroid** glands, anterior **pituitary** gland, and **pancreatic** islet cells. Gastroenteric endocrine tumors, such as gastrinomas, carcinoids, glucagonomas, adrenal adenomas, and prolactinomas, may also develop. Nonendocrine tumors that may be seen include angiofibromas, lipomas, meningiomas, leiomyomas, and others.

MEN II is subdivided into 3 types: (1) **MEN IIa;** all patients with this subtype develop medullary thyroid cancer (MTC); 45% develop pheochromocytoma, and 30% develop parathyroid hyperplasia; (2) **MEN IIb,** same as MEN IIa without hyperparathyroidism; and (3) **familial medullary thyroid cancer** (FMTC), which is more indolent than MEN I and MEN II and does not exhibit any other endocrinopathies.

Etiology MEN I is the result of a mutation of the tumor suppressor *MEN1* gene (also called *menin*), located on the long arm of chromosome 11. MEN II is the result of a mutation of the *RET* gene, located on the long arm of chromosome 10.

Epidemiology MEN I and MEN II are present in 1 in 30,000 to 50,000 individuals in the United States. MEN I patients can develop endocrine tumors as young adults, but symptoms and diagnosis are commonly delayed until patients reach their 40s. Ninety percent of patients develop primary hyperparathyroidism by age 50. The most common pituitary tumor associated with MEN I is prolactinoma, yet pituitary tumors are the least common type seen in MEN I.

MEN II has an incidence similar to MEN I. The most common variety is **MEN IIa,** followed by FMTC, and last, by MEN IIb. Ninety percent of MEN II carriers develop MTC, which is the most common feature of MEN II. Among patients with MEN IIa who develop pheochromocytoma, this tumor is the first manifestation of the syndrome in 25% of cases. The MEN IIb type is rare and is associated with more aggressive pheochromocytoma and MTC presenting at earlier ages.

Symptoms The symptoms are manifestations of the types of tumor(s) that develop. In **MEN I**, then, **parathyroid** tumors present with hypercalcemia, which results in depression, confusion, nausea, kidney stones, and hypertension. **Pituitary tumors** may present with menstrual alterations and galactorrhea in females, and rarely, males may present with gynecomastia if a prolactinoma is present. **Pancreatic islet cell tumors** are the most clinically problematic and result in the greatest morbidity and mortality of the syndrome. **Multifocal tumors are almost always malignant,** and the pancreas typically exhibits diffuse involvement. **Gastrinomas** (Zollinger-Ellison syndrome), which are the most common pancreatic tumors, may produce symptoms of peptic ulcer disease, such as abdominal pain with secretory diarrhea; **glucagonomas** may induce diarrhea, glossitis, and lack of appetite.

In **MEN II,** almost all patients have **medullary thyroid cancer** at the time of diagnosis, although symptoms might be associated with pheochromocytoma or hyperparathyroidism. Symptoms may include hypertension, diarrhea (from elevated calcitonin levels), constipation, and pruritic skin lesions.

Physical Exam and Signs The clinical signs of these syndromes are related to the endocrine alterations or local tumor indicators present and to their malignant evolution. In **MEN I,** malignant tumors may have manifestations secondary to their location, the presence of metastatic disease, and so on. If a patient exhibits cutaneous tumors, awareness of their characteristics in **MEN I** may lead the clinician to investigate and attempt to confirm the presence of the disease.

In patients with **MEN II,** a neck mass or a thyroid nodule may be present. Patients with **MEN IIb** variant may exhibit a Marfanoid habitus, including a high-arched palate, pectus excavatum, and scoliosis. Neuromas on the lips, eyelids, and tongue are frequent findings.

Differential The differential for MEN I and MEN II focuses on the distinction between tumors resulting from inherited genetic mutations and the same tumors presenting as a sporadic case. However, other hereditary conditions must be considered.

MEN 1: Tuberous sclerosis (hamartomas of several organs), Cowden's disease (multiple hamartomas). **MEN 2:** Von Hippel–Lindau syndrome (hereditary pheochromocytoma), neurofibromatosis (pheochromocytoma), familial hyperparathyroidism.

Diagnosis The clinical diagnosis of MEN I is suspected if 2 endocrine tumors are present, such as a parathyroid tumor and a pituitary tumor.

Labs. **MEN I:** ↑Calcium and ↑parathyroid hormone with parathyroid tumors, ↑prolactin with prolactinomas, ↑gastrin with gastrinomas; the *MEN1* mutation is detected with genetic testing in approximately 80% of patients. **MEN II:** Genetic testing for a mutated *RET* gene is indicated because the syndrome can be identified in this way in 98% of patients; ↑calcitonin level strongly suggests MTC; ↑catecholamines excreted in a 24-hour urine collection suggests pheochromocytoma.

Imaging. **MEN I:** MRI for pituitary tumors; octreotide scanning for endocrine tumors; endoscopic ultrasound assists in diagnosing pancreatic endocrine tumors; nuclear scanning for parathyroid tumors (multiple parathyroid adenomas are typical of MEN I). **MEN II:** CT or MRI of adrenals. **MIBG scan** can localize a pheochromocytoma.

Complication(s) Related to the progression of biochemical manifestations or tumor(s) associated with the presentation.

Treatment **MEN I:** Treatment is directed to control the presenting problem as manifested. Hyperparathyroidism is treated surgically, as is the case with most pancreatic tumors. Prolactinoma may be treated with dopamine agonists. Nonsecreting pituitary adenomas are treated with transsphenoidal surgery. **MEN II:** MTC and pheochromocytoma are treated surgically.

BIBLIOGRAPHY

Carey RM. Primary aldosteronism. *J Surg Oncol.* 2012;106(5):575-579.

Moore SW, Appfelstaedt J, Zaahl MG. Familial medullary carcinoma prevention, risk evaluation, and RET in children of families with MEN2. *J Pediatr Surg.* 2007;42(2):326-332.

CLINICAL KEYS: QUESTIONS AND ANSWERS

What is primary aldosteronism?	Hypersecretion of aldosterone, manifesting as resistant hypertension and hypokalemia
What is the most common cause of primary aldosteronism?	Aldosterone-producing adrenal adenomas
How are adrenal adenomas treated?	Surgically
What is adrenal insufficiency?	Insufficient adrenal production of cortisol
What is the most common cause of acute secondary adrenal insufficiency?	Withdrawal of exogenous corticosteroid therapy
What is a significant sign of acute adrenal insufficiency?	Severe hypotension
What are common lab findings of acute adrenal insufficiency?	Hyperkalemia, hyponatremia, decreased cortisol, azotemia, and hypoglycemia
What is a pheochromocytoma?	A catecholamine-producing (mostly norepinephrine and some epinephrine) tumor that may induce life-threatening hypertension
From which part of the adrenal gland do most pheochromocytomas arise?	The adrenal medulla
What are the symptoms of pheochromocytoma?	Headaches, palpitations, diaphoresis, flushing, anxiety
What is the most common sign of pheochromocytoma?	Paroxysmal or sustained severe hypertension
What is the lab test of choice to diagnose pheochromocytoma?	24-hour–urine collection for catecholamines and metanephrines
What is the treatment of choice for pheochromocytoma?	Surgical resection preceded by medical management of hypertension with an alpha-blocker
What is an incidentaloma?	Adrenal tumor(s) >1 cm discovered as an incidental finding on CT

Adrenals, Pituitary, and Multiple Endocrine Neoplasias

What hormone do incidentalomas most commonly secrete?	Cortisol
What is a prolactinoma?	A pituitary prolactin-producing tumor
What are the multiple endocrine neoplasias?	Genetic syndromes that predispose individuals to the development of benign or malignant endocrine and/or neuroendocrine tumors

Topic III
Thoracic

Esophagus 6

The esophagus is a muscular tube connecting the pharynx to the stomach (Fig. 6-1). It has 3 artificial divisions important to the surgeon: the cervical, the thoracic, and the abdominal portions.

At its origin, the cervical esophagus has a high pressure zone known as the **upper esophageal sphincter** (UES), which is partly a result of the action of the crycopharingeus muscle.

The **lower esophageal sphincter** (LES) is a natural constriction that prevents gastric reflux into the esophagus.

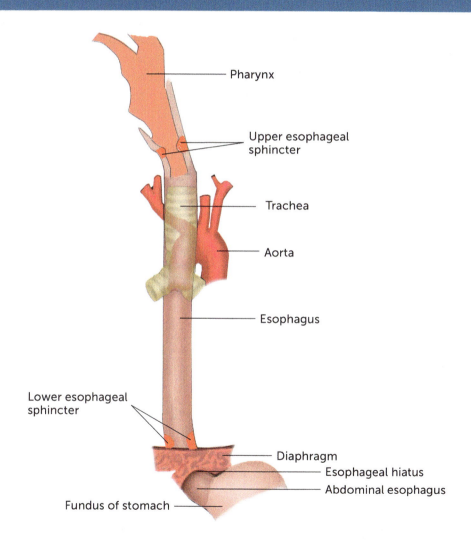

Fig. 6-1. Anatomy of the Esophagus

Hiatal Hernia

Definition A hiatal hernia (HH) is the protrusion of a portion of the stomach through the diaphragmatic esophageal hiatus.

Etiology HH is a result of the weakening of the hiatus muscular structure. Possible causes include obesity, aging, and pressure as result of coughing or straining.

Epidemiology The incidence of HH increases with age, and they are more common in women than in men. There are 2 main types of HHs: type I, or *sliding* (Fig. 6-2), and type II, or *paraesophageal* (Fig. 6-3). **Type I** represents 95% or more of all HHs; in this type, the cardia of the stomach and the GE junction move into the mediastinum. **Type II HH** occurs when the fundus of the stomach protrudes into the chest (to a paraesophageal location) while the GE junction remains in its normal position. A **type III HH** (Fig. 6-4) is a combination of types I and II—the GE junction, cardia, and fundus move into the chest. When other viscera, such as intestine, are associated with the sliding/paraesophageal component, it is known as a **type IV HH** (Fig. 6-5).

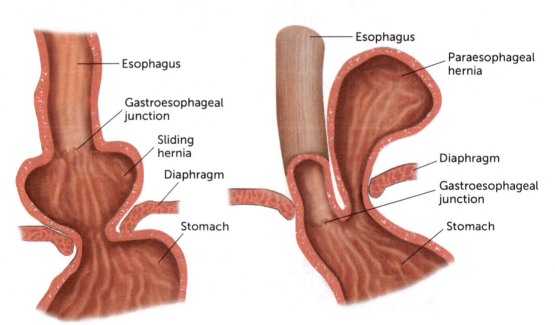

Fig. 6-2. Type I (Sliding) Hiatal Hernia

Fig. 6-3. Type II (Paraesophageal) Hiatal Hernia

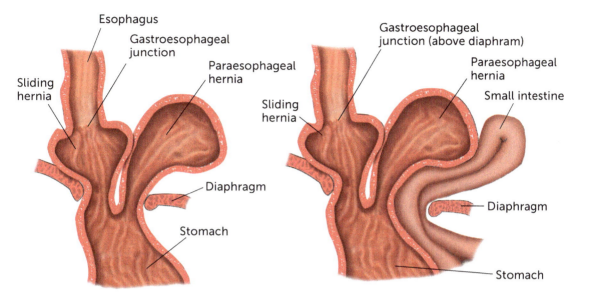

Fig. 6-4. Type III Hiatal Hernia

Fig. 6-5. Type IV Hiatal Hernia

Symptoms The majority of HHs are asymptomatic. However, reflux, bloating, chest pain, and dysphagia may be noted.

Physical Exam and Signs There are no specific physical signs.

Differential If a patient presents with chest pain, angina must be ruled out. Gastroesophageal reflux disease (GERD), esophagitis, peptic ulcer disease, and esophageal carcinoma may be considered.

Diagnosis **Barium swallow** is the test of choice to diagnose HH. It can help differentiate between type I and type II HHs.

Labs. There are no specific laboratory tests. Anemia may be noted if GERD is associated.

Imaging. Chest radiograph may reveal an air-fluid level, which suggests the presence of HH.

Complication(s) Usually, complications are the result of untreated reflux. Erosive esophagitis, ulcerations, or Barrett's esophagus may develop. Incarceration or strangulation of a type II hernia is rare.

Treatment The treatment is guided by symptoms, which are most often caused by reflux. The Society of American Gastrointestinal and Endoscopic Surgeons (SAGES) evidence-based guidelines of management for 2013 include recommendations that **asymptomatic type I HHs** do not require treatment, and that all **symptomatic type II through type IV HHs** should be surgically repaired. Patients with type I HH associated with reflux should undergo medical management.

Gastroesophageal Reflux Disease

Definition Gastroesophageal reflux disease (GERD) occurs when gastric juices reflux into the esophagus and cause symptoms, with or without associated injury to the esophagus.

Etiology Reflux can be transient or persistent. The most common mechanism of reflux involves **mechanical dysfunction of the LES (60%)**. This may result in esophageal or gastric dysfunction, such as decreased esophageal peristalsis or delayed gastric emptying. Alcohol, fatty foods, medications (eg, calcium channel blockers, anticholinergics), hormones (eg, progesterone), and smoking can transiently exacerbate symptoms. A common persistent cause of reflux is the presence of a hiatal hernia.

Epidemiology GERD is a common problem in industrialized countries. In the United States, it affects 30% to 40% of the population at some point, including children and adults, and its prevalence increases with age.

Symptoms **Pyrosis (heartburn)** is the most common symptom of GERD. Patients can present with regurgitation, dysphagia (~25% to 30%), substernal chest pain, coughing, and wheezing (aspiration). Hoarseness may occur.

Physical Exam and Signs There are no specific signs.

Differential Cholelithiasis, esophagitis, gastritis, peptic ulcer disease, and esophageal carcinoma may be considered.

Diagnosis **Upper GI endoscopy** is essential for identifying complications of GERD and for evaluating the anatomic panorama of the disease.

Labs. Anemia may be noted. **Manometry** helps determine LES dysfunction and location, and to rule out motility disorders. It is useful in preparation for surgical therapy. An **ambulatory 24-hour pH probe** may be used when the presentation is atypical, when the endoscopic findings are negative, or when the patient does not respond to appropriate medical therapy. In these situations, pH monitoring is 95% sensitive and 95% specific.

Imaging. Upper GI series can demonstrate spontaneous reflux in only ~40% of patients, but it can reveal HH and complications of GERD, such as strictures and ulcers of the esophagus. Therefore it is an appropriate initial study. A nuclear medicine gastric emptying scan can provide information about gastric function.

Complication(s) The most common complication is **esophagitis**, noted in 50% of patients with GERD. A stricture may be a result of advanced esophagitis and may cause dysphagia. **Barrett's esophagus** is the most clinically important complication of chronic reflux because of its malignant potential.

Treatment **Lifestyle changes** include losing weight, elevating the head of the bed 6 to 8 inches when sleeping, and eating smaller, more frequent meals. Patients are advised to refrain from eating meals 3 hours before bedtime, drinking alcohol, smoking cigarettes, and consuming fatty foods, chocolate, peppermint, and caffeine. **Medical therapy** is recommended when lifestyle changes are ineffective. These include **(1) antacids** to neutralize gastric acids, **(2) H_2-blockers** to lower gastric acidity by decreasing the amount of acid produced, and **(3) proton pump inhibitors (PPIs)** that inhibit the H^+/K^+ pump. PPIs are more effective than H_2-blockers and can reverse esophagitis. **Surgery** is indicated for those who fail medical therapy, those with Barrett's esophagus, and those with extraesophageal manifestations of GERD (eg, respiratory, ear, nose, and throat symptoms). **Laparoscopic fundoplication** (Nissen's fundoplication) results in the best surgical outcomes.

BARRETT'S ESOPHAGUS

Definition Barrett's esophagus is the **replacement of the normal squamous epithelium** of the distal esophagus by **metaplastic columnar epithelium,** resulting in a predisposition to develop carcinoma.

Etiology Chronic GERD is the cause of Barrett's esophagus.

Epidemiology The risk of developing esophageal cancer as a result of Barrett's esophagus is approximately **30 to 40 times higher** than the risk in the general population. Yet mortality from esophageal cancer is low, perhaps because patients with Barrett's esophagus are older and die from other, more common diseases. Barrett's esophagus has a **higher incidence in men,** with a male-to-female ratio of 2:1. It presents as long-segment Barrett's esophagus (LSBE), or short-segment Barrett's esophagus (SSBE). SSBE is the most common of the two types.

Symptoms Similar to GERD. Seventy-five percent of patients have dysphagia and 25% have esophageal bleeding.

Physical Exam and Signs No specific clinical findings.

Differential The differential is the same as in patients with GERD.

Diagnosis **Upper GI endoscopy** is the procedure of choice for diagnosing Barrett's esophagus. **Biopsy** with histologic findings of **intestinal-type metaplasia** anywhere in the esophagus confirms the diagnosis.

Labs. No specific laboratory findings.

Imaging. Radiographs may suggest the presence of Barrett's esophagus by demonstrating the presence of an HH (associated with Barrett's esophagus ~80% of the time).

Complication(s) Strictures, low or high grade dysplasia, esophageal carcinoma.

Treatment Uncomplicated, asymptomatic Barrett's esophagus requires no therapy. However, patients must undergo endoscopy with biopsy annually. Symptomatic patients are advised similarly to patients with GERD—coffee, alcohol, smoking, and nonsteroidal anti-inflammatory drugs (NSAIDs) should be avoided. These patients also benefit from medical or surgical treatment, or both. The current standard of care for high-grade dysplasia is **endoscopic ablation,** which removes dysplastic mucosa and allows regrowth of squamous epithelium. It is used with medical or surgical therapy to control reflux.

Esophageal Cancer

Definition A malignant tumor of the esophagus.

Etiology Factors influencing the development of esophageal carcinoma include obesity, drinking alcohol, cigarette smoking, and GERD.

Epidemiology The incidence of adenocarcinoma compared to the historically more common squamous type has increased in the last 3 decades in the United States—**adenocarcinoma** now represents the most common histologic type of esophageal cancer (~70% of new cases). Adenocarcinoma most commonly involves the **distal esophagus** and **gastroesophageal junction**. Squamous cell carcinoma most frequently involves the middle third of the esophagus. Esophageal cancer is 3 or 4 times more common in men than in women and is currently the seventh most common cause of death in men, with a 5-year aggregate survival rate of 19%. The 5-year survival rate for stage IV esophageal cancer is close to 0%. Esophageal cancer rates in Iran, northern China, India, and southern Africa are 10 to 100 times higher than in the United States, most likely as a result of diet.

Symptoms The most common symptom is **dysphagia**, at first only to solids; then as the disease progresses, to liquids as well. Other symptoms include retrosternal discomfort or pain, cough (from aspiration), or blood in the stool.

Physical Exam and Signs The most common sign is weight loss. Findings from a physical exam are usually negative, unless lymphadenopathy or metastatic liver disease is present.

Differential Other presentations that can cause dysphagia include strictures, achalasia, benign tumors (leiomyomas), and gastric carcinoma.

Diagnosis **Upper GI endoscopy** is the test of choice to diagnose esophageal carcinoma. In addition to visualizing the tumor, a biopsy can be obtained for definitive diagnosis. **Endoscopic ultrasound** (EUS) is useful and sensitive for determining the depth of tumor invasion and the status of periesophageal lymph nodes, both of which allow clinical staging and resectability to be determined. **Bronchoscopy** reveals whether tracheobronchial invasion has occurred.

Labs. There are no specific laboratory tests; however, CBC may reveal anemia, and liver function tests may suggest metastatic disease.

Imaging. CT and PET scans reveal the extent of metastatic disease.

Complication(s) Obstruction of the esophagus with inability to swallow, increasing likelihood of malnutrition, bleeding, and death can occur.

Treatment Options vary depending on the stage of the disease at the time of diagnosis. However, these options center around a combination of surgery, chemotherapy, and radiotherapy. Chemotherapy and radiation followed by surgery offers the best results for patients who can tolerate this regimen. Chemoradiation before surgery has been associated with pathologic complete response (disappearance of the tumor on gross exam) as high as 30% of the time, which is likely to produce better long-term results. Stage IV disease is treated with chemotherapy or palliation according to the specifics of the case.

Achalasia

Definition Achalasia is a primary dysmotility disorder of the esophagus, characterized by **lack of peristalsis in the esophageal body and absent or incomplete relaxation of the LES** in response to swallowing.

Etiology Typical pathology involves a **loss of ganglion cells** from the esophageal wall, which starts at the LES and develops proximally over time. Causation is unknown.

Epidemiology Achalasia is the most common primary dysmotility disorder, but it is rare, representing 1 in 100,000 individuals.

Symptoms Dysphagia to solids followed by dysphagia to liquids is noted by almost all patients. Regurgitation immediately after meals is noted by ~70% of patients. Chest pain and heartburn may be reported.

Physical Exam and Signs There are no specific clinical signs. Weight loss may be reported.

Differential If chest pain is reported, angina must be ruled out.

Diagnosis **Esophageal manometry** is the test of choice for the diagnosis of achalasia.

Labs. There are no specific lab tests.

Imaging. **Chest radiographs** may suggest the diagnosis by revealing an air-fluid level, a widened mediastinum, and the absence of a gastric air bubble. **Barium esophagogram** may show a **"bird's beak"** (tapering) appearance of the distal esophagus and a widening of the proximal esophagus. Hiatal hernia may be present in 10% to 15% of patients. **Esophageal manometry** reveals lack of peristalsis and incomplete or absent LES relaxation with swallowing. Endoscopy is crucial to rule out benign or malignant causes of obstruction.

Complication(s) Stagnation of food may lead to mucosal erythema and friability, and/or ulceration and infection (eg, candidiasis). The risk of developing squamous cell carcinoma of the esophagus is higher in patients with achalasia.

Treatment **Medical therapy** is aimed at decreasing LES tone; **nitrates** or **calcium channel blockers,** such as nifedipine, are given. Botulinum toxin injection into the LES has been used with varying results. **Endoscopic pneumatic dilatation** of the LES has the best long-term results. A postdilatation LES pressure below 10 mm Hg predicts a good outcome, whereas higher pressures do not. A **thoracoscopic** or **laparoscopic surgical myotomy** of the LES appears to confer longer lasting benefits than balloon dilatation. In cases of very advanced disease, when the anatomy is significantly distorted, **esophagectomy** may become necessary.

ESOPHAGEAL PERFORATION

Definition Esophageal perforation is a hole in the esophageal wall.

Etiology The most common cause of esophageal perforation is **trauma from instrumentation** (75%), usually from endoscopy. Less common causes include ingestion of a foreign body or caustic substances, and esophageal carcinoma. Rarely, the perforation is spontaneous—this is known as *Boerhaave's syndrome.* Spontaneous rupture usually follows food or alcohol ingestion and is precipitated by **violent retching** and **vomiting.**

Epidemiology The majority of instrument perforations occur in the cervical esophagus. Most spontaneous perforations occur in the distal esophagus, and a significant number occur in patients with GERD. The incidence of perforation increases when attempts are made to dilate strictures or obstruction caused by radiation or tumors. Incidence is also higher when associated pathologic conditions are present, such as hiatal hernia or esophageal diverticula. The mortality rate following esophageal perforation is approximately 20%.

Symptoms Initially, symptoms may include **severe and acute pain in the chest, neck, or epigastric area, and dysphagia.** A history of vomiting or retching, or both, suggests Boerhaave's syndrome.

Physical Exam and Signs Subcutaneous emphysema and crepitus may be noted in 50% to 60% of patients, but this sign might not be immediately apparent. **Mackler's triad**—vomiting, pain, and subcutaneous emphysema—is present in 14% to 40% of patients. If the perforation is intra-abdominal, peritonitis is typically noted.

Differential Myocardial infarction, pneumonia, pneumothorax, and aortic dissection may be considered.

Diagnosis Chest radiograph is helpful, often suggesting esophageal perforation.

Labs. No laboratory tests are specific.

Imaging. Chest radiograph may show pneumomediastinum, pleural effusion, atelectasis, soft tissue emphysema, hydrothorax or hydropneumothorax, or air outlining the diaphragm and the mediastinal border, forming a **V** shape. The imaging procedure of choice to diagnose esophageal perforation is an **esophagogram,** which initially must be performed with water-soluble contrast (Gastrografin). If negative, the study can be done using barium, which has a higher sensitivity. Barium, however, can cause a severe inflammatory response if it leaks into the mediastinum, so the study should be performed with the patient in right lateral decubitus position. If an esophagogram cannot be performed or if findings are negative despite a likely clinical presentation, a CT scan should be performed.

Complication(s) If untreated, an esophageal perforation may lead to mediastinitis, empyema, shock, respiratory failure, and death in the acute period. Long-term complications after patients survive the initial insult may include formation of esophageal strictures, which requires intervention.

Treatment Initially, patients are kept on a nothing-by-mouth (NPO) status. IV fluids and antibiotics are administered, and a nasogastric tube is inserted. If no manifestations of sepsis are present, and if the leak is contained and not in the abdomen, the patient may be treated nonsurgically and carefully followed. Otherwise, a surgical approach of variable intensity must be performed depending on the presentation and location of the perforation.

BIBLIOGRAPHY

Spechler SJ. Barrett esophagus and risk of esophageal cancer: a clinical review. *JAMA*. 2013;310(6):627-636.

Stefanidis D, Richardson W, Farrell TM, et al; for Society of American Gastrointestinal and Endoscopic Surgeons. SAGES guidelines for the surgical treatment of esophageal achalasia. *Surg Endosc*. 2012;26(2):296-311.

CLINICAL KEYS: QUESTIONS AND ANSWERS

What is a hiatal hernia?	A protrusion of a portion of the stomach through the diaphragmatic esophageal hiatus
What are the symptoms of a hiatal hernia?	Most are asymptomatic—in some cases, reflux, bloating, chest pain, and dysphagia may occur
What is the test of choice to diagnose a hiatal hernia?	Barium swallow
What is the treatment for asymptomatic type I hiatal hernia?	No treatment is required
What is gastroesophageal disease (GERD)?	Reflux of gastric juice into the esophagus that causes symptoms with or without associated injury to the esophagus
What are the symptoms of GERD?	Pyrosis, substernal burning chest pain, dysphagia, coughing
What is the treatment for GERD?	Lifestyle changes include elevating the head of the bed when sleeping, and avoiding coffee, cigarettes, alcohol, NSAIDs, and fatty foods; medical therapy includes antacids, H_2-blockers, and proton pump inhibitors
What is Barrett's esophagus?	Replacement of the normal squamous epithelium of the distal esophagus by metaplastic columnar epithelium
What is the cause of Barrett's esophagus?	Chronic GERD
What is the test of choice for diagnosing Barrett's esophagus?	Upper GI endoscopy; biopsy with histologic findings of intestinal-type metaplasia confirms the diagnosis

Which is the most common type of esophageal cancer?	Adenocarcinoma
What is the most common symptom of esophageal cancer?	Dysphagia
What is achalasia?	A primary dysmotility disorder of the esophagus resulting in lack of peristalsis in the esophageal body and incomplete or absent relaxation of the LES
What are the symptoms of achalasia?	Dysphagia, regurgitation
What is the most common cause of esophageal perforation?	Instrumentation, such as endoscopic tools
What is Boerhaave's syndrome?	Spontaneous esophageal rupture usually followed by violent retching
What is Mackler's triad?	Vomiting, pain, and subcutaneous emphysema (associated with esophageal perforation)

Lung 7

The lungs are within the chest cavity, and the chest wall protects the anterior, lateral, and posterior lung surfaces. The inner chest wall is lined with parietal pleural membrane, and the lung surface is covered with visceral pleural membrane (Fig. 7-1). These linings create a near frictionless surface for the lung to move without harm.

The trachea is the largest conducting airway in the body and branches into the left and right main bronchi. These give rise to bronchopulmonary segments that divide the lung parenchyma into approximately 10 segments in the right lung and 8 segments in the left lung.

As the airways branch into smaller units, their function changes from gas conduction to gas exchange. At the level of the bronchioles, alveolar ducts, and alveolar sacs, the deoxygenated blood arriving from the right side of the heart and flowing through the capillaries adjacent to the alveolar wall is converted into oxygenated blood (see detail, Fig. 7-1).

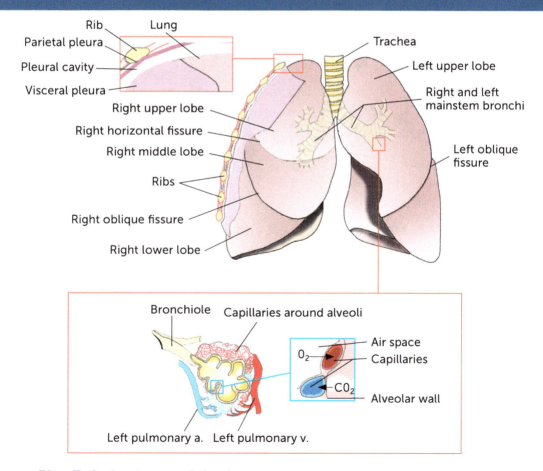

Fig. 7-1. Anatomy of the Lung

The right lung has 3 lobes: the upper, middle, and lower lobes, which are separated by 2 fissures, the horizontal and oblique fissures (Fig. 7-2).

The left lung has 1 upper and 1 lower lobe, which are separated by the oblique fissure.

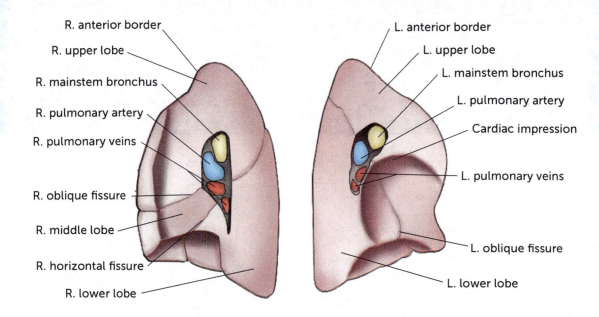

Fig. 7-2. Medial View of Left and Right Lungs

SOLITARY PULMONARY NODULE

Definition Solitary pulmonary nodules are lung nodules that are **less than 3 cm** in diameter and are found through diagnostic imaging. The nodules may be benign or malignant.

Etiology A **granuloma** is the most common type of **benign nodule.** It is an inflammatory nodule from a previous or ongoing lung infection, such as tuberculosis or mycetoma (a bacterial or fungal infection). Hamartomas (abnormal formations of normal tissue) are common benign nodules. A malignant nodule can arise as metastatic disease from malignant tumors in other organs.

Epidemiology Among the benign types of solitary nodules, 70% are granulomas. **Calcification** of the nodule correlates well with **benign disease.** The nodule is malignant in 30% to 40% of cases.

Symptoms Most nodules are asymptomatic and found incidentally. However, hemoptysis, cough, and dyspnea can occur.

Physical Exam and Signs Findings from a physical exam are nonspecific.

Differential Tuberculosis: History of travel to endemic areas, hemoptysis, weight loss, ±time spent homeless, incarceration, +sputum culture, +PPD, calcifications on chest radiograph. **Mycetoma:** Fever, nonproductive cough, ±sputum culture, calcifications on chest radiograph. **Lung cancer:** ±History of smoking tobacco, weight loss, no calcifications on chest radiograph, mass with irregular borders on CT. **Metastatic disease:** History of previous cancer, weight loss, no calcifications on chest radiograph. **Postpneumonia granuloma:** History of pneumonia, smooth nodule borders on CT, calcifications on chest radiograph.

Diagnosis The size and characteristics of the lesion must be considered in the evaluation. Micropulmonary nodules, macropulmonary nodules, indeterminate nodules, and suspicious nodules are categories assigned to nodules based on size (Fig. 7-3 and Fig. 7-4).

Labs. Obtain sputum cultures and cytologic evaluation, PPD test to assess exposure to tuberculosis, and ±leukocytosis if infectious etiology is suspected.

Imaging. Chest radiograph demonstrates lesion. Previous chest radiographs can help determine if the lesion is stable or growing.

Absence of growth for 2 years indicates benign disease. Smooth borders and calcification that is diffuse, is centrally located, and looks like onion skin or popcorn indicates **benign disease.** Lesions with **stippled calcifications** or **irregular borders** may indicate **malignancy. CT scan** with IV contrast yields better resolution and can help identify mediastinal lymphadenopathy. **PET scan** for lesions larger than 1 cm can help differentiate malignant from benign lesions.

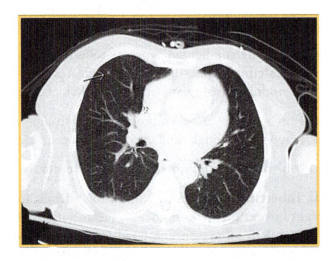

Fig. 7-3. Isolated Micropulmonary Nodule in Right Lung on CT

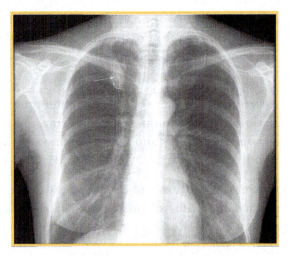

Fig. 7-4. Isolated Macropulmonary Nodule of Right Upper Lobe

Treatment Etiology determines treatment of solitary pulmonary nodules. Tuberculosis is treated with antibiotics and close follow-up. Fungal infections are treated with antifungal agents. Treatment of malignant nodules is determined by their presentation and stage.

HEMOPTYSIS

Definition Hemoptysis is the coughing up of blood or bloody sputum from the lungs or airway.

Etiology The most common cause of hemoptysis is **bronchitis.** Other causes include pneumonia, tuberculosis, and lung cancer. The most common cause in the pediatric age group is the presence of a foreign body. Other causes seen in surgical patients include airway trauma, pulmonary contusion, pulmonary embolism, and anticoagulant use.

Epidemiology In the United States, **bacterial sources** are the most common cause of hemoptysis, accounting for 70% of cases. Worldwide, tuberculosis is the most common cause of hemoptysis, followed by lung cancer in approximately 25% of cases.

Symptoms Hemoptysis is associated with **coughing.** Fever is typically associated with occult infection. Obtaining a detailed history often identifies the underlying cause of the hemoptysis, and it should include questions related to foreign travel, incarceration, and time spent homeless.

Physical Exam and Signs Cachexia and pallor should be assessed during inspection. If hemoptysis is massive, airway compromise and hemodynamic instability may be seen.

Differential The origin of blood from epistaxis or expectoration without cough could arise from a gastrointestinal or nasopharyngeal source, both of which are more common than hemoptysis. **Bronchitis:** Chronic cough, ±tobacco use. **Pneumonia:** Fever, leukocytosis, dullness to percussion and rales, infiltrate(s) on chest radiograph, +sputum cultures. **Tuberculosis:** History of foreign travel, incarceration, ±time spent homeless, fever, +PPD, chest radiograph reveals cavitary lesions. **Foreign body:** Pediatric patient, history of aspiration, stridor, chest radiograph reveals foreign body. **Lung cancer:** Weight loss, peripheral lymphadenopathy, nodule on chest radiograph, ±tobacco use. **Mycetoma:** Fever, nonproductive cough, travel to endemic areas, solitary nodule on chest radiograph.

Diagnosis

Labs. ±Leukocytosis, ±PPD, sputum cultures to identify infectious etiology, sputum cytology to identify neoplasm. Anemia present in chronic or massive hemoptysis; PT/INR/pTT derangements if patient is receiving anticoagulants.

Imaging. Chest radiograph reveals infiltrates, cavitary lesions, pulmonary nodules, and/or hilar adenopathy. Chest CT with IV contrast delineates between different causes of hemoptysis with better resolution than chest radiograph. Arterial angiography is useful in massive hemoptysis as a diagnostic and therapeutic tool (coil embolization of bleeding bronchial vessels).

Treatment The amount of initial bleeding and its cause guides treatment. Infectious causes are treated with antibiotics selected according to culture results. Suspicious lesions are biopsied after an acute episode resolves. Hemorrhage of greater than 200 mL/day is classified as massive hemorrhage. Goals of therapy in massive hemorrhage adhere to the ABCs of resuscitation. Airway is maintained with endotracheal intubation to prevent asphyxiation. Patients may need to undergo intubation of the mainstem bronchus of the unaffected lung to prevent this outcome. Once airway, breathing, and circulation have been addressed, patients are transfused as needed. At this point, bronchoscopic interventions to stop bleeding can be implemented if the patient is stable and bleeding doesn't obscure visualization. If bronchoscopic management fails, the next step is to perform angiographic embolization of the bleeding bronchial artery. The last resort is surgical resection of the affected lobe, a choice associated with much higher morbidity and mortality than less invasive options.

LUNG CANCER

Definition Lung cancer is the uncontrolled and malignant growth of lung cells. The 2 major subtypes of lung cancer are **non–small cell lung carcinoma (NSCLC)** and **small cell lung carcinoma (SCLC).**

Etiology The most significant risk factor associated with lung cancer is **smoking tobacco products,** which is responsible for a 10- to 20-fold increase in the risk of developing the disease. Environmental causes of lung cancer include exposure to radon gas and asbestos. These risk exposures are magnified in smokers. The most common lung cancer in smokers originates from **squamous cells.**

Epidemiology NSCLCs are the most common types of lung cancer (Table 7-1). The 3 most common subtypes are **adenocarcinoma, squamous cell,** and **large cell.** Lung cancer is the leading cause of cancer deaths worldwide.

Table 7-1. Common Lung Cancers

Non–small cell lung carcinoma (80%)
Adenocarcinoma (30%–50%)
Squamous cell (20%–35%)
Large cell (4%–15%)
Small cell lung carcinoma (20%)

Symptoms The most common symptom of lung cancer is **cough.** Symptoms such as anorexia, fatigue, dyspnea, and hemoptysis are not uncommon. Brain metastasis can present with a range of symptoms, including confusion or focal neurologic deficits, vision changes, and headaches. Bone metastasis may induce pathologic fractures and arthritis.

Physical Exam and Signs The most common physical findings include weight loss or cachexia, wheezing on auscultation, and clubbing of the digits in advanced disease; this last finding is similar to what is seen in patients with chronic obstructive pulmonary disease (COPD). Dullness to percussion in lower lung fields suggests the presence of pleural effusions, whereas muffled heart sounds suggest pericardial effusion. **Pancoast tumors,** which are apical lung tumors, may invade the cervical sympathetic ganglia and cause ipsilateral **Horner's syndrome** (anhidrosis, miosis, and ptosis). Lung cancer may induce **paraneoplastic syndromes** caused by the release of hormone-like substances from tumor cells (Table 7-2).

Table 7-2. Paraneoplastic Syndromes of Lung Cancer

Syndrome	Cancer Type	Endocrine Molecule	Signs
SIADH[a]	Small cell	ADH[b]	Seizures, altered mental status
Cushing's syndrome	Small cell	ACTH[c]	Moon facies, cushingoid habitus
Hypercalcemia	Squamous cell	PTHrP[d]	Moans, groans, psychiatric overtones

[a]Syndrome of inappropriate antidiuretic hormone
[b]Antidiuretic hormone
[c]Adrenocorticotropic hormone
[d]Parathyroid hormone–related peptide

Differential **Bronchitis/pneumonia:** Fever, rales/wheezing, chest radiograph reveals lobar infiltrate and no mass. **COPD:** History of smoking, wheezing, no mass on chest radiograph. **Pulmonary contusion:** History of trauma, chest radiograph reveals diffuse infiltrate, no mass. **Mycetoma:** History of travel to endemic area, fever, chest radiograph reveals calcified nodule, ±fungus sputum cultures, +fungus on biopsy. **Tuberculosis:** History of travel to endemic area, ±time spent homeless, incarceration. Fever, hemoptysis, +PPD, chest radiograph reveals calcified nodule, +acid-fast bacillus on sputum culture.

Diagnosis Definitive diagnosis of lung cancer is obtained with **biopsy,** which can be done by a percutaneous image-guided approach, by bronchoscopy, or surgically, depending on tumor location. SCLC usually presents **centrally.** This is true also for squamous cell lung cancer, but unlike SCLC, it commonly has central cavitation. Most peripheral NSCLCs are adenocarcinomas.

Labs. Sputum is assessed cytologically.

Imaging. Chest radiograph demonstrates a **noncalcified nodule(s)** and adenopathy. CT chest with IV contrast details lesion(s) and adenopathy. CT or brain MRI locates brain metastasis. PET scan is used to stage disease and to find occult metastases.

Complication(s) The most common complication of lung cancer is pleural effusion, in which malignant cells seed the pleural space. **Malignant pleural effusion** indicates stage 4 (advanced) disease, which is not curable. It is diagnosed with cytology and chest radiograph findings. Pericardial effusion may be seen occasionally.

Treatment A way to remember the steps necessary to treat any malignancy is "name it, stage it, treat it." Once the diagnosis is made, the next goal is to characterize the tumor based on TNM staging criteria (Table 7-4). This is accomplished by using imaging to identify metastases and lymph node involvement. This may lead to biopsy of suspicious lesions found elsewhere. Treatment according to stage may include surgery (Fig. 7-5), chemotherapy, and radiation. NSCLC stages 1 to 2b and select stage 3a malignancies are treated surgically, with or without chemotherapy or radiation. NSCLC stage 3b to 4 and SCLC are treated with chemotherapy or radiation. **Malignant pleural effusion** is treated by inserting a chest tube or obliterating the pleural space by injecting an adhesion-forming agent (pleurodesis).

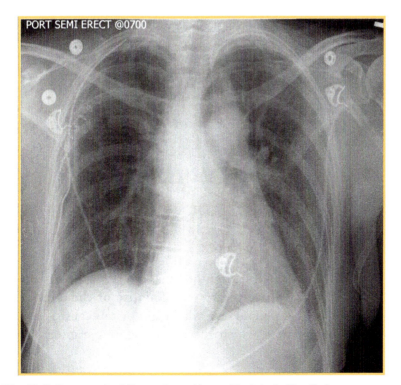

Fig. 7-5. Postsurgical Resection of Lung Nodule in Fig. 7-4

Table 7-4. TNM Definitions (Abbreviated List)

T1a	Tumor <2 cm
T1b	Tumor >2 cm
T2a	Tumor >3 cm and <5 cm
T2b	Tumor >5 cm and <7 cm
T3	Tumor >7 cm; invades resectable structure
T4	Tumor invades unresectable structure
N0	No nodal metastasis
N1	Ipsilateral nonmediastinal lymph node involvement
N2	Ipsilateral mediastinal lymph node involvement
N3	Contralateral lymph node involvement
M0	No metastasis
M1a	Pleural or pericardial effusion
M1b	Distant metastasis

SPONTANEOUS PNEUMOTHORAX

Definition Spontaneous pneumothorax (PTX) is a collection of air within the pleural space that causes **collapse of the affected lung.** PTX is classified as **primary,** in which an obvious cause is not apparent, or **secondary,** in which there is recognizable underlying lung disease.

Etiology The most common cause of primary spontaneous PTX is the **rupture of an apical pulmonary bleb.** The most common cause of secondary spontaneous PTX results from emphysematous changes of the lung—almost always as a result of cigarette smoking. Other, less common causes are seen occasionally (Table 7-5).

Table 7-5. Classification and Causes of Pneumothoraces

Spontaneous	Cause(s)
Primary	Apical bleb
Secondary	COPD, cystic fibrosis, cancer, tuberculosis, endometriosis
Nonspontaneous	**Cause(s)**
Trauma	Blunt, penetrating, or barometric pressure
Iatrogenic	Central venous access, thoracentesis

Epidemiology Spontaneous PTX occurs approximately 20,000 times a year in the United States. Primary spontaneous PTX is approximately 3 to 4 times more common in men than in women, and usually occurs in teenagers or young adults. It is commonly associated with tall, thin men. Secondary spontaneous PTX is more common in the elderly because of its association with COPD. Recurrence rates are approximately 30%, and rise to 60% after 1 episode.

Symptoms The most common symptoms of spontaneous PTX are sudden onset of **pleuritic chest pain and dyspnea,** which is present at rest and exertion.

Physical Exam and Signs The most common sign is **tachycardia.** Other signs include unilateral decreased chest wall motion, hyperresonance to percussion, and decreased or absent breath sounds on auscultation.

Differential Traumatic and iatrogenic causes of PTX are inferred from the history. **Acute coronary syndrome/myocardial infarction:** Usually substernal chest pain that can cause dyspnea. Breath sounds are present, chest radiograph and ECG are helpful. **Pulmonary**

embolism: Tachycardia, dyspnea, ±pleuritic pain, breath sounds present, chest radiograph and chest CT angiogram helpful. **Aortic dissection:** Tearing pain in the back, hypertensive patients, breath sounds present, usually older age, chest radiograph and chest CT angiogram helpful. **Rib fracture:** History of trauma, pain on palpation, breath sounds present, chest radiograph helpful.

Diagnosis Findings on chest radiograph guide diagnosis.

Labs. None specific.

Imaging. Chest radiograph demonstrates a visceral pleural line parallel to the chest wall (Fig. 7-6). If the pleural line is greater than 2 cm from the chest wall, the PTX occupies greater than 30% of lung volume. Chest CT can be performed if the diagnosis is unclear (Fig. 7-7).

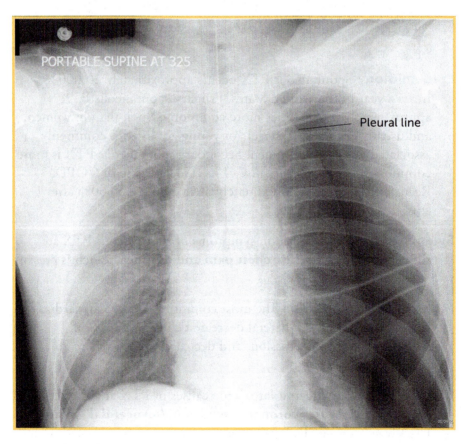

Fig. 7-6. Iatrogenic Tension Pneumothorax of Left Lung

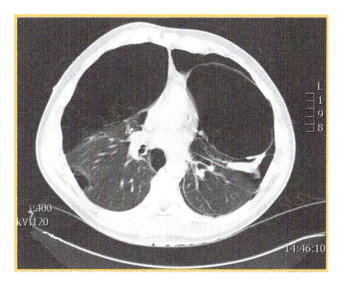

Fig. 7-7. Spontaneous Bilateral Secondary Pneumothorax Caused by Emphysema

Complication(s) Tension PTX is the progression of a pneumothorax as a result of continued leakage of air. Trapped air increases pressure within the pleural space and may compress the mediastinum, shifting it away from the affected side. This mechanical shift may induce kink formation in the superior vena cava, blocking venous return to the heart. Hemodynamic compromise ensues, which can be fatal. Tension PTX is less common in spontaneous PTX than it is in the traumatic and iatrogenic types. Tension PTX presents with **neck vein distention, tracheal deviation,** and **hypotension.**

Treatment Initial treatment of **spontaneous PTX** is based on the size of the PTX. PTX with less than 30% collapse can be observed while administering O_2 therapy. PTX greater than 30% collapse requires **tube thoracostomy (chest tube insertion). Recurrent PTX** is typically treated with **video-assisted thoracoscopic surgery (VATS)** and resection of the apical pleural bleb. **Mechanical pleurodesis** creates adhesions between visceral and parietal pleura and decreases recurrence rates. Special consideration is given to people who have occupations with atmospheric pressure changes or those in remote locations. In these cases, patients may be treated more aggressively when they first develop a PTX. **Tension PTX** is treated with **emergent needle decompression followed by thoracostomy.**

Bibliography

Aberle DR, Gamsu G, Henschke CI, Naidich DP, Swensen SJ. A consensus statement of the Society of Thoracic Radiology: screening for lung cancer with helical computed tomography. *J Thorac Imaging.* 2001;16(1):65-68.

Bidwell JL, Pachner RW. Hemoptysis: diagnosis and management. *Am Fam Physician.* 2005;72(7):1253-1260.

Ettinger DS, Akerley W, Borghaei H, et al; National Comprehensive Cancer Network. Non-small cell lung cancer, version 2.2013. *J Natl Compr Canc Netw.* 2013;11(6):645-653.

Melton LJ III, Hepper NG, Offord KP. Incidence of spontaneous pneumothorax in Olmsted County, Minnesota: 1950-1974. *Am Rev Respir Dis.* 1979;120(6):1379-1382.

Schramel FM, Postmus PE, Vanderschueren RG. Current aspects of spontaneous pneumothorax. *Eur Respir J.* 1997;10(6):1372-1379.

Clinical Recall: Questions and Answers

What is a solitary pulmonary nodule?	A nodule less than 3 cm; may be benign or malignant
What is the most common type of solitary pulmonary nodule?	A granuloma
Which is the most common type of lung cancer?	Non-small cell lung carcinoma
What is the most common type of non-small cell lung carcinoma?	Adenocarcinoma
How is lung cancer diagnosed?	Biopsy
What findings on imaging suggest a benign lung lesion?	Lesion has smooth borders and calcification that is diffuse, is centrally located, and looks like onion skin or popcorn

What findings on imaging suggest a malignant lung lesion?	Noncalcified nodule
What is the greatest risk factor for the development of lung cancer?	Smoking tobacco
How does small cell lung carcinoma appear on imaging?	Commonly as a hilar or mediastinal mass on chest X-ray (central location)
How does non–small cell lung carcinoma appear on imaging?	Pulmonary nodule, mass, or infiltrate (peripheral location)
What is hemoptysis?	Coughing up blood
What is a spontaneous pneumothorax?	Collection of air within the pleural space that causes collapse of the affected lung
What is the most common cause of primary spontaneous pneumothorax?	Rupture of an apical pulmonary bleb, typically seen in tall, thin male
What are the most common symptoms of spontaneous pneumothorax?	Pleuritic chest pain and dyspnea
How is a spontaneous pneumothorax treated?	Observation or tube thoracostomy depending on size of the pneumothorax
What is a tension pneumothorax?	Pneumothorax classically associated with hypotension and hypoxia
How is a tension pneumothorax treated?	Needle decompression followed by thoracostomy

Topic IV

Breast, Skin, and Soft Tissue

Breast

8

The breast (Fig. 8-1) is a modified apocrine sweat gland covered by adipose tissue. The mature female breast extends from the clavicle superiorly to the insertion of the anterior recti muscles inferiorly, and from the sternum medially to approximately the midaxillary line laterally.

A cross section of the female breast reveals glandular epithelial tissue, a fibrous stroma with supporting structures, and adipose tissue. The glandular tissue is contained in approximately 15 to 20 lobes, distributed radially and each composed of several lobules.

Myoepithelial cells with contractile properties that serve to propel milk toward the nipple surround the luminal epithelium of the ducts.

The breast is tear-shaped because its superolateral portion extends into the axilla, forming what is known as the *tail of Spence*.

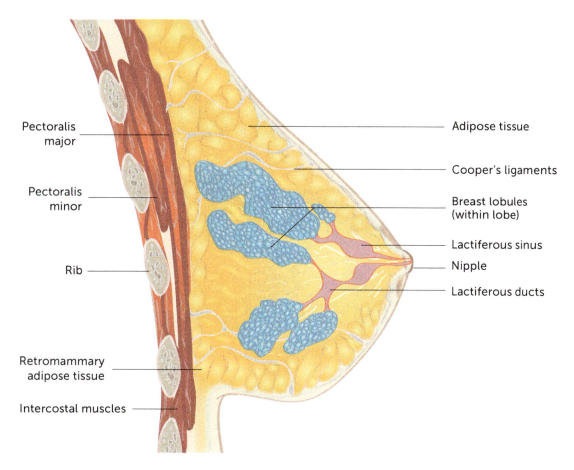

Fig. 8-1. Cross Section of Female Breast

Surgery 113

The axilla (Fig. 8-2) is shaped like a pyramid, with its base located at the lateral edge of the pectoralis major and its apex located roughly where the clavicle and the first rib cross.

Most of the lymphatic flow of the breast, an important route of cancer spread, drains into the axillary lymph nodes (~80%), and a small percentage reaches the internal mammary chain of nodes.

Nodes lateral to the lateral edge of the pectoralis minor are categorized as level I nodes; level II nodes are posterior to the pectoralis minor, and nodes medial to the medial edge of the pectoralis minor are categorized as level III nodes.

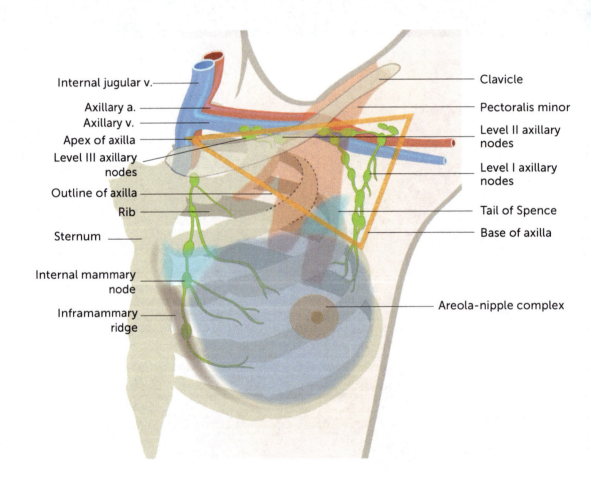

Fig. 8-2. Axilla and Lymphatic Drainage of Breast

During the seventh week of embryologic development, paired milk lines (Fig. 8-3) appear and run from the axillae to the groins.

Lack of complete involution along these lines may give rise to supernumerary nipples with or without associated ectopic breast tissue.

The presence of supernumerary nipples is called polythelia. Rarely, these ectopic sites may develop the same inflammatory or neoplastic processes that occur in primary breast tissue.

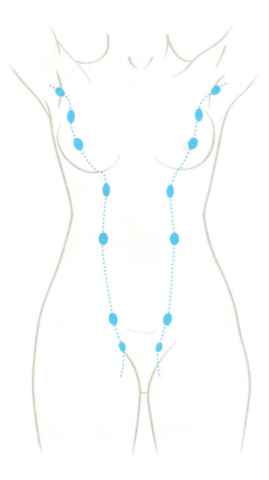

Fig. 8-3. Embryonic Milk Lines

The normal development of the breast is under hormonal control, as is its function during lactation (Fig. 8-4). Estrogens and progesterone play a central role in the complex interplay that governs breast physiology from menarche to menopause.

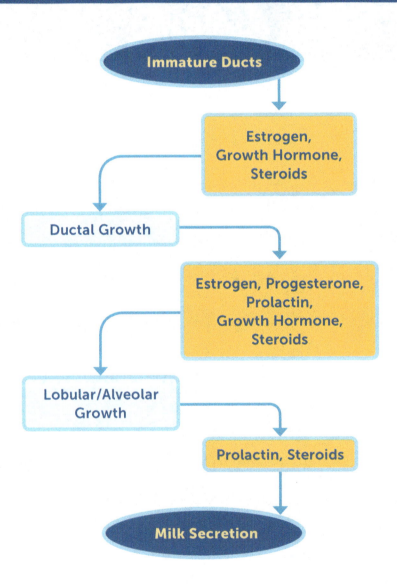

Fig. 8-4. Hormonal Effects on Breast Development and Function

Common Benign Breast Disorders

Definition Fibrocystic disease (FD) and some of its subsets are a common problem affecting females in almost every age group. In effect, FD is a "condition" rather than a disease because many of its histologic features are part of the normal architecture of the breast. FD is defined mainly by its histologic appearance, but it encompasses a range of clinical, radiologic, and histopathologic findings. Among its subtypes, **cysts** are one of the most common presentations. Another common disorder of the nonlactating breast is the development of **fibroadenomas**—benign tumors of the breast most commonly seen in young women. FD is divided histologically into proliferative and nonproliferative types, and some subcategories of the proliferative fibrocystic condition increase the risk for breast cancer substantially. This is specifically the case with **atypical ductal hyperplasia (ADH) and atypical lobular hyperplasia (ALH).**

Etiology Unknown. The popularly cited connection between caffeine intake and FD is not supported by evidence. However, a connection between hormones and the presence of symptoms related to FD is likely.

Epidemiology FD is most common in women 30 to 60 years of age, although it can be seen at any age. On ultrasonography, it has been noted that as many as two-thirds of women over 35 years of age have demonstrable cysts. **Fibroadenomas** are the second most common breast tumor after carcinoma, and they are most common in women younger than 30 years of age.

Symptoms A common symptom of FD is breast pain, or *mastalgia*. However, to say that pain without other demonstrable stigmata is due to FD is incorrect and confusing. Pain alone does not support the diagnosis of FD. Other presenting symptoms of FD may include nipple discharge.

Physical Exam and Signs Commonly, cysts and fibroadenomas present as a **palpable mass.** (It is important to recognize that normal breast tissue is nodular.) The breast has an area of denser tissue in the upper outer quadrant and at the inframammary fold, where a ridge is commonly palpated. These areas must not be interpreted as abnormal during palpation, unless clear findings different from those in the rest of the breast are noted. The clinician must differentiate between the normal nodularity of the breast and what is termed a **"dominant mass,"** which is simply an area that feels different from normal breast tissue. This may present as a distinct mass or as a thickened fold. A fibroadenoma is typically **round** or **ovoid, rubbery** in consistency, **mobile,** and **nontender.** Fibroadenomas are usually 1 cm to 3 cm in diameter, but occasionally they can be of considerable size (>5 cm in diameter), in which case they are called *giant fibroadenomas.* When fibroadenomas are large, it is important to rule out the possibility of a phyllodes tumor, which has fibroadenoma-like characteristics and may be malignant. If nipple discharge is present, it must be noted whether the discharge is spontaneous or not, uniductal or multiductal, and unilateral or bilateral; and the presence or absence of blood must be ascertained. The most common cause of a unilateral, spontaneous, uniductal serosanguinous discharge is an **intraductal papilloma.**

Differential The main differential of a dominant mass in the breast is carcinoma. Some benign conditions may mimic cancer, most notably fat necrosis and sclerosing adenosis; the latter condition is a histologic subtype of FD.

Diagnosis The definitive diagnosis of an abnormal finding in the breast is made by obtaining a **tissue biopsy,** also referred to as a *core biopsy.* In this type of biopsy, samples of tissue are extracted and analyzed histologically. A fine needle aspiration biopsy (FNAB) recovers only cellular material, which is analyzed cytologically. A **solid mass,** palpable or not, must be biopsied. A negative FNAB must not be accepted as the final diagnosis when a solid mass is being investigated, as the false-negative rate is approximately 25% to 30%. Most biopsies of nonpalpable mammographic abnormalities are currently done with a sampling needle under mammographic or ultrasonographic guidance. A **cystic mass** may simply be needle aspirated, which proves the cystic nature of this finding. Cystic fluid may be clear, green, or turbid. It may be discarded without further workup unless it contains blood or, if palpable, it does not disappear completely after aspiration.

Labs. None specific.

Imaging. Mammography is the primary type of imaging used to screen women without symptoms. Its purpose is to identify abnormalities not detectable on clinical exam. The degree of suspicion elicited by a mammographic finding is graded using the Breast Imaging Reporting and Data System (BI-RADS) scale, with the higher numbers indicating greater likelihood of a cancer diagnosis. **Ultrasonography** is commonly used to assess whether a **breast lesion is solid or cystic**. MRI is now used more often as a modality of breast imaging. Newer imaging techniques are becoming more prevalent, such as CT synthesis.

Complication(s) FD has few associated complications, but patients may present with pain and infection. When infection does occur, it is seen mostly in the periareolar or subareolar area.

Treatment FD is treated according to its presentation. A cyst may be simply observed if imaging is unequivocal that it is indeed a cyst. A complex cyst and, frequently, simple cysts are best aspirated, as they may enlarge over time. A fibroadenoma should be biopsied to confirm the diagnosis. In some cases, excision is a reasonable approach. When infection is present, antibiotics are usually effective, but recurrent infections might require excision of the underlying tissue. Patients initially diagnosed with ADH or ALH by core biopsy must be treated with subsequent surgical excision, as approximately 20% of patients with this finding have an associated carcinoma.

FEMALE BREAST CANCER

Definition Malignant tumor(s) of the breast(s).

Etiology Unknown. However, a variety of risk factors that increase risk are recognized (Tables 8-1 and 8-2). Some, such as mutations of *BRCA1* and *BRCA2* genes, **lobular carcinoma in situ** (LCIS), and histologic atypia, increase the risk significantly. The probability of mutated *BRCA* genes increases with a family history of breast and ovarian cancer diagnosed before age 50; screening of these genes should be reserved for patients with this type of history. The prevalence of *BRCA* mutations varies among ethnic groups (Table 8-3).

Table 8-1. Factors That Increase the Relative Risk (RR; 2.1–8.0) of Developing Breast Cancer

Risk Factor	Comments
Mutation of *BRCA1* and *BRCA2* genes	5%–10% of all breast cancer cases; women with *BRCA1* mutation have 85% risk of developing breast cancer by age 70
Therapeutic radiation to chest (eg, Hodgkin's lymphoma)	Risk increased for young women
ADH or ALH	RR ≥4.0 for some subsets
LCIS	RR >8
First-degree relative with breast cancer (5%–7% of women with breast cancer have family history of disease)	RR 2.0–3.0; higher if 2 or more relatives; higher if relative was premenopausal with bilateral cancer
Personal history of breast cancer	RR 3.0–4.0 for contralateral breast; absolute risk is 0.5%–1% per year, depending on population subset

Table 8-2. Factors That Increase the Relative Risk (1.1–2.0) of Developing Breast Cancer

Risk Factor	Comments
Early menarche (before age 12 y)	Longer exposure to estrogen
Late menopause (after age 55 y)	Longer exposure to estrogen
Late first live birth (after age 30 y)	Pregnancy increases cellular proliferation; risk increase is transient
Nulliparity	Less cell differentiation
Hormonal replacement therapy	Combined estrogen and progesterone use
Postmenopausal obesity	No evidence available for premenopausal obesity
Lifestyle factors	Sedentary lifestyle; alcohol use

Table 8-3. Prevalence of *BRCA1* Mutation Among Ethnic Groups

Population	Prevalence
Jewish Ashkenazi	8.3%
Hispanic	3.5%
African American	1.3%
Asian American	0.5%

Epidemiology Breast cancer is the most common female cancer and the second most common cause of cancer death in women. In the 1970s, the incidence of breast cancer in the United States was 1 in 15; in 2011 it rose to 1 in 8, which can also be expressed as an absolute lifetime risk of 12%. African American women have a lower incidence of breast cancer than white women do, except for those in the premenopausal group, where the incidence is higher. However, the mortality rate is higher in African Americans than in other groups. The mortality rate has been decreasing steadily since the 1990s, and the largest decrease in mortality has been seen in women younger than age 50 years. These observed mortality decreases are attributed to early detection methods and improved treatment options.

The most common histologic type of breast cancer is **invasive ductal carcinoma,** which accounts for approximately 50% to 70% of all invasive cancers. The second most common type is **ductal carcinoma in situ** (DCIS). Invasive lobular carcinoma accounts for approximately 15% of breast cancers, and the combined ductal-lobular type is becoming more frequent. Noninvasive, or in situ lesions, are classified as such because they have not invaded the basement membrane of the mammary ducts or lobules. It is important to note that **LCIS is a risk factor for developing breast cancer;** it is not considered a malignancy.

The traditional histomorphologic classification of breast cancers is complemented by a molecular classification system based on expression of receptors to hormones and other markers. Estrogen receptor (ER)–positive and progesterone receptor (PR)–positive breast cancers have a better prognosis. Expression of the Her2/neu protein serves as the basis for tumors classified as luminal A and luminal B, Her2/neu–positive, and basal-like subtypes. This classification is significant because it guides treatment possibilities.

Symptoms Pain is seldom a symptom of breast cancer, presenting in less than approximately 4% of patients with carcinoma.

Physical Exam and Signs It is best to examine patients in both seated and supine positions. While the patient is seated, breasts should be examined for erythema, edema, dimpling, or other deformitites. Palpation is best accomplished while the patient is supine, with the breast evenly distributed over the costal cage. An examination of the axillary, supraclavicular, and infraclavicular areas must always be performed. An experienced examiner who considers a palpable axillary node(s) clinically malignant will be correct 85% of the time.

The most common presenting sign is a palpable mass or a mammographic finding. Patients may consult because of nipple discharge or skin changes. Nipple discharge containing blood must lead to a tissue biopsy. Retraction of the nipple might be noted if a central lesion is present, and skin ulceration might be noted in advanced stages. Most breast cancers present in the **upper outer quadrant** of the breast, followed in frequency by a central location.

An uncommon and aggressive type of breast cancer, called **inflammatory cancer,** presents with skin erythema and edema; it must not be confused with an infection and erroneously treated as such. Skin erythema and edema—known as *peau d'orange*—of this ominous type of cancer are the result of involvement of the underlying lymphatics. *Paget's disease* of the breast is an in situ or invasive breast carcinoma that presents with an eczema-like lesion of the areola-nipple complex, which is easy to confuse with a benign skin lesion. Paget's disease represents less than 1% of all breast malignancies.

Differential The differential of any finding in the breast requires that such a finding must be identified as benign or malignant. The clinician must be well aware of the clinical and radiologic findings that can mimic carcinoma. A **radial scar** is a lesion found on mammography that has a central component of sclerosis. Although benign, it is associated with increased risk of cancer in both breasts. Fat necrosis may mimic carcinoma on exam and on imaging, and a biopsy may be necessary to rule out malignancy.

Diagnosis The definitive diagnosis of a breast lesion is made by obtaining a **tissue biopsy.** Initially, tissue must be collected with a core needle biopsy. Occasionally, these cores are not histologically concordant with the finding seen on imaging. When this is the case, the area in question should be rebiopsied to confirm that the tissue analyzed is indeed the one detected by mammography or ultrasonography. A palpable lesion may be biopsied with or without the assistance of mammography or ultrasonography.

Labs. No specific blood findings are expected, unless a patient has advanced or metastatic disease, in which case the laboratory abnormalities depend on the organs affected and the magnitude of the tumor burden. A patient with bone or liver metastases may present with elevation of alkaline phosphatase or with hypercalcemia. Pathologic analysis of the tissue obtained must include measurement of estrogen, progesterone, Her2/neu protein receptors, and proliferation indices such as Ki-67.

Imaging. A malignant lesion is not always seen on mammography, and the incidence of false-negative films is approximately 15%. This is particularly true for, but is not exclusive to, patients with LCIS. **Nonpalpable** mammographic abnormalities usually appear as microcalcifications or areas of abnormal density. A **carcinoma** detected on **mammography** commonly appears as a **density with an irregular** and sometimes **spiculated contour.** A **malignancy** seen on **ultrasonography** typically appears as a **hypoechoic (black) mass** that is taller than it is wide and has an **irregular contour** (Fig. 8-5).

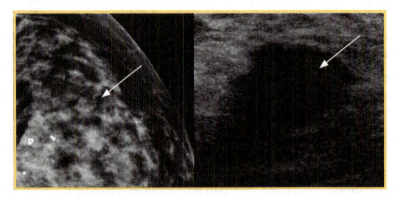

Fig. 8-5. *Left Panel:* Microcalcifications (DCIS) on Mammography
Right Panel: Density (Invasive Carcinoma) on Ultrasound

Complication(s) Breast cancer complications are linked to local and/or distant progression of the disease. Survival rates depend on the stage of the cancer at the time treatment is initiated. Stage at the time of diagnosis is the most consistent indicator of prognosis.

Treatment Breast cancer therapy depends on the type and stage of disease at the time of diagnosis. In general, surgical treatment may initiate the sequence of treatment in early stages. Surgical options include breast conserving surgery (BCS), known as *lumpectomy* or *segmental mastectomy*, and mastectomy, in which the whole breast is removed. A lumpectomy implies that the tissue removed from the breast must have its margins clear of cancer cells, and this procedure should be followed by radiation therapy (RT) to the remaining breast to decrease the rate of local recurrence. When the cancer is invasive, whether the patient undergoes a lumpectomy or a mastectomy, the procedure is almost always accompanied by sampling of the sentinel node (SN). **The SN is the first node in the chain of lymphatics draining the breast in which cancer cells are expected to appear**. When the SN is negative for the presence of malignant cells, it is anticipated that the rest of the nodes in the axillary basin also will be negative. If the SN contains malignant cells, usually the patient will undergo an axillary node dissection, during which the rest of the nodes in the axilla are removed. This concept is currently under scrutiny, as questions have been raised about its necessity. Information accumulated by analyzing the tumor and the lymph node(s) is used to establish whether the patient needs further therapy. Some patients may receive chemotherapy after surgery (also known as *adjuvant chemotherapy*), as well as RT and/or endocrine therapy. **Adjuvant chemotherapy** is used to eliminate possible occult micrometastases responsible for late recurrences. Currently, the molecular signature of certain tumors is used to determine the possibility of a late systemic recurrence, and this information is applied to the decision of whether to initiate chemotherapy.

Surgery, chemotherapy, and RT may be used in different sequences in advanced stages or with aggressive cancers. A patient who presents with a large tumor might be treated first with chemotherapy followed by surgery, with the SN biopsied before chemotherapy is initiated or afterward, during the chosen surgical procedure. Chemotherapy, RT, and surgery—alone or combined—can be used as palliative treatment.

BIBLIOGRAPHY

John EM, Miron A, Gong G, et al. Prevalence of pathogenic *BRCA1* mutation carriers in 5 US racial/ethnic groups. *JAMA*. 2007;298(24):2869-2876.

Parker JS, Mullins M, Cheang MCU, et al. Supervised risk predictor of breast cancer based on intrinsic subtypes. *J Clin Oncol*. 2009;27(8):1160-1167.

Clinical Keys: Questions and Answers

What 2 histologic types of fibrocystic breast disease increase the risk for breast cancer?	ADH and ALH
What are the most common mammographic abnormalities?	Microcalcifications and densities
What percentage of the population has a mutated *BRCA* gene?	Approximately 8%
How often is localized breast cancer associated with pain?	Very infrequently
How is the diagnosis of breast cancer made?	Tissue biopsy
What is a common reason to perform a breast ultrasound?	To differentiate a solid lesion from a cystic one
How often is breast cancer not seen on mammography?	Approximately 15% of the time
Which type of breast finding must always be biopsied?	Solid tumors
What is the most common type of breast cancer?	Invasive ductal carcinoma
What is the second most common type of breast cancer?	Ductal carcinoma in situ (DCIS)
What is a fibroadenoma?	A benign breast tumor
What is the sentinel node?	The first node in the chain of lymphatics draining the breast in which a breast malignancy is expected to appear
Which type of tumor is typically round or ovoid, mobile, rubbery, and nontender?	Fibroadenoma

Melanoma, Soft Tissue Infection, and Skin Cancer

9

The skin is the largest organ of the body, with a surface area of 2 square meters supplied by approximately 4.5 meters of blood vessels per square inch.

The epidermis is the outermost layer of the skin (Fig. 9-1). Underneath the epidermis lies the dermis, a layer of the skin between the epidermis and the subcutaneous tissues, comprising a superficial papillary region and a deeper, thicker region known as the reticular dermis.

The subcutaneous tissue, or *hypodermis*, contains fat, connective tissue, and lymphatic and blood vessels.

Beneath the subcutaneous tissue is a thin layer of extremely strong, fibrous tissue called the fascia, which can surround muscles, vessels, or nerves.

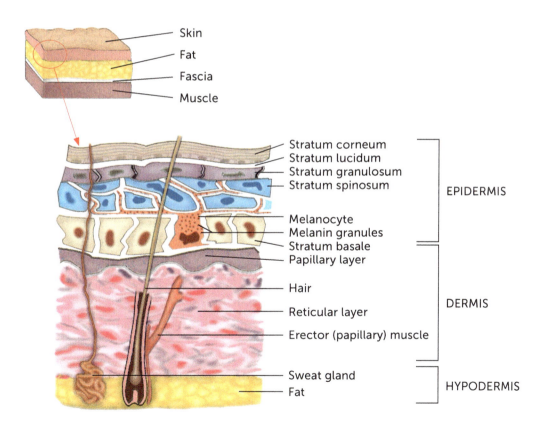

Fig. 9-1. Anatomy of the Skin

Basal Cell Carcinoma

Definition Basal cell carcinomas (BCCs) are skin cancers arising from the **basal epithelial layer.** Although they have low metastatic potential, they can be locally invasive and aggressive.

Etiology The development of BCCs is influenced by environmental factors, with ultraviolet (UV) light exposure thought to be most important. Other risk factors include chronic arsenic exposure and therapeutic radiation.

Epidemiology BCCs are particularly common in whites and uncommon in darker-skinned individuals. Within the white population in the United States, the incidence of BCCs has increased and the lifetime risk of developing BCC is 30%. The frequency is 30% higher in males than females. The incidence varies, with higher reported rates in areas near the equator, such as Hawaii and California. The incidence also increases with age: individuals older than 55 years have a 100-fold increased risk compared to those younger than 20 years.

Symptoms Many BCC lesions are noted visually and lack presenting symptoms. Approximately 70% of BCCs occur on the face, supporting the theory that UV-related exposure is a primary cause.

Physical Exam and Signs Most BCCs appear as **smooth, superficial, flesh-colored papules** or **nodules.** They can be ulcerated and/or have visible telangiectasias.

Differential Squamous cell carcinoma, melanoma, dermal nevi, inclusion cysts, and molluscum contagiosum may be considered.

Diagnosis Biopsy is needed for definitive diagnosis of BCC.

Labs. There are no specific labs needed for diagnosis.

Imaging. Imaging is not routinely needed for these lesions.

Complication(s) These lesions may be locally invasive and aggressive, resulting in significant soft tissue and bony destruction when advanced.

Treatment Most BCCs are treated with **resection or ablation.** BCCs can be managed by wide local excision (WLE) with 5 mm margins. Alternatively, Mohs micrographic surgery can be used, a technique that allows for intraoperative margin assessment; this minimizes the amount of normal tissue resected. Other treatment options include topical therapies, such as **5-fluorouracil** (5-FU), which interferes with DNA synthesis, or **imiquimod,** which modifies the immune response to lesions. Under rare circumstances, these lesions can be treated with radiation or photodynamic therapy in patients who are not surgical candidates.

SQUAMOUS CELL CARCINOMA

Definition Squamous cell carcinomas (SCCs) are abnormal overgrowths of squamous cells from the epidermis.

Etiology Contributing factors to the formation of SCCs are exposure to UV radiation and chronic inflammation. **Chronic sun exposure** is responsible for the majority of SCCs, but they can also develop in sites of previous burns, scars, ulcers, or sores. Additionally, immunosuppression can also lead to an increased risk of developing SCCs. Premalignant lesions, called actinic keratoses, can be found on sun-exposed regions of the body and may later develop into SCC.

Epidemiology SCCs are twice as common in men than women and are more common in patients over the age of 50 years. In African American patients, the majority of skin cancers are SCCs.

Symptoms These lesions are rarely symptomatic and generally are only a cosmetic issue.

Physical Exam and Signs On physical exam, SCCs appear as scaly, crusted areas that often bleed.

Differential Basal cell carcinoma, melanoma, pyoderma gangrenosum, papilloma induced by human papillomavirus, dermatitis, and scars/burns/traumatic injuries may be considered. SCCs may be mistaken for a nonhealing wound.

Diagnosis There are no labs or specific imaging studies, because this is a clinical and pathologic diagnosis. The use of imaging should be guided by symptoms (eg, palpable lymphadenopathy, neurologic symptoms).

Complication(s) The complications vary depending on lesion location and are usually related to local invasion/extension.

Treatment The majority of SCCs can be treated by WLE with 0.5 cm margins or with ablative techniques. For low-risk lesions, resection (via WLE or Mohs microsurgery), cryotherapy, or electrosurgery may be used. Radiation therapy is sometimes employed for patients who are not candidates for other treatments. Topical 5-FU has been approved by the US Food and Drug Administration for the treatment of actinic keratoses and can be used by patients who are not surgical candidates.

MELANOMA

Definition Melanoma is the most aggressive skin cancer and arises from **melanocytes** (pigmented cells) within the skin. It occurs most commonly in the skin but can develop in other tissues that arise from the neural crest, such as the GI tract.

Etiology These tumors arise from malignant transformation of melanocytes.

Epidemiology Close to 77,000 people were diagnosed with melanoma in 2013, and more than 9000 patients died of this disease. Overall, the incidence of melanoma is increasing worldwide; in the United States the incidence has been rising by an average of 2.6% per year. Increasing awareness has led to earlier detection and treatment of melanoma. The major environmental risk factor is exposure to **UV radiation** (specifically UV-B). Rates of melanoma vary worldwide and are correlated with sun exposure and ethnic patterns. Tanning bed use has been associated with increased risk of melanoma. Whites are 10 times more likely to develop melanoma than African Americans. Additionally, people with red or blond hair, light skin, and/or blue eyes are at a higher risk. The incidence of melanoma increases with age. Patients who have a history of melanoma are at increased risk for the development of a subsequent melanoma and should be carefully monitored. There are also some genetic predispositions to melanoma and a correlation with family history.

Symptoms These lesions are often noted on visual inspection by the patient or screening physician. Clinical features of concern include the **ABCDs:** asymmetry, border irregularity, color variegation, and diameter greater than 6 mm. Lesions should raise concern if they increase in size or are associated with symptoms such as pruritus.

Patients should be questioned about other symptoms that suggest evidence of metastatic disease.

Physical Exam and Signs Close inspection of the lesion and a head-to-toe skin exam for other suspicious lesions is required. Cervical, axillary, and inguinal lymph node basins should be clinically inspected and palpated for evidence of regional disease.

Differential Basal cell carcinoma, actinic keratoses, squamous cell carcinoma, common melanocytic nevus, lentigo, Spitz nevus, and seborrheic keratosis may be considered.

Diagnosis Biopsy of any suspicious lesion is critical for diagnosis. Techniques include punch biopsy, core biopsy, or excisional biopsy. Fine needle aspiration (FNA) should never be used to biopsy these lesions. Shave biopsies can be done; however, these can lead to downstaging if the entire thickness of the lesion is not adequately sampled.

Labs. Lactate dehydrogenase (LDH) level should be checked in the setting of more advanced or suspected metastatic disease, because it is a component of the American Joint Committee on Cancer (AJCC) staging criteria. There is no indication for checking the LDH level in early-stage melanoma.

Imaging. Imaging should be guided by clinical history and concern. There is no role for screening imaging in patients with early-stage melanoma.

Complication(s) The complications of disease treatments vary and depend on the initial stage of disease and the required subsequent treatment approaches. For patients who undergo lymph node dissection, there is the risk of developing lymphedema of the involved extremity. These patients should be counseled regarding lymphedema risk factors and prevention. Additionally, complications of systemic therapies offered in the setting of metastatic disease will vary according to the agents used.

Treatment Decisions regarding treatment are primarily based upon the **Breslow thickness** (Table 9-1, Fig. 9-2), which is reported in millimeters (mm). Although it is an important pathologic variable, Clark's level is no longer part of the AJCC staging criteria and does not factor into treatment decisions. Thin melanomas are treated with a WLE with margins determined by the Breslow thickness.

Table 9-1. Appropriate Surgical Margins of Excised Melanomas

Primary Tumor Thickness (mm)[a]	Excision Margin (cm)
In situ	0.5–1
0–1	1
1–2	1 cm in anatomically restricted areas; otherwise 2 cm margin preferred
2–4	2
>4	2

[a] Breslow's classification

The decision to sample lymph nodes via **sentinel lymph node biopsy** (SLNB) depends on the clinical stage and the presence of concerning pathologic features of the primary lesion, such as ulceration or the number of mitotic figures. For stage Ia disease (melanomas <1 mm thick with no concerning or high-risk features), SLNB is usually not offered. Patients with stage Ib disease (melanoma <1 mm with ulceration or mitotic figures), SLNB is generally recommended. For patients with intermediate-thickness or thick tumors, SLNB is performed routinely. However, in the presence of clinically detectable lymph node disease (palpation of suspicious lymph nodes and verification with FNA), SLNB can be deferred in favor of therapeutic lymph node dissection.

For melanomas on the torso, head, or neck (sites that may have more than one draining lymph node basin), patients should undergo preoperative lymphoscintigraphy to determine draining nodal basins. In this procedure, radiolabeled isotope is injected at the site of melanoma and traced to the sentinel lymph nodes or sites of early lymph node drainage. SLNB is then used to assess these sites for early, clinically occult disease at the time of WLE.

Currently, there are molecular targeted therapies available for patients who have a specific mutation in the *BRAF* gene. Drugs that target the immune system may also be included in treatment. These therapies are offered only to patients with evidence of metastatic disease, and the choice of therapy depends on characteristics of the patient and the tumor.

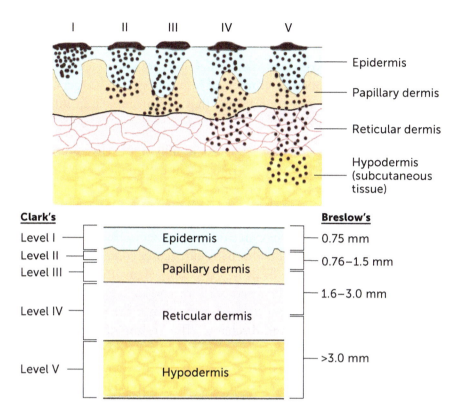

Fig. 9-2. Classification of Melanoma

NECROTIZING FASCIITIS AND FOURNIER'S GANGRENE

Definition Necrotizing soft tissue infections include various forms of cellulitis and fasciitis that vary clinically based on the site of disease. Fournier's gangrene specifically refers to a necrotizing infection of the perineum.

Etiology These infections can be divided into 2 types. **Type I are polymicrobial infections,** and **type II are group A streptococcal infections.** Susceptibility to infection is related to bacterial presence and host response. Necrotizing fasciitis (NF) is more commonly seen in patients with a **compromised immune system.** For type I NF, usually caused by aerobic and anaerobic bacteria, host factors such as diabetes, peripheral vascular disease, immune compromise, or recent surgery may play a contributing role. Type II NF can occur in healthy individuals of all ages.

Epidemiology Necrotizing soft tissue infections are associated with diabetes, IV drug use, obesity, suppressed immune system, surgery, traumatic wounds, and other conditions that compromise skin integrity (eg, burns, childbirth).

Symptoms These infections can progress rapidly and may lead to systemic manifestations. Symptoms of concern include fever and/or any evidence of systemic toxicity or hemodynamic instability.

Physical Exam and Signs The physical examination is extremely important. The typical patient has an area of erythema that is extremely painful when palpated, and the pain extends beyond the erythema into tissue that appears healthy. Alarming signs include rapidly changing erythema or skin discoloration, and/or crepitus (suggesting the presence of gas-forming organisms within the wound). There may be foul smelling wound discharge. The finding of subcutaneous emphysema, while rare, is a clear indication of a necrotizing infection and should prompt immediate operative débridement. These same findings occur with Fournier's gangrene (FG) but are localized to the perineum.

Differential Cellulitis, ecchymosis, normal postoperative changes, hematoma, deep venous thrombosis, and brown recluse spider bite may be considered.

Diagnosis NF is diagnosed clinically, and surgical intervention should not be delayed for laboratory assessment or possible need for imaging.

Labs. Surgical exploration and biopsy analysis are the only definitive means of diagnosis. However, necrotizing soft tissue infections are usually accompanied by an elevated creatine kinase (CK) level, an elevated WBC count, and acidosis. Blood cultures may yield positive results in the setting of septicemia, but cultures must also be obtained from the wound—both preoperatively and intraoperatively to assess the extent of the infection.

Imaging. Radiographic studies may be helpful in determining the extent of involvement (subcutaneous tissue versus muscle layer) and can verify the presence of gas in the soft tissue. If radiographic studies are used, CT scanning is the study of choice.

Complication(s) Necrotizing soft tissue infections are associated with many complications that depend on the location and extent of disease and the timeliness of surgical intervention. In the most severe cases, these infections can rapidly lead to multiorgan failure and death.

Treatment **Early recognition and aggressive treatment of this disease is critical. Surgical débridement** is the mainstay of treatment and the most crucial element in removing the source of infection. Multiple serial débridements are often needed along with intraoperative biopsies of the peripheral and deep margins to precisely assess extent of infection. Serial débridements must be performed until all sites of infection have been cleared. Simultaneously, all patients should begin a regimen of broad-spectrum antibiotics that cover gram-positive, gram-negative, and anaerobic organisms. Choice of antibiotics should be guided by the results of blood cultures. Antibiotic treatment should be continued until no further débridements are needed. Under most circumstances, these infections are associated with tissue loss that requires skin and/or muscle flaps for tissue replacement once the infection has been managed. Limb amputation is sometimes necessary.

BIBLIOGRAPHY

Feig BW, Ching DC. *The M.D. Anderson Surgical Oncology Handbook.* 5th edition. Philadelphia, PA: Lippincott Williams & Wilkins; 2011.

CLINICAL KEYS: QUESTIONS AND ANSWERS

What is the lifetime risk of developing basal cell carcinoma?	30%
What is the most common location of basal cell carcinoma?	Face
What factors increase the risk of developing basal cell carcinoma?	Exposure to UV light, radiation, and arsenic
How are most cases of basal cell carcinoma treated?	Surgical resection or ablation

What topical therapies can be used to treat basal cell carcinoma?	Imiquimod or 5-fluorouracil (5-FU)
What is the typical appearance of squamous cell carcinoma?	Scaly, crusty lesions
What are actinic keratoses?	Premalignant lesions that can develop into squamous cell carcinoma
How are the majority of squamous cell carcinomas treated?	Wide local excision with 0.5 cm margins or ablative techniques
Which is the most aggressive skin cancer?	Melanoma
What characteristics of a skin lesion are concerning for melanoma?	ABCDs: asymmetry, border irregularity, color variegation, and diameter >6 mm
What is the most common type of melanoma?	Superficial spreading type (75%)
What is the most common type of melanoma in African Americans?	Acral lentiginous type
Where is acral lentiginous melanoma commonly located?	Palms, soles, under toenails and fingernails, mucous membranes
Why should a melanoma not be biopsied using a shaving technique?	Because the thickness cannot be assessed
What is a Hutchinson freckle?	Noninvasive lentigo maligna (in situ)
What is the second most common location of melanoma?	Eyes
What lab changes can be seen in necrotizing fasciitis?	Elevated creatine kinase, elevated WBC count, and acidosis
Which organisms should be targeted by antibiotics to treat necrotizing fasciitis?	Gram-positive, gram-negative, and anaerobic bacteria
How is necrotizing fasciitis diagnosed?	Clinically
How is necrotizing fasciitis treated?	Surgical débridement

Topic V

Cardiac and Vascular

Heart

10

The four-chambered heart lies in the middle mediastinum within the pericardium.

The right atrium (RA) receives systemic venous drainage via the superior vena cava (SVC) and the inferior vena cava (IVC). Deoxygenated blood then passes across the tricuspid valve (TV) into the right ventricle (RV), where it is ejected through the pulmonic valve (PV) into the lungs to be oxygenated. The oxygenated blood then flows into the left atrium (LA) via four pulmonary veins, two each from the left and right lungs. Blood then travels across the mitral valve (MV) into the left ventricle (LV), where it is ejected through the aortic valve (AV) into the systemic arterial circulation.

The myocardium is supplied by the right coronary artery (RCA) and the left main (LM) coronary artery, both of which arise from the sinuses of Valsalva in the proximal portion of the ascending aorta.

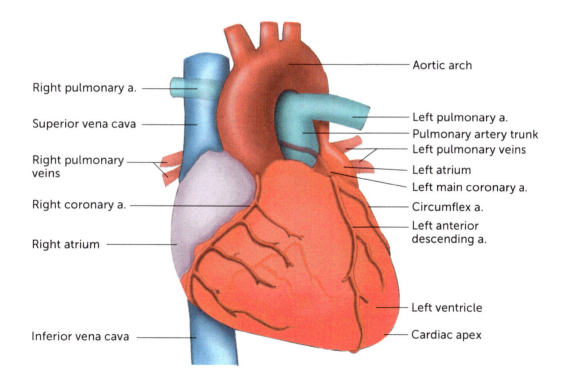

Fig. 10-1. Anatomy of the Heart: External View

The TV is composed of 3 leaflets, whereas the MV has 2 leaflets. The TV and the MV are supported by a subvalvular apparatus composed of papillary muscles and chordae tendineae (Fig. 10-2). The AV and the PV are composed of 3 semilunar cusps, and unlike the TV and MV, they do not have a true annulus nor a subvalvular apparatus.

The conduction system of the heart includes the sinoatrial node, at the junction of the RA and SVC, laterally. The atrioventricular node sends signals to the bundle of His, which penetrates the interventricular septum and branches into right and left bundles.

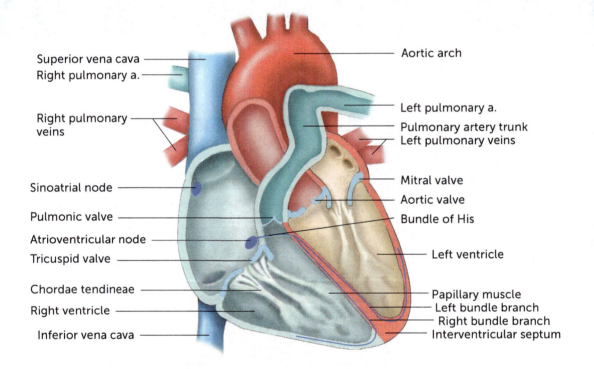

Fig. 10-2. Anatomy of the Heart: Internal View

Cardiac Diagnostic Testing

Patients with cardiac disease are often referred for evaluation of chest pain, palpitations, and dyspnea. Workup begins with a thorough history and physical examination focused on heart rate, rhythm, and auscultation for murmurs. The **electrocardiogram (ECG)** is often the first diagnostic test in the evaluation of heart disease. The ECG will demonstrate rhythm disturbances, signs of acute or chronic ischemia, ventricular hypertrophy, and pulmonary hypertension. **Transthoracic echocardiography (TTE)** and **transesophageal echocardiography (TEE)** are useful in the assessment of structural heart defects such as valvular heart disease, congenital defects, and ventricular function. TEE is very useful in estimating the LV ejection fraction (EF), an important prognostic indicator of mortality and operative risk. Suspected cardiac ischemia and the severity of valvular heart disease can be evaluated by **stress testing.** Patients suspected of having coronary ischemia are often referred for **left heart catheterization** (LHC). LHC consists of selective contrast injection of the left and right coronary arteries as well as left ventriculography. Stenotic lesions and anatomic anomalies of the coronary arteries are readily demonstrated with these techniques. Left ventriculography demonstrate MV regurgitation and provides an estimate of left ventricular function. Simultaneous pressure recordings in the LV and aorta can be performed during LHC in order to assist in the diagnosis of aortic stenosis. **Right heart catheterization** (RHC) is performed to measure pressures and oxygen saturations at various points on the right side of the heart and is useful for making the diagnosis of pulmonary hypertension and detecting intracardiac shunts such as atrial or ventricular septal defects. Additional information about coronary calcification can be obtained by **computed tomography. Cardiac magnetic resonance imaging** is becoming an increasingly important modality to evaluate left ventricular ejection fraction (LVEF), congenital defects, valvular heart disease, and myocardial viability. Normal intracardiac pressures obtained during RHC are listed in Table 10-1.

Table 10-1. Normal Intracardiac Pressures Measured During Right Heart Catheterization

Heart Chamber or Vessel	Normal Intracardiac Pressures
Right atrium	<5 mm Hg
Right ventricle	Systolic pressure: <25 mm Hg Diastolic pressure: <5 mm Hg
Pulmonary artery	Systolic pressure: <25 mm Hg Diastolic pressure: <10 mm Hg Mean pressure: <15 mm Hg
Left atrium	<12 mm Hg (measured via pulmonary capillary wedge pressure [PCWP])
Left ventricle	Systolic pressure: 100–140 mm Hg Diastolic pressure: 0–10 mm Hg (prediastole), 0–20 mm Hg (postdiastole)
Aorta	Systolic pressure: 100–140 mm Hg Diastolic pressure: 60–90 mm Hg

CORONARY ARTERY DISEASE

Definition Coronary artery disease (CAD) is a decrease in coronary blood flow resulting from disease of the coronary arteries.

Etiology Atherosclerosis is the main cause of CAD, in which atherosclerotic changes are present within the walls of the coronary arteries. CAD results in buildup of lipids and cholesterol within the intima of the arterial wall. This results in plaque formation, obstruction, and decreased oxygen supply to the parts of the heart supplied by these vessels. This can lead to **stable angina. Acute coronary syndrome** (ACS) results from **severe vessel stenosis** or **acute vessel occlusion.** ACS can manifest as (1) **ST elevation myocardial infarction (STEMI)**, (2) **non–ST elevation MI (NSTEMI)**, or (3) **unstable angina** (UA) (Fig. 10-3). A STEMI is the result of atherosclerotic plaque rupture and formation of a thrombus that occludes the vessel. NSTEMI can occur as a consequence of plaque rupture and thrombosis, coronary spasm, progressive coronary obstruction, or increased myocardial oxygen demand (eg, during exercise).

Epidemiology CAD is the leading cause of death in adults in the United States. Prevalence of CAD (but not incidence) is higher in men. Risk factors include cigarette smoking, hypertension, obesity, and diabetes.

Symptoms In **stable angina,** patients may report episodes of chronic, recurring chest pain that is brought on by activity and relieved with rest. **UA** refers to chest pain that occurs at rest or pain that increases in frequency, duration, or severity over time. The most common symptom of an MI is chest pain, which may be associated with nausea, sweating, or shortness of breath.

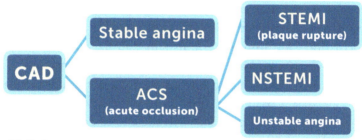

Fig 10-3. Presentations of Coronary Artery Disease

Abbreviations: CAD, coronary artery disease. ACS, acute coronary syndrome. STEMI, ST elevation myocardial infarction. NSTEMI, non–ST elevation myocardial infarction.

Physical Exam and Signs An MI may be associated with dyspnea, nausea, diaphoresis, and unexplained fatigue.

Differential Other causes of chest pain or cardiac dysfunction, such as cardiomyopathy, hypertensive heart disease, pericarditis, and the different presentations of CAD mentioned already should be considered.

Diagnosis Initial workup for CAD includes lab work and performing an ECG. Other diagnostic measures include cardiac catheterization, echocardiography, stress testing, nuclear imaging, and cardiac MRI (see previous section, "Cardiac Diagnostic Testing").

Labs. In patients with suspected cardiac events, troponins (I or T), creatine kinase MB (CK-MB) isozymes, lactate dehydrogenase (LDH), and serum aspartate aminotransferase levels must be measured. A STEMI and an NSTEMI are associated with an **increase in cardiac enzymes,** whereas UA is not.

Imaging. ECG findings include ST-segment elevation, T-wave inversion, and the development of Q waves.

Complication(s) Myocardial ischemia can cause a decline in myocardial function and depressed ejection fraction resulting in pulmonary edema or congestive heart failure (CHF). Mechanical complications of an acute MI include ventricular free wall rupture, postinfarction ventricular septal defects, and papillary muscle rupture. These result in cardiogenic shock and constitute surgical emergencies.

Treatment Depending on the number, location, and severity of the stenoses, patients may be offered **medical therapy** or **revascularization** with either **percutaneous coronary intervention** (PCI) or **coronary artery bypass grafting** (CABG). PCI includes **angiography** and **coronary angioplasty** and usually coronary stenting for stenotic coronary lesions. CABG is generally performed through a median sternotomy. It can be done with or without use of the cardiopulmonary bypass (CPB) pump. Off-pump coronary artery bypass grafting (OPCAB) gained popularity in the 1990s because of a presumed decreased morbidity compared to CPB. Proponents of CPB argue that revascularization is more complete than with OPCAB. Several prospective studies have failed to demonstrate a clear benefit of one technique over the other. Both techniques can prove useful, depending on the clinical circumstances.

CABG requires use of **autologous conduits** to bypass the stenoses, which typically occur in the proximal portion of the coronary arteries. The most common conduits used are the **left internal mammary artery** (LIMA) and **greater saphenous vein grafts** (SVG). The LIMA has been shown to be the **most durable conduit.** The right internal mammary artery, radial artery, and the gastroepiploic artery are also used, in decreasing order of frequency. PCI and CABG have similar survival rates, but the incidence of required revascularization is higher with PCI. Overall mortality from CABG is 1% to 3%.

AORTIC AND MITRAL VALVULAR DISEASE

Definition Valvular heart disease is defined as damage to or a defect in one of the 4 heart valves: the mitral, aortic, tricuspid, or pulmonary.

The 2 main pathologies associated with the aortic valve are **aortic stenosis** (AS) (valvular narrowing) and **aortic insufficiency** (AI), and the same is true for the mitral valve (MV), which can develop **mitral regurgitation** (MR) or **mitral stenosis** (MS).

Etiology (See Fig. 10-4.) The most common cause of **AS** is **calcific degeneration.** Other causes of AS include congenital valve abnormalities (eg, bicuspid valve) or rheumatic heart disease.

AI is secondary to poor valve cusp coaptation due to cusp pathology, or a dilated aortic root. This results in regurgitant flow from the aorta back into the LV during diastole. The most common causes of acute AI are bacterial endocarditis and aortic dissection.

MR is a result of the impaired ability of the valve to close properly during ventricular contraction, causing retrograde blood flow from the LV into the LA during systole. The etiologies of MR are subcategorized into **ischemic mitral regurgitation** (IMR) and **nonischemic MR.** Nonischemic causes include degenerative myxomatous disease, which leads to elongation of the chordae tendineae and subsequent leaflet prolapse with annular calcification. IMR results from annular dilation and retraction of the subvalvular apparatus secondary to the LV dilation that accompanies CAD and chronic ischemia. MR may also occur as a sequela of endocarditis, a process that causes perforation of the infected leaflet tissue and rupture of infected chordae tendineae. Another cause of nonischemic MR is **rheumatic heart disease** (RHD), which results in very thickened, rolled edges of the mitral leaflets with fusion and retraction of the subvalvular apparatus. The valve takes on a slit-like appearance, the so-called **fish mouth deformity.**

MS is the result of severe inflammatory changes and subsequent fusion of the MV commissures. The increase in LA pressure causes LA dilation (a factor predisposing to atrial fibrillation) and increased pulmonary pressure (causing dyspnea and pulmonary edema). Other causes of MS are often associated with age, congenital anomalies, radiation to the chest, mucopolysaccharidosis causing amyloid deposition in the mitral valve, mitral annular calcification, left atrial myxoma, and infective endocarditis with large vegetations.

Epidemiology **MR** is the most common valvular abnormality, accounting for 20% of the cases of valve disease. The major cause of MR in Western countries is degenerative myxomatous disease, which accounts for approximately 60% of cases. Myxomatous degeneration of the mitral valve is more commonly seen in women and elderly patients. Endocarditis and RHD are each responsible for 2% to 5% of cases. In developing regions of the world, RHD remains a leading cause. The most common cause of **MS** (worldwide) is RHD; 60% of patients with MS report a history of **rheumatic fever** (RF). It is estimated that the incidence of RF in the United States is less than 1 out of 100,000 people. In developing countries, the prevalence of RF is estimated to be between 100 to 150 out of 100,000 people and 5 to 15 out of 1000 children. RHD may affect the aortic valve and, less often, the tricuspid valve.

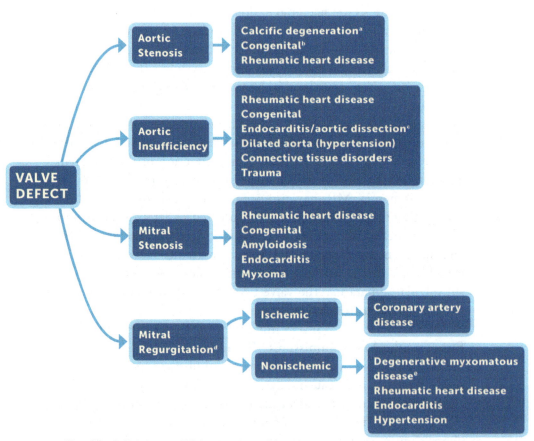

Fig. 10-4. Etiology of Valvular Heart Disease
[a]Most common cause of aortic stenosis, especially in patients with bicuspid aortic valve.
[b]Bicuspid aortic valve is the most common congenital abnormality of the human heart.
[c]Most common causes of acute aortic insufficiency.
[d]Most common valvular disease.
[e]Most common cause of nonischemic mitral regurgitation.

Symptoms AS is associated with angina, syncope, and dyspnea. The onset of **chronic AI** is insidious and progression of the disease is slow. Patients may remain relatively asymptomatic for many years. In contrast, **acute AI** leads to rapidly decreased cardiac output and symptoms of decompensated CHF. Symptoms of **MR** often depend on the amount of regurgitation and the acuity of the disease process. Most patients with MR are asymptomatic with normal exercise tolerance and rarely develop serious complications. Patients with acute onset of severe MR exhibit symptoms of CHF, including dyspnea or orthopnea. The latency of MS following an episode of RF is 5 to 10 years, with the onset of symptoms occurring many years later. **MS** is associated with a gradual decrease in activity secondary to worsening dyspnea on exertion and fatigue. Symptoms during exercise usually develop when the valve area decreases to below 2.5 cm^2 and to below 1.5 cm^2 at rest.

Physical Exam and Signs AS: A crescendo-decrescendo murmur can be heard best at the second intercostal space. AS is associated with CHF. **AI:** A **soft blowing early diastolic decrescendo murmur** and possibly a **systolic flow murmur with diastolic rumble** (Austin Flint) can be heard best at the second intercostal space. **MR: A high-pitched holosystolic murmur** can be heard best at the cardiac apex, with radiation to the back. The classic murmur of MR is caused by turbulent blood flow backward into the left atrium during ventricular contraction. Signs of MR include pulmonary edema or cardiogenic shock. **MS:** Exam findings include a **laterally displaced cardiac apex, loud first heart sound,** and a **mid-late diastolic murmur** best heard in the **left lateral decubitus position.** With advanced disease, signs of right-sided heart failure, including hepatomegaly, ascites, and peripheral edema may occur.

Differential The differential focuses mostly on the various types and causes of valvular disease.

Diagnosis Aortic valve pathology is typically diagnosed with echocardiogram, which can be used to estimate aortic valve area (AVA) and the gradient between the aorta and LV. A complete medical history and physical exam are used in various combinations to guide diagnosis.

Labs. In acute presentations, measurement of cardiac troponins and CK-MB levels can be helpful and are more specific for cardiac causes.

Imaging. AS is graded as mild (AVA >1.5 cm^2), moderate (AVA 1 to 1.5 cm^2), or severe (<1 cm^2). A mean gradient across the aortic valve greater than 40 mm Hg is considered severe.

AI is graded based on the severity of the regurgitant jet. Severe AI is defined by a regurgitant fraction greater than or equal to 50%, regurgitant volume greater than 60 mL, pressure half-time of the regurgitant jet less than 250 msec, Doppler vena contracta width greater than 0.6 cm, and regurgitant orifice area greater than 0.3 cm^2.

In MR, secondary effects of the regurgitant flow may include LA enlargement, which in severe disease can be seen as an enlarged heart on chest X-ray. An echo readily demonstrates the regurgitant blood flow from the LV to the LA during ventricular contraction.

The classification of MS is based on the valve area and gradient across the valve. Echocardiography provides information about the mitral leaflet structure, annular size, LA size, LV function, and transvalvular gradient. Additional testing includes chest X-ray, which may demonstrate interstitial edema; MV calcification; prominent pulmonary vessels with pulmonary congestion; and significant cardiomegaly due to LA enlargement. Atrial fibrillation (AF) is often present.

Complication(s) The median survival for untreated **AS** is 5 years if associated with angina, 3 years if associated with syncope, and 1 to 2 years if associated with CHF. These patients typically die from left ventricular failure. The prognosis of patients with **AI** is determined by symptoms, as well as the extent of LV dilation and dysfunction. Patients with chronic **MR** often develop atrial fibrillation. Patients with **MS** may develop CHF, AF, and embolic events.

Treatment Symptomatic patients with AS (syncope, angina, dyspnea) should undergo **aortic valve replacement** (AVR). Asymptomatic patients with severe AS plus LV systolic dysfunction or those undergoing cardiac surgery for other cardiac pathologies should also have concomitant AVR. Currently, aortic valve pathology can be treated by inserting an expandable stented bioprosthetic valve using transcatheter techniques. A **mechanical AV** is the most durable option and can last a lifetime; however, it requires lifelong anticoagulation therapy. **Bioprosthetic valves** do not require anticoagulation therapy and can last 15 years or longer. Many patients older than 70 years are candidates for bioprosthetic valves. Younger patients (<60 years) with a near-normal life expectancy should be considered for mechanical valve replacement.

In symptomatic patients with severe AI, and some subsets of asymptomatic patients, AVR is indicated. Unlike AS where AVR is always required, the AV or aortic root can be repaired in AI to restore competency in some cases. Acute AI is generally considered a surgical emergency.

Treatment of MR is determined by the presence and severity of symptoms, clinical status, cause of the regurgitation, and time course of the disease. In the absence of symptoms, patients with mild to moderate regurgitation may not require treatment. Medical therapy for MR is noncurative and is often used in patients with mild to moderate disease and those unable to tolerate surgical correction. Patients with chronic MR are often **medically managed** with the use of diuretics, vasodilators, and angiotensin-converting enzyme (ACE) inhibitors in an effort to decrease cardiac afterload and, therefore, decrease MR. **Surgical intervention** is recommended in patients with severe MR who are symptomatic or show signs of LV dysfunction. Cardiac surgery is the treatment of choice in patients with acute MR secondary to a mechanical defect such as rupture of a papillary muscle or chordae tendineae and signs or symptoms of cardiogenic shock. MV repair or replacement is indicated in endocarditis with large vegetations, severe MR, evidence of systemic emboli, or persistent positive blood cultures despite appropriate antibiotic therapy. Surgical repair is preferred over replacement because survival has been shown to be superior.

Asymptomatic or mildly symptomatic MS may not require treatment. Intervention is recommended for patients with moderate to severe MS and symptomatic disease, signs of pulmonary hypertension, or new-onset AF. Therapeutic options include percutaneous mitral balloon valvotomy (MBV) or cardiac surgery. MBV has become the first-line treatment for most patients with MS. When it is unsuccessful or contraindicated, surgery should be considered early. RHD results in such severe destruction of the valve that replacement is often required.

AORTIC DISSECTION

Definition Aortic dissection is a **disruption in the intima of the aorta,** resulting in separation of the layers of the aortic wall. Aortic dissection is classified using the **DeBakey** or **Stanford** (Fig. 10-5) classification systems, based on the anatomic location and/or distal extent of the dissection. Stanford type A includes aortic dissections that involve the ascending aorta, with or without involvement of the transverse and descending thoracic aorta. Stanford type B aortic dissections originate in the descending and thoracoabdominal aorta and do not involve the ascending aorta. DeBakey type I and type II dissections involve the ascending aorta; however, Debakey type II dissections are confined to the ascending aorta. DeBakey type III dissections are confined to the descending aorta. The Stanford system is used most often.

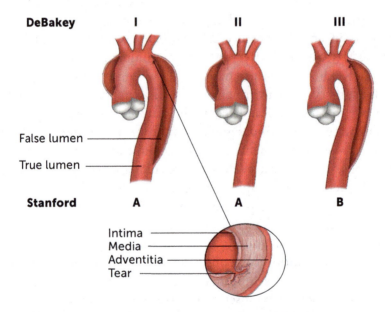

Fig. 10-5. DeBakey and Stanford Classification of Aortic Dissections

Etiology A tear of the intima and media results in a **false lumen,** a blood-filled space within the aortic wall that continues to expand as the blood flow propagates the dissection both proximally and distally from the initial tear site. Dissection may result from trauma, iatrogenic injury, or excessive strain (eg, lifting heavy weights). The most common cause is **chronic hypertension** and **atherosclerotic disease,** resulting in spontaneous dissection. Patients with connective tissue disorders such as Marfan's, Loeys-Dietz, and Ehlers-Danlos syndromes have an increased risk for aortic dissection, and at a younger age. Patients with uncontrolled hypertension and bicuspid aortic valve also have a higher incidence.

Epidemiology Aortic dissection occurs most commonly in the sixth and seventh decades of life, and the male-to-female ratio is 5:1. It occurs in approximately 3 in 100,000 persons per year.

Symptoms Most commonly, **pain in the chest or back** develops abruptly and is described as tearing. Ascending aortic involvement usually presents with anterior pain, with or without radiation to the jaw, neck, and arm. If a descending aortic component is present, the pain is usually described between the scapulae.

Physical Exam and Signs Hypertension is present in two-thirds of those with type B dissections, but only in one-fourth of those with ascending aortic dissections. Hemoptysis, dyspnea, dysphagia, and altered mental status may be present. Arm or leg ischemia may be present if malperfusion of the extremity occurs.

Differential Aneurysms with thrombosed false lumens are difficult to differentiate from dissections. In a penetrating peptic ulcer, pain is present without evidence of dissection on imaging. In intramural hematoma, there is absence of an entry tear. A myocardial infarction must be ruled out.

Diagnosis Computed tomography angiography (CTA) with intravenous contrast is the test of choice for diagnosing aortic dissection.

Labs. Malperfusion may result in laboratory derangements, but they are not diagnostic. In patients with renal or visceral malperfusion, an increased creatinine level and lactic acidosis may be present.

Imaging. CTA is used to identify the entry and exit points of the dissection and any aneurysmal changes. It has limitations in cases involving the ascending aorta. MRI has over 90% sensitivity and specificity, but it is limited because it is not immediately available and takes longer to perform. TEE is performed mostly in cases involving the ascending aorta, but sensitivity and specificity are highly variable (reported from 30% to 40% and 80% to 90% for both parameters). Unstable patients with a high index of suspicion for dissection can be taken directly to the operating room for surgical repair without first performing a CTA. In these cases, TEE is used routinely to assess the location of the dissection, evaluate the AV for the presence of AI, evaluate LV function, and assess the operative repair at conclusion of surgery. TEE can be performed while the patient is prepped for surgery. Chest radiograph may demonstrate a widened mediastinum.

Complication(s) Acute or chronic aortic dissection can result in impairment of blood flow in branch arteries within the range of the dissection. Stroke may occur if the great vessels are involved. Paraplegia complicates up to 10% of type B dissections. If the dissection results in rupture of the aorta, shock and death ensue rapidly as a result of hemorrhage or cardiac tamponade.

Treatment The cornerstone of initial treatment includes **blood pressure control** to prevent further propagation of the dissection. **Intravenous beta-blockade** to achieve a heart rate less than 60 bpm and vasodilators to maintain a systolic blood pressure at less than 120 mm Hg is imperative. In hypotensive patients, a thorough investigation for cardiac tamponade is required. Type A dissections require immediate surgical reconstructions with graft replacement. This group of patients exhibit over a 50% mortality rate when treated only medically. Operative mortality for type A dissections is 10% to 20%. Type B should be first treated medically, but if surgical therapy is required the mortality ranges between 6% and 45%.

PERICARDITIS

Definition Pericarditis is an inflammation of the pericardium.

Etiology Pericarditis is often idiopathic. Some common causes include viral or bacterial infections, metabolic abnormalities, and systemic inflammatory disorders. The most common viral agents are coxsackieviruses and echoviruses. Pericarditis can also result as a complication of MI. **Dressler syndrome** describes inflammation caused by an immune response to cardiac tissue damaged from an MI, open-heart surgery, or trauma. Other less common but important causes of pericarditis include side effects of medications or radiation therapy.

Epidemiology The true incidence of pericarditis is unknown, yet approximately 6% of all patients on postmortem examination have signs of pericardial inflammation. The disorder has an increased prevalence in men and older adults.

Symptoms The most common symptom of pericarditis is chest pain. Classically the pain is described as a sharp, stabbing sensation that is **relieved by leaning forward** and worsened with deep inspiration or lying supine. When pericarditis is caused by infection, symptoms tend to appear quickly, whereas inflammation resulting from chronic disease is more gradual in onset and usually painless.

Physical Exam and Signs Chronic pericarditis may present with signs of right- or left-sided heart failure, including dyspnea, fatigue, and peripheral edema. The most common sign is a **pericardial friction rub** that results from the two layers of the pericardium rubbing against each other with each heartbeat.

Differential Esophageal disorders, costochondritis, or other causes of noncardiac chest pain may need to be ruled out.

Diagnosis The diagnosis of pericarditis is made by obtaining a history and physical examination and begins with a thorough review of chest pain characteristics.

Labs. No specific lab tests are available.

Imaging. ECG or chest X-ray are commonly normal. However, if a large amount of fluid accumulates within the pericardial sac, the heart may appear larger on chest X-ray and is classically described as having a **water-bottle appearance.** Diffuse ST segment elevation is often seen on ECG in acute pericarditis. Echocardiography and chest CT may help to clarify the diagnosis. Echocardiography is useful in quantifying the pericardial effusion. Cardiac catheterization with intracardiac pressure measurements can help confirm the diagnosis of constrictive pericarditis.

Complication(s) Cardiac tamponade can be a life-threatening complication of pericarditis. It is the result of fluid accumulation in the pericardial sac, causing a rise in pericardial pressure. The increased pressure constricts normal cardiac movement and impedes venous return. This leads to decreased cardiac output and hypotension. The classic exam findings of cardiac tamponade are known as **Beck's triad,** which includes hypotension, distended neck veins, and muffled heart sounds.

Treatment The treatment of the underlying cause(s) is essential. Most often therapy is aimed at decreasing inflammation and controlling pain with **nonsteroidal anti-inflammatory drugs.** The treatment of **constrictive pericarditis** is sternotomy with pericardiectomy. **Acute cardiac tamponade** is a true emergency that requires immediate intervention, usually by **pericardiocentesis.** This relieves the pressure by aspirating the fluid through a long needle inserted through the chest wall into the pericardial sac. The fluid can also be drained via surgical approach through a small subxiphoid incision.

BIBLIOGRAPHY

Bonow RO, Carabello BA, Chatterjee K, et al; 2006 Writing Committee Members; American College of Cardiology/American Heart Association Task Force. 2008 Focused update incorporated into the ACC/AHA 2006 guidelines for the management of patients with valvular heart disease: a report of the American College of Cardiology/American Heart Association Task Force on Practice Guidelines. *Circulation.* 2008;118:e523-661.

Carabello BA. Valvular heart disease. In: Goldman L, Schafer AI, eds. *Goldman's Cecil Medicine.* 24th ed. Philadelphia, PA: Saunders Elsevier; 2011:chap 75.

Cohn LH, Byrne JG. Minimally invasive mitral valve surgery: current status. *Tex Heart Inst J.* 2013;40(5):575-576.

Le Huu A, Shum-Tim D. Tissue engineering of autologous heart valves: a focused update. *Future Cardiol.* 2014;10(1):93-104

CLINICAL KEYS: QUESTIONS AND ANSWERS

What major veins drain into the right atrium?	Superior and inferior vena cava
From where do the coronary arteries arise?	Ascending aorta
What is a STEMI?	ST elevation myocardial infarction
What causes a STEMI?	Atherosclerotic plaque rupture
How does unstable angina present?	Unremitting chest pain without increasing cardiac enzymes or ST changes on ECG
What is the difference between an NSTEMI and unstable angina?	NSTEMI is associated with enzyme elevation
What is the mortality rate of CABG?	1% to 3%
What is the most common cause of aortic stenosis?	Calcific degeneration
What is aortic stenosis?	Increased valve stiffness, reduced cusp excursion, and progressive valve orifice narrowing
What are the most common causes of acute aortic insufficiency?	Bacterial endocarditis and aortic dissection
What is aortic insufficiency?	Regurgitant blood flow from the aorta back into the left ventricle during diastole
What is mitral regurgitation?	The mitral valve does not close properly during ventricular contraction, causing retrograde blood flow from the left ventricle into the left atrium during systole.
What is the most common cause of mitral stenosis?	Rheumatic heart disease (60% of cases are associated with rheumatic fever)

What is mitral stenosis?	The narrowing of the mitral valve area with subsequent left atrial pressure elevation and dilatation
What is the most common valvular disease?	Mitral regurgitation
What is the most common congenital abnormality of the human heart?	Bicuspid aortic valve
What is a common complication of mitral regurgitation?	Atrial fibrillation
Which type of valve replacement requires lifelong anticoagulation therapy?	Mechanical valve
What is aortic dissection?	A tear in the intima that results in a false lumen
What is the test of choice for diagnosing aortic dissection?	CTA with IV contrast
What is the most common cause of aortic dissection?	Chronic hypertension and atherosclerotic disease
What is the initial treatment for aortic dissection?	Blood pressure control with IV beta-blockers
What are the symptoms of pericarditis?	Chest pain that is typically relieved when leaning forward
Which is a life-threatening complication of pericarditis?	Cardiac tamponade

Vascular Surgery 11

The **thoracic aorta** has an ascending portion and a descending portion (Fig. 11-1). The ascending segment gives off the right and left coronary arteries. The **aortic arch** has 3 arterial branches: (1) **the brachiocephalic trunk** or the *innominate artery*, (2) **the left common carotid artery**, and (2) **the left subclavian artery.**

One of the first branches of the brachiocephalic trunk is the **right common carotid artery.**

As the aorta crosses the diaphragm into the abdomen it becomes known as the **abdominal aorta.** It is the origin of 3 important arterial branches—the **celiac axis,** the **superior mesenteric artery** (SMA), and the **inferior mesenteric artery** (IMA), which supplies blood flow to the colon.

The **renal arteries** originate from the abdominal aorta below the SMA.

The aorta bifurcates to form the **common iliac arteries** at the level of the umbilicus.

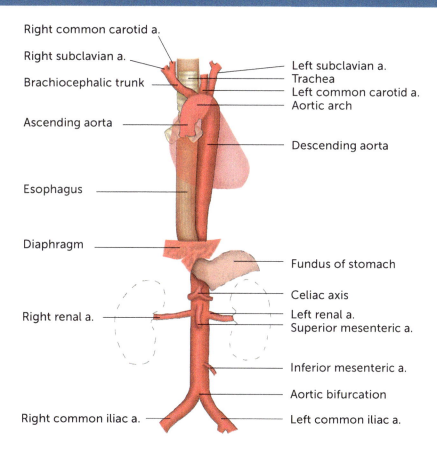

Fig. 11-1. Thoracic and Abdominal Aorta

Surgery 157

Carotid Artery Occlusive Disease

Definition Carotid artery occlusive disease (CAOD) is characterized by the **narrowing of the carotid artery.** It is categorized by the severity of the narrowing (reported as percent stenosis, which is a measure of the decrease in diameter at the level of occlusion compared to the normal vessel) and the presence or absence of symptoms. Four levels of stenosis are described: (1) mild (<50%), (2) moderate (50% to 79%), (3) severe (80% to 99%), and (4) occluded (100%).

Etiology Atherosclerosis is the most common cause of CAOD. The atherosclerotic plaque is most common at the **bifurcation of the common carotid arteries,** with plaque extension into the proximal internal carotid arteries. Associated risk factors for atherosclerotic disease include tobacco use, hypertension, diabetes mellitus, family history, and hyperlipidemia.

Epidemiology CAOD is responsible for 20% to 25% of cerebrovascular accidents (CVAs), or stroke, which is the fourth leading cause of death in the United States. Disease of the carotid bifurcation is thought to be the cause of nearly all CVAs from CAOD, which is responsible for 20% to 25% of neurologic events.

Symptoms Most patients with carotid artery stenosis are **asymptomatic.** If symptoms arise, they manifest as **neurologic deficits.** Amaurosis fugax are episode(s) of transient monocular blindness. They are often described as a shade being pulled down over one eye. Hemispheric symptoms include speech deficits or transient ischemic attacks (TIAs). TIAs may last from seconds to several hours, but focal neurologic deficits restore to baseline within 24 hours of symptom occurrence. Completed strokes are characterized by persistent neurologic impairment.

Physical Exam and Signs An ocular examination may demonstrate cholesterol crystals in the retina (Hollenhorst plaques), and these findings typically suggest the presence of carotid lesions. The presence of a **carotid bruit** on exam necessitates diagnostic imaging. The findings are equally likely to fall in 1 of 3 categories (the one-third rule): one-third of patients will have normal carotids, one-third will have mild disease, and one-third will have significant disease. Stroke may be associated with facial drooping opposite to the hemisphere affected, leg weakness, and speech disturbances.

Differential Neurologic symptoms might not be a result of CAOD, so the differential revolves around other causes. Embolic events, (eg, from atrial fibrillation), thrombotic events (eg, from hypercoagulability syndromes), or hemorrhagic events (eg, from hypertension or brain aneurysms) must be considered.

Diagnosis CAOD is diagnosed via imaging.

Labs. None specific.

Imaging. **Carotid artery duplex scanning** is the initial test of choice, and it is the recommended modality for surveillance. Duplex imaging provides anatomic characteristics of the plaque. Soft low echoes indicate that the plaque is homogeneous; echogenic plaque is hard with significant calcifications, and a heterogeneous appearance is characteristic of plaques with soft and hard components. Reporting is based on established Doppler criteria. False positives or false negatives occur in 10% to 15% of carotid duplex scans, and they have the largest technical variation between institutions. CT and MRI with intravenous contrast are noninvasive modalities that provide better accuracy than duplex scanning alone, but drawbacks associated with these studies include added toxicity from intravenous contrast agents and radiation exposure. For patients requiring surgery, **digital subtraction angiography** (DSA) is the gold standard to study CAOD, in which the narrowed ICA is compared to the normal distal ICA. However, catheter-based angiography is associated with a 1% risk of neurologic events and at least a 1% risk of an access-related complication (site of arterial puncture). Therefore, DSA is not performed instead of ultrasonography unless study results are conflicting or an intervention is entertained (eg, carotid stenting).

Complication(s) Surgery for CAOD is associated with a mortality rate of 1%. It is associated with myocardial infarction in up to 10% of patients, stroke in less than 5% of symptomatic patients, cranial nerve injury in up to 15%, neck hematoma in less than 5% of patients, and recurrent stenosis in up to 10% of patients at 10 years.

Treatment

Asymptomatic CAOD: These patients are managed with risk factor modification, which includes smoking cessation, control of hypertension, management of lipid disorders, strict blood glucose control, and the implementation of a weight loss and exercise regimen.

Asymptomatic CAOD with 60% to 79% stenosis: These patients are managed with antiplatelet agents, such as aspirin, dipyridamole, and clopidogrel. Contemporary management of asymptomatic stenosis requires an 80% narrowing before considering surgical repair by carotid endarterectomy (CEA)—the removal of the culprit carotid lesion via a neck incision.

Asymptomatic CAOD with 80% stenosis or more: CEA.

Symptomatic stenosis greater than 50%: CEA. Included in this category are patients with a documented TIA or stroke and those with an ipsilateral ICA stenosis greater than 50%. If the stenosis is greater than 70%, the absolute stroke reduction after surgery approaches 20% at 2 years.

Peripheral Vascular Disease

Definition Peripheral vascular disease (PVD) is characterized by narrowing of the arteries of the extremities. This refers mostly to lower extremity arteries, because upper extremity disease is uncommon. The length of the stenotic segment and the severity of symptoms should be used to qualify the extent of disease. An example is a symptomatic 4-cm segment of the common iliac artery with 75% stenosis, resulting in debilitating pain of the lower extremity.

Etiology Atherosclerosis is the main cause of PVD (Fig. 11-2). Tobacco use is a significant risk factor for aortoiliac and femoral disease, and infrapopliteal disease is associated with long-standing diabetes mellitus.

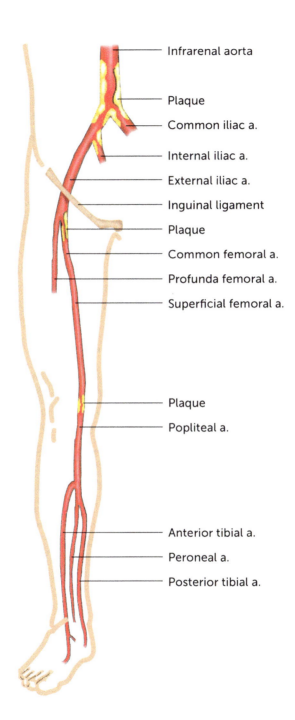

Fig. 11-2. Peripheral Arterial Anatomy and Common Plaque Locations

Epidemiology The prevalence of PVD increases with age. PVD is noted in 10% of those aged 65 years and in more than 25% of those aged 80 and older.

Symptoms The main symptom of PVD is **claudication** (Table 11-1), which is described as cramping pain or heaviness in the affected extremity that occurs after physical exertion and is relieved by rest. As the disease progresses, the pain in muscle groups below the disease causes symptoms after walking shorter distances, and once the disease reaches a critical level, patients develop **rest pain.** Ischemic rest pain generally occurs at an absolute resting ankle pressure of less than 50 mm Hg and occurs in the toes or dorsum of the foot when supine. Rest pain often awakens the patient from sleep and may improve by placing the foot in a dependent position, allowing gravity to augment perfusion. **Leriche syndrome** (decreased femoral pulses, impotence, leg pallor, buttock and leg claudication, and leg musculature atrophy) is a constellation of symptoms that occurs in men as a result of occlusion of the terminal aorta.

Physical Exam and Signs Pulses should be examined at the femoral, popliteal, dorsalis pedis, and posterior tibial arteries. A normal palpable pulse is designated 2+, a diminished but palpable pulse is designated 1+, and a pulse that cannot be palpated is designated as nonpalpable. If the pulse is absent, the artery should be assessed with continuous wave Doppler ultrasound using a handheld device. Inspection of the limb in patients with arterial insufficiency reveals decreased hair growth below the calf region. Critical ischemia causes erythema of the foot in a dependent position (dependent rubor) that becomes pale with elevation. Tissue loss, including ulceration and gangrene, is seen with critical limb ischemia.

Table 11-1. Rutherford Classification of Peripheral Arterial Disease

Grade	Category	Clinical Presentation
0	0	Asymptomatic
I	1	Mild claudication
I	2	Moderate claudication
I	3	Severe claudication
II	4	Ischemic rest pain
III	5	Minor tissue loss
III	6	Major tissue loss

Differential The differential revolves around the causes of pseudoclaudication. **Spinal stenosis:** ±Leg pain with standing and/or ambulation, posterior limb and hip paresthesia, often positional. **Venous insufficiency:** Leg pain worsens while standing, leg swelling, varicosities that worsen as the day progresses. **Neuropathy:** Foot rest pain, typically burning and in a "sock-like distribution." **Musculoskeletal pain:** Muscle strain or tear.

Diagnosis Initial evaluation includes measurement of the **ankle brachial index** (ABI). ABI is the ratio of the systolic blood pressure of the leg compared to the brachial systolic blood pressure of either arm (Table 11-2). In general, patients with claudication have an ABI of less than 0.8, and patients with rest pain have an ABI of less than 0.4. **Peripheral arterial duplex** is the diagnostic **noninvasive** test of choice for patients with or without planned intervention and for surveillance following interventions.

Labs. No specific labs.

Imaging. Digital subtraction angiography (DSA) is the gold standard for disease assessment before planned revascularization. It requires arterial catheter placement and intra-arterial contrast administration. Computed tomography angiography (CTA) and magnetic resonance angiography (MRA) with intravenous contrast are used to map the location and severity of disease. However, calcifications sometimes make interpretation of CTA difficult, and MRA is known to overestimate the degree of stenosis.

Table 11-2. ABI Severity Classification

Arterial Disease	Ankle Brachial Index Value
Noncompressible	>1.30
Normal	1.0–1.29
Borderline	0.90–0.99
Mild	0.70–0.89
Moderate	0.40–0.69
Severe	<0.40

Complication(s) **Cardiac-related death** is the most common complication of PVD. Pain or discomfort in mild to moderate PVD can limit an individual's quality of life, and chronic limb pain can worsen as the disease progresses. Progressive disease—measured by a declining ABI—can result in limb loss (1% to 2% of patients with claudication develop critical limb ischemia at 5 years, and 10% to 15% of patients with limb loss ultimately require a contralateral amputation.)

Treatment For patients with claudication, the best therapy is to prescribe a supervised **exercise program,** which may increase the development of collateral arteries. **Medical management** can be accomplished with antiplatelet agents (aspirin and/or clopidogrel), strict control of hypertension and diabetes, and statin therapy. **Cilostazol** is a phosphodiesterase inhibitor that has been shown in clinical studies to nearly double walking distance in approximately 50% of patients. **Endovascular intervention,** such as angioplasty, atherectomy, or stenting is the first line of treatment for patients with debilitating claudication and for rest pain and tissue loss in most short to moderate lesions (Fig. 11-3).

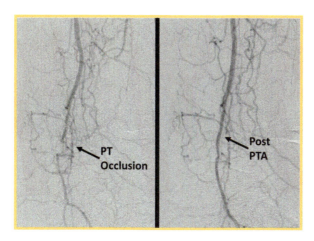

Fig. 11-3. Angiogram of the Posterior Tibial Artery. *Left:* Posterior Tibial Occlusion *Right:* Post Percutaneous Transluminal Angioplasty

Surgery is considered for patients with failed endovascular treatment, extensive disease, or disease locations inaccessible to an endovascular approach. Surgery may include **endarterectomy** or **surgical bypass** to provide distal blood flow around the obstructions.

THORACIC AORTIC ANEURYSM

Definition Thoracic aortic aneurysm (TAA) is a dilation of the thoracic aorta that exceeds **1.5 times the diameter of the normal adjacent aorta.** The ascending aorta and/or aortic root are involved in 60% of aneurysms, the descending aorta in 40% of cases, and the aortic arch in 10% (Fig. 11-4). Aneurysms of the thoracic and abdominal aorta, described as *thoracoabdominal aneurysms*, occur in 10% of cases.

Etiology Smoking tobacco products, personal or family history of atherosclerosis, and hypertension are risk factors for the development of aneurysms. Less common causes include connective tissue disorders (eg, Marfan's syndrome), a bicuspid aortic valve, syphilis, arteritis, and trauma.

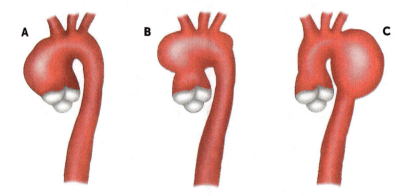

Fig. 11-4. Types of Thoracic Aortic Aneurysms **A.** Ascending Aortic Aneurysm **B.** Aortic Arch Aneurysm **C.** Descending Aortic Aneurysm

Epidemiology TAAs are less common than abdominal aortic aneurysms (AAAs), though both have similar risk factors and are more common in whites and men. Over one-fourth of those with a TAA have a history of or an associated AAA. The mean age of diagnosis is in the sixth decade.

Symptoms Most patients are asymptomatic. Patients may experience hoarseness or hematochezia related to nerve compression or erosion into the esophagus. If a TAA ruptures, chest and back pain may be reported. Hemoptysis as a result of erosion of the aneurysm into the airway is rare.

Physical Exam and Signs There are no appreciable physical findings unless the TAA has ruptured or is rapidly enlarging. TAAs cannot be palpated.

Differential Aortic dissection with thrombosis of the false lumen might present with similar findings.

Diagnosis The gold standard for the diagnosis of TAA is **CTA with intravenous contrast.**

Labs. Lab tests are nonspecific.

Imaging. CTA reveals the maximum aortic diameter and delineates the proximal and distal extent of the aneurysm. Chest X-ray occasionally detects a TAA incidentally by revealing a calcium silhouette within the aortic wall or a widened mediastinum.

Complication(s) Intrathoracic hemorrhage with rupture is nearly always fatal. Rates of rupture increase when the aneurysm exceeds 6 cm in diameter. Annual risk of rupture is directly related to the maximum thoracic aortic diameter (Table 11-3). Compression of the recurrent laryngeal nerve resulting in hoarseness or erosion into the esophagus or trachea can occur. Paraplegia occurs in less than 10% of cases. Complications such as renal failure and stroke occur in less than 5% of cases.

Table 11-3. Annual Rupture Risk Based on Thoracic Aortic Aneurysm Diameter

Diameter of Aneurysm	Annual Rate of Rupture
<4 cm	<1%
4–6 cm[a]	<3%
6–7 cm	<10%

[a]Repair offered when aneurysm reaches 6 cm in diameter.

Treatment **Surgical reconstruction** is the treatment of choice for ascending aorta and aortic arch aneurysms. Aneurysms of the descending aorta are best treated with **stenting.** Annual exams are recommended until repair is performed. The annual growth rate increases as the aneurysm grows and is faster for aneurysms involving the descending aorta. Surgery or stenting has an operative 30-day mortality of less than 10%.

ABDOMINAL AORTIC ANEURYSM

Definition Similar to TAA, abdominal aortic aneurysm (AAA) is a dilation of the abdominal aorta that exceeds **1.5 times the diameter of the normal adjacent aorta.** Aneurysms that begin at least 1 cm below the renal arteries are considered **infrarenal** (Fig. 11-5); 90% of AAAs are in this category. Less commonly, the border of the aneurysms is within 1 cm of the renal arteries; these are designated **juxtarenal.** Or the aneurysm may include the renal arteries, in which case it is designated **pararenal.** If the aneurysm involves the visceral arteries, it is categorized as a **suprarenal** aortic aneurysm. Aneurysms may be **fusiform** or **saccular**. Fusiform aneurysms are diffusely dilated, whereas saccular aneurysms are focal dilations. Most AAAs are **true aneurysms** (dilation of all three layers of the arterial wall). **Pseudoaneurysms** resulting from contained ruptures, though less common, can develop.

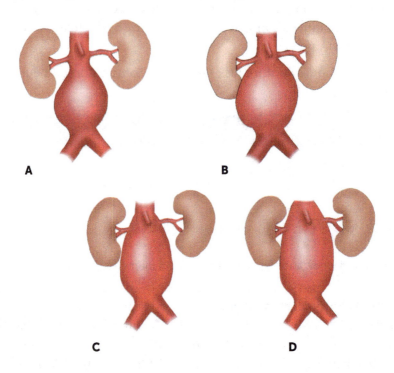

Fig. 11-5. Types of Abdominal Aortic Aneurysms **A.** Infrarenal **B.** Juxtarenal **C.** Pararenal **D.** Suprarenal

Etiology Causes are multifactorial, and most patients have cardiovascular atherosclerotic disease associated with a TAA. The 2 most important risk factors are a history of smoking tobacco products and a family history of aneurysms.

Epidemiology The highest incidence occurs in men older than 65 years of age (male-to-female ratio is 5:1) with a history of tobacco use (approximately 5% incidence by ultrasound). It is one of the top 10 causes of death in men over 55 years of age. Approximately 40,000 repair procedures are performed annually. Approximately 20% of first-degree relatives have an AAA.

Symptoms AAAs are generally asymptomatic, and most are diagnosed incidentally. The most common symptomatic presentation is a result of rupture with intra-abdominal or retroperitoneal hemorrhage. Although rare, rupture can occur into the vena cava, creating a large arteriovenous fistula.

Physical Exam and Signs A **pulsatile abdominal mass** (located between the xiphoid process and the umbilicus) is palpable in less than 50% of patients with AAAs greater than 5 cm in diameter. Rupture may present with the classic triad of abdominal and/or back pain, pulsatile mass, and hypotension/shock.

Differential Since an AAA can rarely be diagnosed on physical examination, the differential applies to a patient presenting with a ruptured AAA. In this case, the differential includes a ureteral stone (most common misdiagnosis of leaking aneurysms) with flank pain and hematuria (present in 20% of patients with a ruptured AAA). Musculoskeletal injury with back pain must be considered.

Diagnosis The initial screening and surveillance method of choice is an **abdominal ultrasound.**

Labs. No laboratory values are predictive of an AAA in asymptomatic patients. In patients with rupture, anemia secondary to acute blood loss, elevated creatinine, and lactic acidosis may be present.

Imaging. Ultrasound demonstrates enlargement of the abdominal aorta. **CTA with contrast** is the gold standard of imaging and is reserved for patients planning to undergo repair and for surveillance following endovascular stent repair. DSA does not demonstrate the mural thrombus and actual aortic diameter, so accurate size measurements typically cannot be determined with DSA.

Complication(s) The most common complication is rupture, with an associated mortality of nearly 75%. Risk of rupture is correlated to aneurysm size (Table 11-4). Thromboembolization with an ischemic limb is present in greater than 5% of cases. Compression of adjacent structures may cause hydronephrosis, congestive heart failure (CHF), and venous hypertension.

Table 11-4. Annual Rupture Risk Based on Abdominal Aneurysm Diameter

Abdominal Aneurysm Diameter (cm)	Annual Rupture Risk (%)
<4.0	<1
4.0–4.9	12
5.0–5.9	5–10
6.0–6.9	10–20
7.0–7.9	20–40
>8.0	30–50

Treatment An AAA greater than 4 cm should be imaged every 1 to 3 years, one that measures 4 to 4.5 cm should be imaged annually, and one that is greater than 4.5 to 5.5 cm should be imaged every 6 months. Once the aneurysm exceeds 5.5 cm, or if the aneurysm enlarges rapidly (≥1 cm in 1 year by the same imaging technique), repair should be performed. The usual expansion rate is 10% of the aortic diameter per year. A rupture is always an emergency. Treatment is done either by inserting covered stents or by performing open surgery. Currently, over 75% of aneurysms are treated with stent grafts. Pararenal aneurysms require either surgical reimplantation of 1 or both of the renal arteries or fenestrated stent grafting.

DEEP VEIN THROMBOSIS

Definition A deep vein thrombosis (DVT) is the thrombotic occlusion of the deep venous system, predominantly in the legs. The constellation of presentations is currently described as venous thromboembolism (VTE). The lower extremities have a superficial venous system above the fascia, a deep system below it, and the connecting veins, which join the superficial and deep systems.

Etiology **Virchow's triad** is often used to explain the development of perioperative DVT. It consists of **vascular stasis, hypercoagulability,** and **endothelial damage.** Risk factors include advanced age, immobility, pregnancy, recent major surgery (within 4 weeks), cancer, previous DVT, spinal cord injury, factor V Leiden, and other predisposing factors.

Epidemiology DVT/VTE is considered the number one preventable cause of in-hospital deaths, and it is a common cause of morbidity and mortality. The incidence of VTE exceeds 1 in 1000 persons, with almost 400,000 new cases annually in the United States. Of patients who survive the initial event of VTE, 30% have a recurrence and 30% develop a postphlebitic syndrome within 10 years.

Symptoms Leg swelling and pain may be noted, or it may be asymptomatic.

Physical Exam and Signs A tender swollen extremity with red discoloration in any patient with risk factors should raise concern for acute DVT. **Homan's sign** (calf tenderness on dorsiflexion of the foot) may be present with DVT, but this is not a reliable finding. Fever and erythema are uncommon.

Differential Muscle strain, lymphedema, valvular venous insufficiency, cellulitis, other causes of limb edema such as CHF, liver or renal failure, nutritional deficiency (hypoalbuminemia), and myxedema must be considered.

Diagnosis Compression ultrasonography is the test of choice.

Labs. The D-dimer assay is a very sensitive but nonspecific blood test that can rule out DVT in 97% of cases. Therefore, it is most useful if negative.

Imaging. Lack of compressibility of a vein with the ultrasound probe is highly sensitive (>95%) and specific (>95%) for a proximal DVT, versus 35% accuracy for a tibial DVT. Impedance plethysmography measures blood volume changes and can indirectly evaluate for the presence of DVT.

Complication(s) The most common complication of DVT is pulmonary embolism (PE).

PULMONARY EMBOLISM A PE develops when an embolus lodges in the pulmonary circulation, resulting in hypoxia, hemodynamic compromise, pulmonary hypertension, and increased right ventricular afterload, which may lead to right-sided ventricular failure. The true prevalence of perioperative PE is unknown; it varies according to the type of surgery. Estimates indicate that without prophylaxis, fatal PE occurs in 0.1% to 0.8% of patients undergoing elective general surgery, 2% to 3% of those undergoing elective hip replacement, and 4% to 7% of those undergoing surgery for a fractured hip.

Symptoms. Shortness of breath/wheezing, chest pain, cough, and hemoptysis can occur.

Physical Exam and Signs. Tachycardia, fever, hypotension, cold, clammy skin, cyanosis (a result of low oxygen saturation) may be noted. **Westermark's sign** on imaging, although seldom present, consists of dilatation of the pulmonary vessels proximal to an embolism along with collapse of distal vessels.

Differential. Tension pneumothorax: Decreased lung sounds and deviation of mediastinal structures on chest X-ray. **Massive pericardial effusion with muffled heart sounds:** Chest pain, pressure, discomfort. Echocardiogram confirms effusion. **Septic shock:** Bacteremia, low systemic vascular resistance, tachycardia. **Myocardial infarction:** Chest pain, ECG changes.

Diagnosis. Spiral chest CTA with thinner slices is the test of choice. Pulmonary embolism rule-out criteria (PERC) are sensitive for the diagnosis of PE. They include age greater than 50 years, heart rate greater than 100 bpm, O_2 saturation on room air less than 95%, and a prior DVT or PE. If all are negative, the risk of PE is less than 2%. The most commonly used criterion is the modified Wells score (Table 11-5).

Table 11-5. Modified Wells Score

Criteria	Point Value
Previous history of PE or DVT	1.5 points
Clinical suspicion of DVT	3 points
Tachycardia	3 points
Alternative diagnosis is less likely than PE	3 points
Active or previous diagnosis of cancer within 6 months	1 point
Recent surgery and ± immobilization within 4 weeks	1.5 points
Recent history of hemoptysis	1 point
Score	**Probability of PE**
<2 points	Low probability
2–6 points	Moderate probability
>6 points	High probability

Labs. The D-dimer assay is sensitive but nonspecific for PE. As with DVT, negative findings from a D-dimer test excludes the presence of PE with great certainty.

Imaging. Classic findings on ECG include a large S wave in lead I, a large Q wave in lead III, and an inverted T wave in lead III ($S_1 Q_3 P_3$.), but they are not always present. Chest radiograph is typically normal but may serve to rule out other causes. Ventilation-perfusion scan (V/Q scan) detects areas of the lung that are ventilated but not perfused. This test can be used in certain patients with an iodine allergy and possibly in pregnant women, because radiation exposure is significantly lower than with CTA.

Treatment

DVT: One of the following methods of anticoagulation must be considered, depending on the clinical circumstances.

1. IV unfractionated heparin with a target activated partial thromboplastin time (aPTT) of 1.5 to 2.5 times the control. Warfarin treatment is overlapped for 5 to 10 days until the target international normalized ratio (INR) of 2.0 to 3.0 is achieved, at which point heparin may be discontinued.
2. Subcutaneous low-molecular-weight heparin (LMWH) to achieve a range of anti–factor Xa activity between 0.6 IU/mL and 1.0 IU/mL (normal range is 0.3 IU/mL to 0.7 IU/mL). Warfarin treatment is overlapped for 5 to 10 days until the target INR of 2.0 to 3.0 is achieved, at which point LMWH may be discontinued.
3. Oral anticoagulant with rivaroxaban, an oral factor Xa inhibitor may be considered.

The length of therapy varies, as follows:

- Known risk factor with DVT: 3 months (American College of Chest Physicians guidelines)
- Idiopathic: 6 to 12 months. If 2 or more episodes occur or a hypercoagulable state is present, lifelong treatment is recommended.

Thrombolytic therapy is considered for patients with severe clinical manifestations (eg, phlegmasia alba dolens or phlegmasia cerulea dolens). Consider in patients with PE and right-sided ventricular strain or large saddle PE. An inferior vena cava (IVC) filter is recommended for patients with acute DVT or a PE and an absolute contraindication for anticoagulation (eg, GI bleeding).

> **PE:** Therapy consists of anticoagulation, thrombolytics, or an IVC filter as for DVT. Occasionally, transcatheter clot removal is required.

BIBLIOGRAPHY

Botham CM, Bennett WL, Cooke JP. Clinical trials of adult stem cell therapy for peripheral artery disease. *Methodist DeBakey Cardiovasc J.* 2013;9(4):201-205.

Ferguson GG, Eliasziw M, Barr HW, et al. The North American Symptomatic Carotid Endarterectomy Trial: surgical results in 1415 patients. *Stroke.* 1999;30(9):1751-1758

Wennberg PW. Approach to the patient with peripheral arterial disease. *Circulation.* 2013;128(20):2241-2250.

CLINICAL KEYS: QUESTIONS AND ANSWERS

How many arterial branches does the aortic arch have?	Three: the brachiocephalic trunk, the left common carotid, and the left subclavian
How is the internal carotid artery differentiated from the external carotid artery?	The internal carotid has no extracranial branches
What is the most common cause of carotid artery occlusive disease?	Atherosclerosis
What is the most common location for carotid artery plaque formation?	The carotid bifurcation
What is the difference between a transient ischemic attack and a stroke?	Transient ischemic attack: neurologic deficits restore to baseline after 24 hours of symptom occurrence Stroke: characterized by persistent neurologic impairment

What is the initial test of choice for diagnosing carotid artery occlusive disease?	Carotid artery duplex ultrasonography
What constitutes severe carotid stenosis?	80%–99% stenosis
What are some of the risk factors for carotid artery occlusive disease?	Tobacco use, hypertension, diabetes, family history, and hyperlipidemia
What is the mortality rate of stroke in the United States?	It is the fourth leading cause of death
What is peripheral vascular disease?	Stenosis of the arteries of the extremities, typically the lower extremities
What is the most common symptom of peripheral arterial disease?	Claudication
What is claudication?	Pain or heaviness in the affected extremity that occurs after physical exertion and is relieved by rest
What is an aortic aneurysm?	Dilatation of the aorta that exceeds 1.5 times the diameter of the normal aorta
What is the test of choice to diagnose a thoracic aorta aneurysm?	CTA with IV contrast
What is the risk of rupture of an abdominal aortic aneurysm less than 4 cm in diameter?	<1%
What is the mortality of a ruptured abdominal aortic aneurysm?	75%
What is a palpable exam finding that may be present with an abdominal aortic aneurysm?	Pulsatile abdominal mass

What is the treatment of an abdominal aortic aneurysm that exceeds 5.5 cm in diameter?	Surgical repair
What is a deep vein thrombosis (DVT)?	Thrombotic occlusion of the venous system, primarily in the lower extremities
If no contraindications, what is the recommended therapy for a DVT?	Anticoagulation therapy
What percentage of patients with an episode of DVT will have a recurrence?	30%
What is Homan's sign?	Calf pain with dorsiflexion of the foot
What is the recommended management of a DVT and GI bleeding?	IVC filter
What is a pulmonary embolism?	An embolus that lodges in the pulmonary circulation, typically originating from a DVT
What imaging technique is used to diagnose a PE?	Spiral chest CTA with thin cuts

Topic VI

Abdomen

Stomach And Duodenum

12

The stomach is located mostly in the LUQ of the abdomen and can be anatomically divided into 5 segments: (1) **the cardia**—the most proximal segment just distal to the gastroesophageal (GE) junction; (2) **the fundus**—the most superior segment; it is partly cephalad to the GE junction and is mobile and distensible; (3) **the body** or *corpus*—the largest segment, bordered by the fundus superiorly and the pylorus inferiorly; (4) **the antrum**—the segment that occupies approximately the distal third of the stomach; and (5) **the pylorus**—an area that contains the pyloric sphincter; this sphincter regulates passage of food into the duodenum.

The duodenum, or the first portion of the small intestine, is C-shaped and frames the head of the pancreas. It consists of 4 segments: (1) **the superior segment** or *duodenal bulb*, (2) **the descending** or *second* segment, (3) **the horizontal** or *third* segment, and (4) **the ascending** or *fourth* segment.

The common bile duct (CBD) and the pancreatic duct open into the second portion of the duodenum.

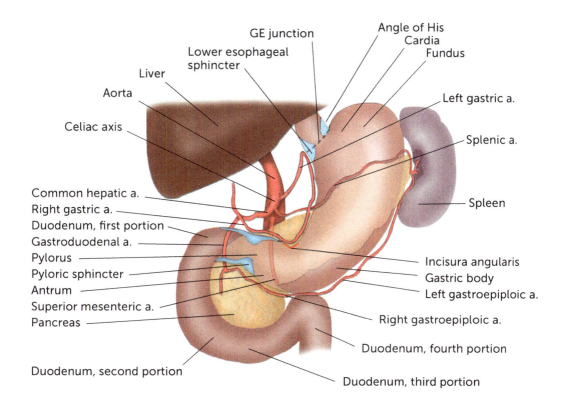

Fig. 12-1. Anatomy of the Stomach and Associated Arteries

Physiology of Digestion

Various types of gastric cells in the gastric epithelia produce secretions that aid in digestion (Table 12-1).

Table 12-1. Gastric Cells and Their Products

Cell Type	Location	Product	Action
Chief cells	Fundus and corpus	Pepsinogen	Cleave to pepsin when gastric pH <5; break down protein into amino acids
Parietal cells	Fundus and corpus	HCl and intrinsic factor (IF)	HCl creates an acidic environment so pepsinogen can be cleaved to pepsin. IF is a mucoprotein responsible for the absorption of vitamin B_{12}
Mucous neck cells	Fundus, corpus, and antrum/pylorus	Mucus and HCO_3^-	Create a pH of 7 at the mucosal surface of the stomach
Enterochromaffin-like cells (ECLs)	Corpus	Histamine	Trigger production of HCl

Gastric hormones, too, play a role in digestion. An abbreviated list of gastric hormones is provided in Table 12-2.

Table 12-2. Gastric Hormones and Their Functions

Hormone	Cell Type	Anatomic Source	Action
Gastrin	G cells	Primarily antrum; some from duodenum	Primarily responsible for gastric HCl secretion. HCl secretion is inhibited by a drop in antral pH to <2.5
Somatostatin	D cells	Antrum	Inhibits GI motility and release of all GI hormones and secretions
Cholecystokinin (CCK)	I cells	Primarily duodenum; also from jejunum and ileum	Regulates gastroduodenal and gallbladder motility. Inhibits gastric emptying
Secretin	S cells	Duodenum	Stimulates release of HCO_3^- and H_2O to create an alkaline environment. Inhibits gastric HCl secretion

PEPTIC ULCER DISEASE

Definition Peptic ulcer disease (PUD) refers to **erosion of the gastric or duodenal mucosa greater than 5 mm.**

Etiology Peptic ulcer disease is the result of the erosive action of gastric acid on compromised epithelium of the stomach or duodenum. Four main causes are responsible for PUD. The 2 most common causes are (1) infection with *Helicobacter pylori* (HP), a flagellated spiral-shaped gram-negative rod that is responsible for approximately 90% of duodenal ulcers and 75% of gastric ulcers; and (2) the use of **NSAIDs,** which are more commonly responsible for gastric ulcers than duodenal ulcers. Tobacco and alcohol use also contributes to the development of PUD. Acid hypersecretion, another cause of PUD, leads to the development of most duodenal ulcers. Other causes of peptic ulcer include steroid use, stasis (eg, chronic pyloric obstruction), and stress.

Epidemiology Approximately 2% of the US population present with ulcer disease every year. Men are affected more frequently than women. Duodenal ulcers are more common than gastric ulcers in young patients, and after age 40 the incidence of gastric and duodenal ulceration is about the same. The peak incidence of gastric ulcer is seen between 55 and 65 years of age. **Type I** gastric ulcers (60%–70%) are located in the distal portion of the lesser curvature, near the incisura angularis. **Type II** gastric ulcers (~15%) are located in the distal portion of the lesser curvature and in the duodenum. **Type III** gastric ulcers (~20%) are prepyloric, and type IV gastric ulcers are located in the proximal portion of the lesser curvature near the GE junction. **Type V** gastric ulcers are medication induced and can be found anywhere in the stomach (see Fig. 12-2 for ulcer types I–IV). Ninety-five percent of duodenal ulcers are found in the first portion of the duodenum; most measure less than 1 cm in diameter.

Symptoms Invariably, **midepigastric burning episodic pain** is the presenting symptom. In patients with **gastric ulcers,** the pain tends to be **exacerbated by meals,** whereas in patients with **duodenal ulcers,** meals and antacids **relieve the pain.** If the pain becomes constant, it is likely that an ulcer has penetrated more deeply, and if the pain radiates to the back, it is possible that a gastric ulcer has eroded through to the pancreas. With well-established disease, the pain may awaken the patient in the middle of the night.

Physical Exam and Signs No specific findings are noted.

Differential Cholelithiasis/cholecystitis: +Gallstones by u/s. **Pancreatitis:** ↑Amylase, ↑lipase. **Reflux esophagitis:** +Endoscopy, ±UGI series. **Gastritis:** +Endoscopy findings. **Gastric carcinoma:** +Biopsy.

Diagnosis UGI endoscopy is the test of choice for diagnosing PUD. A gastric ulcer must always be biopsied to rule out carcinoma.

Labs. *H pylori* detection is the mainstay of lab testing. It can be performed with or without a sample of gastric mucosa. If an endoscopy is performed, antral tissue obtained is histologically examined, and a **rapid urease assay** is performed to detect the presence of *H pylori* in the tissue. This assay has a sensitivity of 90% and a specificity of 98%.

Imaging. **Upper GI endoscopy** will show ulceration, usually in the lesser curvature of the stomach, when a gastric ulcer is present. The duodenal bulb is the most common location of duodenal ulcers.

Complication(s) Hemorrhaging, perforation, and obstruction are complications of PUD. Most cases of massive upper GI hemorrhage are due to duodenal ulcers, although most patients with duodenal ulcers present with only minor bleeding detected by melena or guaiac-positive stool. Perforation is an uncommon complication of PUD, occurring more commonly in patients with gastric ulcers and in 5% of patients with duodenal ulcers. Approximately 15% of patients with perforated ulcers die, usually because of a combination of delayed diagnosis, advanced age, and comorbidities. Obstruction results in the typical symptoms of nausea and vomiting. Weight loss and malnutrition are common in chronic stages of the disease.

Treatment

Uncomplicated PUD: *H pylori* infection is managed with triple therapy, which consists of a combination of **2 antibiotics** (such as metronidazole with clarithromycin or amoxicillin) and a **proton pump inhibitor** (PPI). PPIs inhibit acid secretion and are more effective than H_2-blockers, with a 96% healing rate after 8 weeks of treatment. H_2-blockers differ in effectiveness, with healing rates of 80% to 90% after 8 weeks of treatment. **Famotidine** is probably the most potent H_2-blocker. In patients who fail triple therapy, quadruple therapy can be provided by adding bismuth to the medication regimen. After treatment, the **urea breath test** is used to detect eradication of *H pylori*. NSAID-induced PUD is treated by discontinuing the offending agent and initiating the use of an H_2-blocker or a PPI. Lifestyle changes include decreasing consumption of coffee—which stimulates gastric acid secretion—and decreasing intake of alcohol—which damages the gastric mucosa.

Complicated PUD: Approximately 80% of bleeding from PUD stops spontaneously. Endoscopy that reveals the presence of a visible vessel in the ulcer base suggests that the possibility of rebleeding is 50%. Endoscopy remains the diagnostic test of choice because it can be used to diagnose and treat. Endoscopic therapy can employ thermotherapy (heater probe, electrocoagulation), injection therapy (epinephrine or ethanol), or clips. An obstruction can sometimes be treated by means of endoscopic dilatation. When medical therapy and endoscopic interventions are unsuccessful, or if a perforation occurs, surgery is indicated. The goal of surgical therapy is to correct the cause of the complication and, if possible, reduce gastric acid secretion. A variety of approaches have been used with different rates of success and recurrence. The most commonly performed operation for a duodenal ulcer for which medical and endoscopic interventions have failed is a **truncal vagotomy,** usually associated with a **pyloroplasty** because the pylorus closes in response to a vagotomy. Sometimes, a duodenal or gastric ulcer requires an **antrectomy**, in which case removing the antrum eliminates the gastrin-producing section of the stomach. In these cases, the remaining stomach is anastomosed to the duodenum (**Billroth I** operation) or to the jejunum (**Billroth II** operation). A **highly selective vagotomy,** also known as a *parietal cell vagotomy*, can be used to suppress the acid-producing section of the stomach while preserving pyloric innervation, resulting in no or little alteration of antral pyloric motor function.

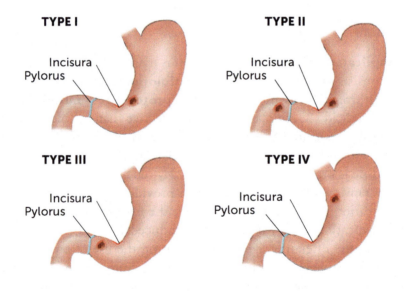

Fig. 12-2. Ulcer Types I–IV

Mallory-Weiss Syndrome

Definition Upper GI bleeding caused by a **gastroesophageal tear**.

Etiology Gastroesophageal tears most often result from severe retching, vomiting, or coughing. Typically, these tears are seen in alcoholic patients, but they may occur in any patient as a result of forceful contractions of the abdominal musculature in the presence of an unrelaxed cardia. Approximately 65% to 75% of patients with a Mallory-Weiss tear have an associated hiatal hernia.

Epidemiology Mallory-Weiss syndrome is responsible for 15% of episodes of upper GI bleeding. Approximately one-quarter of patients may have 2 tears.

Symptoms Bleeding, nausea, and vomiting are common.

Physical Exam and Signs No specific signs are known.

Differential All causes of upper GI bleeding (see Algorithm 3) may be considered.

Diagnosis The diagnostic test of choice for Mallory-Weiss syndrome is an upper GI endoscopy.

Labs. Findings related to the severity of the bleeding, such as ↓hemoglobin.

Imaging. An endoscopy will show a linear laceration extending between 1 and 3 cm, usually along the lesser curvature, involving the mucosa and frequently the submucosa. Most lesions are seen on the gastric side alone, and about 20% span both the stomach and the esophagus.

Complication(s) Severe bleeding, which is uncommon.

Treatment Bleeding stops spontaneously in 9 out of 10 patients. Initial therapy is an ice water lavage of the stomach. The next step is an endoscopic attempt to control the bleeding using electrocautery and/or vasopressor injection. If bleeding persists, surgical repair is the next step.

ZOLLINGER-ELLISON SYNDROME

Definition Zollinger-Ellison syndrome (ZES) is a clinical syndrome presenting with gastrin-mediated gastric acid hypersecretion, PUD, and non–β islet cell gastrin-producing tumors of the pancreas, known as *gastrinomas*, which are the hallmark of the disease.

Etiology Unknown.

Epidemiology Gastrinomas are most often found in the **gastrinoma triangle,** bound by the head of the pancreas, the porta hepatis, and the third portion of the duodenum. In 60% of cases, gastrinomas are found in the duodenum. Fifty percent of cases involve multiple gastrinomas; 60% to 65% of gastrinomas are malignant, and in about 30% of cases, patients present with ZES associated with multiple endocrine neoplasia syndrome type I (MEN I). When this is the case, patients usually have multiple benign gastrinomas. In general, gastrinomas may be as small as 2 to 3 mm and may be difficult to find.

Symptoms Gastric acid hypersecretion, which is caused by gastrinomas, results in the development of severe PUD. The most common symptom is abdominal pain (80% of cases). Fifty percent of patients have diarrhea, and the increased acid load to the duodenum may inhibit lipase and produce secondary steatorrhea. Symptoms are often unresponsive to large doses of antacids or standard doses of H_2-blocking agents.

Physical Exam and Signs No specific findings are noted.

Differential Atrophic gastritis: Chronic gastric mucosa inflammation, ±*H pylori*–associated, ±autoimmune-associated gastritis, ±megaloblastic anemia, ±iron deficiency anemia, definitive diagnosis by histology, secretin test negative. **Pernicious anemia:** ±Beefy tongue, neurologic symptoms in severe cases (eg, paresthesias, unsteady gait), macrocytic anemia, thrombocytopenia, ↑LDH, ↑bilirubin, +Schilling's test (cobalamin deficiency). **Gastric outlet obstruction:** See PUD. **MEN I syndrome:** Hyperparathyroidism (hyperplasia of 4 glands), parathyroid tumors, pituitary tumors (prolactinomas), pancreatic tumors (gastrinomas).

Diagnosis Hypergastrinemia and gastric acid hypersecretion are almost always diagnostic. H_2-blockers, antacids, and PPIs should be avoided for several days before gastrin levels are measured, because these agents tend to increase gastrin levels.

Labs. Fasting gastrin levels ≥200 pg/mL (normal fasting gastrin levels <200 pg/mL). Marked acid hypersecretion is defined as more than 15 mEq H^+ per hour in patients with an intact stomach. Borderline gastrin values and borderline values derived from acid secretion tests may require a secretin provocative test, which is most sensitive and specific. The test is performed by measuring fasting gastrin levels before IV secretin is administered at 2 U/kg. If serum gastrin levels rise to more than 200 pg/mL above basal levels within 15 minutes, the test is diagnostic for ZES because it identifies gastrinoma as the cause of hypergastrinemia as opposed to other potential causes, such as gastric outlet obstruction, atrophic gastritis, or retained antrum after gastric surgery. Serum calcium levels must always be measured because hyperparathyroidism associated with MEN I can cause hypergastrinemia.

Imaging. CT is the initial test of choice for diagnosing gastrinoma, but it may fail to localize as many as 50% of tumors. MRI may be of use, but it has a higher failure rate than CT. Endoscopic ultrasound is reported to have a sensitivity of 80% and a specificity of 95%. Octreotide (a somatostatin analog) scan is fairly sensitive for localization of primary and metastatic sites. If imaging methods are unsuccessful, the most effective invasive test is selective angiography, but it may fail to diagnose small tumors.

Complication(s) Similar to PUD.

Treatment Initial treatment consists of **medical management** with an H_2-blocker or a PPI, such as **omeprazole.** Ideally, tumors that can be localized should be resected. If gastrinomas are malignant, resection of metastases, when possible, may lead to remission. For advanced malignant cases, chemotherapy with **streptozocin** is most effective. Total gastrectomy is rarely indicated in patients when the tumors cannot be found.

GASTRIC CANCER

Definition **Adenocarcinoma**, the most common type of gastric cancer, is a malignant tumor of the stomach.

Etiology Several risk factors have been associated with gastric adenocarcinoma, including a diet high in complex carbohydrates, salted meats, fish, and nitrates. *H pylori* infection, chronic gastric inflammation—such as that found in patients with pernicious anemia and atrophic gastritis—blood type A, gastric polyps, alcohol consumption, and tobacco use appear to play a role in the development of gastric cancer as well.

Epidemiology The incidence of gastric cancer peaks in the seventh decade of life, and its incidence has been decreasing over the past 75 years. However, the incidence of cancer in the gastric cardia has been increasing steadily, despite the overall decrease in the number of gastric cancer cases. Gastric cancer is more common in men than in women, at a ratio of 2:1, and the incidence is higher in African American men than in white men. Morphologically, gastric cancer may present as an ulcer (25%), as a polypoid tumor (25%), as a superficial spreading type of tumor, which is confined to mucosa and submucosa (15%), or as linitis plastica, in which all layers of the stomach are involved (10%). The advanced type (35%) consists of a large tumor, a portion of which is outside the stomach. The survival rate of gastric cancer remains low, and detection at an early stage is uncommon.

Symptoms Early in the course of the disease, patients may experience vague epigastric discomfort and indigestion. Later, patients may experience fatigue, lack of appetite, early satiety, and constant pain with vomiting. The pain is not relieved by food intake, and approximately 15% of patients develop hematemesis.

Physical Exam and Signs Typically, signs appear late in the progression of the disease and are usually associated with advanced local or metastatic disease. Patients may exhibit a palpable abdominal mass, palpable nodes in the supraclavicular region known as *Virchow's nodes*, or periumbilical nodes known as *Sister Mary Joseph's nodes*. Jaundice, ascites, and malnutrition may be noted.

Differential Peptic ulcers and other gastric malignancies may be considered.

Diagnosis **Upper endoscopy** is the test of choice for the diagnosis of gastric cancer. **Multiple biopsies** should be obtained.

Labs. Forty percent of patients are anemic.

Imaging. Upper endoscopy reveals an ulceration or a mass. CT of the abdomen and pelvis may show metastases. Endoscopic ultrasound is useful for staging the disease.

Complication(s) Bleeding, obstruction, and perforation, which are usually seen in advanced disease, are possible complications.

Treatment Cure is possible only with **resection**. Fifty percent of operable lesions are resectable, and about half of these have no signs of spread beyond the resected area. At least a 6-cm margin must be achieved when surgery is done with curative intention. Proximal lesions require a total gastrectomy.

BIBLIOGRAPHY

González CA, López-Carrillo L. *Helicobacter pylori*, nutrition and smoking interactions: their impact in gastric carcinogenesis. *Scand J Gastroenterol.* 2010;45(1):6-14.

Smolka AJ, Backert S. How *Helicobacter pylori* infection controls gastric acid secretion. *J Gastroenterol.* 2012;47(6):609-618.

CLINICAL KEYS: QUESTIONS AND ANSWERS

Which arteries supply the greater curvature of the stomach?	The right and left gastroepiploic arteries
Which cells secrete intrinsic factor?	Parietal cells
What tests can be used to detect *H pylori*?	Rapid urease assay and the urea breath test
Which types of peptic ulcers are more commonly caused by *H pylori*?	Duodenal ulcers
How is *H pylori* treated?	Triple therapy, consisting of 2 antibiotics (such as metronidazole with clarithromycin or amoxicillin) and a PPI
Where are type I gastric ulcers located?	In the distal portion of the lesser curvature

Food intake exacerbates the pain from which type of peptic ulcer?	Gastric ulcer
What is the diagnostic test of choice for peptic ulcer disease?	Upper GI endoscopy
Which part of the small intestine is anastomosed to the stomach in a Billroth I operation?	Duodenum
What are the symptoms of Zollinger-Ellison syndrome?	Abdominal pain, diarrhea, and steatorrhea
Where are gastrinomas commonly found?	In the gastrinoma triangle
What is the normal value for fasting gastrin serum levels?	Less than 200 pg/mL
Which test is most sensitive and specific for diagnosing Zollinger-Ellison syndrome?	Secretin provocative test
What is the most common type of gastric cancer?	Adenocarcinoma
What is Mallory-Weiss syndrome?	Upper GI bleeding caused by a gastroesophageal tear

Small Intestine

The small intestine begins at the pylorus and ends at the cecum and consists of the duodenum, the jejunum, and the ileum (Fig. 13-1). The total length varies but ranges from 18 to 21 feet.

The jejunum begins at the ligament of Treitz, a musculotendinous structure that originates from the diaphragm and the connective tissue surrounding the celiac artery before attaching to the duodenojejunal junction. The lumen narrows in the distal segments of the intestine.

The small bowel attaches to the posterior abdominal wall by a double layer of peritoneum, called the *mesentery*, which contains fat, vessels, lymph nodes, and nerves. The mucosa of the small intestine is distinguished by plicae circulares (transverse folds also called *valvulae conniventes*), which are more pronounced in the duodenum and jejunum. The blood supply to the jejunum and ileum is derived from the superior mesenteric artery (SMA).

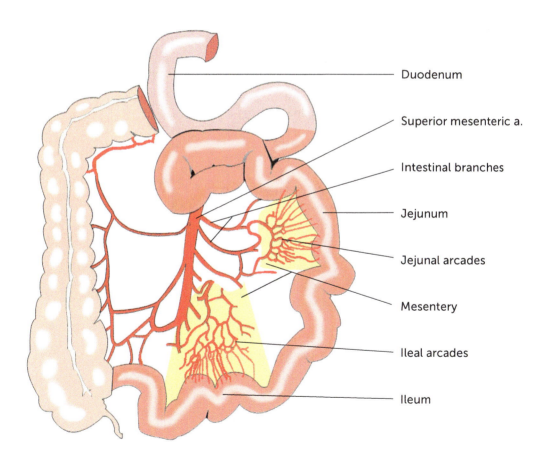

Fig. 13-1. Anatomy of the Small Intestine

The layers of the small bowel (Fig. 13-2) are similar to the layers in other segments of the GI tract. The mucosa of the small bowel is covered with villi and microvilli, the latter of which significantly increase the absorptive capacity of the bowel.

The main function of the small intestine is absorption of dietary nutrients and water; regulation of motility, secretion, and absorption is complex and is delicately balanced by neuroendocrine factors.

Carbohydrates are hydrolyzed by salivary and pancreatic amylases and other enzymes into monosaccharides, and from the small intestine, these compounds are delivered into the portal circulation through active transport. Protein is broken down into amino acids; most ingested fat is absorbed in the duodenum and the jejunum, with the help of bile acids.

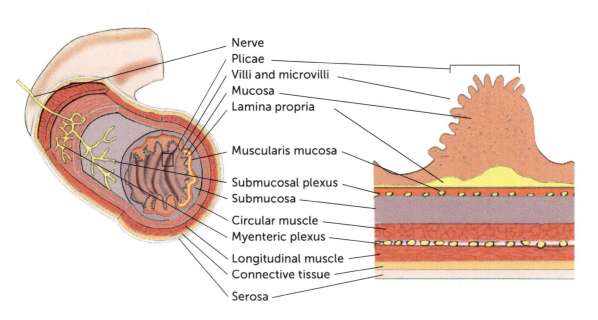

Fig. 13-2. Layers of the Small Intestine

Small Bowel Obstruction

Definition A small bowel obstruction (SBO) is a **partial or complete blockage** of the small intestine that interrupts passage of its contents. SBO can be extrinsic or intrinsic to the bowel wall, and it may be high (proximal) or low (distal). In general, SBO refers to a mechanical obstruction, in contrast to an **adynamic ileus,** which usually occurs as a secondary functional response to a variety of disease processes and/or drugs.

Etiology The most common cause of SBO is the presence of **adhesions (60%),** which usually are the result of **previous operations,** although they can form in response to an inflammatory process. The second most common cause of SBO is **neoplasm** (20%)—intrinsic or extrinsic to the bowel wall—and the third most common cause of SBO is a **hernia** (10%). These problems are followed in frequency by disorders of the bowel wall, such as Crohn's disease, and by miscellaneous events, such as intussusception, the presence of foreign bodies, and other causes.

Epidemiology The incidence of SBO varies depending on the etiology, but it is estimated that the most common type—that caused by adhesions—can lead to postoperative obstruction in 2% to 17% of cases. These statistics apply to patients who present early (within 30 days) and late (within 2 years) in their postoperative course.

Symptoms Depending on whether the obstruction is proximal or distal, symptoms vary. Proximal obstruction usually presents with repeated, unrelieved vomiting and "abdominal discomfort" as opposed to cramping pain. Obstruction that is located distally causes less vomiting and presents initially with periumbilical or diffuse cramping abdominal pain. Vomiting occurs after the onset of pain, and it may become feculent if the obstruction is distal. Initially, the patient might still be able to expel gas and feces per rectum, but obstipation occurs when the obstruction becomes complete.

Physical Exam and Signs SBO may be simple, in which the bowel is simply blocked, or it may be strangulated, in which the blood supply to the small intestine is compromised. The presentation varies accordingly. In simple obstruction, vital signs may be normal initially, or the patient may present with some degree of tachycardia proportionate to the dehydration level. Abdominal distention is not significant with proximal obstruction, but it becomes obvious with distal obstruction. Early in the course of SBO, auscultation of the abdomen reveals peristaltic rushes during episodes of pain, as well as gurgles and high-pitched tinkles. As SBO progresses, these **hyperactive bowel sounds** are replaced by a relative auscultatory silence—with few or no bowel sounds—suggesting that the small bowel has lost its tone. The exam must include an evaluation for the presence of hernias and surgical scars. Strangulation is not suspected in 30% of cases, but fever and constant pain should put strangulation high on the differential. As ischemia progresses, signs of peritoneal irritation, such as guarding and rebound tenderness, make strangulation likely. Strangulation is commonly seen in cases of closed loop obstruction, in which an intestinal segment is occluded in two places, as is the case in a volvulus. Rectal exam does not usually reveal any specific findings.

Differential **Paralytic ileus:** Pain is not severe, +distention, symptoms of a primary problem (eg, appendicitis), plain abdominal films +gas commonly in both small and large intestine. **Large bowel obstruction:** +Gas in colon up to obstructing point, abdominal distention, ±vomiting, +small bowel dilatation if ileocecal valve is incompetent (see Chapter 14).

Diagnosis The diagnosis is based on clinical and radiologic findings. A **plain radiograph** of the abdomen is the test of choice in diagnosing SBO, and it should be performed first (Fig. 13-3). The value of a small bowel barium study compared with that of a CT scan is debatable; a barium study is the first choice for testing in a patient with an incomplete obstruction but should not be performed if the obstruction is believed to be complete, or if peritoneal signs are noted. CT provides reliable information regarding both the level and the cause of the obstruction, but it is more sensitive in patients with complete rather than partial SBO.

Labs. Early on, findings may be normal. As the syndrome progresses, ±↑Hct (due to hemoconcentration), ↑BUN, ↑creatinine, ±leukocytosis and/or ±electrolyte abnormalities, ±↑serum amylase. With strangulation, leukocytosis becomes severe and lactic acidosis is present; this does not correct with fluid resuscitation.

Imaging. Supine radiographs of the abdomen show dilated loops of small bowel. Gas seldom reaches the colon when obstruction is complete. Upright radiographs demonstrate a ladder-like pattern of air-fluid levels, commonly centrally located, with swelling and enlargement of the valvulae conniventes. This appearance has been described as a **"stack of coins."** The air-fluid levels simply represent the nonfunctional fluid that has accumulated inside the bowel and is not advancing distally because of the obstruction. These air-fluid levels might not be visible on a supine radiograph. Barium may show a delay in transit and a "snakehead" appearance caused by bulbous dilatation of the bowel immediately proximal to the obstructing point. This occurs secondary to peristaltic efforts to overcome the obstruction.

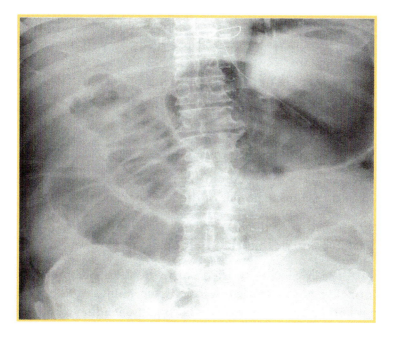

Fig. 13-3. Small Bowel Obstruction on X-ray

Complication(s) Vascular compromise evolves as the obstruction remains untreated and can lead to ischemia, perforation, and death.

Treatment SBO alters the absorptive function of the intestine. The bowel proximal to the obstruction distends with gas (mainly from swallowed air) and fluid, which may accumulate in large amounts within the lumen. This third-space fluid loss can be large enough to result in hypovolemia, leading eventually to multiorgan failure if unrecognized and left untreated. Therefore, treatment begins with **fluid resuscitation.** Fluid losses are generally isotonic, so lactated Ringer's is typically administered. **Nasogastric suction** must be part of the initial therapy because it reduces vomiting, prevents aspiration, and decreases the amount of swallowed air. Electrolytes should be corrected on the basis of results of blood chemistry and blood gas testing. Operation for obstruction should be performed promptly, but judicious observation must be exercised in some situations, as in patients with incomplete obstruction or in those who have had numerous previous operations for obstruction. Postoperative patients and those with inflammatory bowel disease, prior radiation treatment, or carcinomatosis may need to be treated conservatively. Mortality due to obstruction is highest in cases of associated ischemia; in these cases, mortality increases the longer the surgery is postponed. Mortality for a strangulated obstruction can be as high as 25% if surgery is performed more than 36 hours after initial presentation. Even with an incomplete obstruction, surgery might be needed at some point.

MECKEL'S DIVERTICULUM

Definition Meckel's diverticulum refers to a **congenital diverticulum** of the antimesenteric border of the terminal ileum.

Etiology Meckel's diverticulum is the result of incomplete closure of the omphalomesenteric duct, or **vitelline duct**.

Epidemiology Meckel's diverticulum is the most common congenital abnormality of the small intestine. Commonly, Meckel's diverticulum is known as the **"disease of 2s"** because it adheres approximately to the following statistics: it is present in 2% of the population, it is 2 inches long, it is 2 cm wide, it is 2 feet from the ileocecal valve, 2% of patients are symptomatic, it most commonly presents at age 2, and 2 types of ectopic tissue—gastric and pancreatic—may be present in Meckel's diverticulum. Although it has been reported that men are 2 times more likely to be affected than women, the prevalence is approximately the same in men and in women. Ectopic gastric mucosa is present in 50% of cases of Meckel's diverticula, and 5% of cases reveal ectopic pancreatic tissue.

Symptoms Patients may be asymptomatic. Symptoms are described only in patients presenting with a complication; the most common is

GI bleeding, which is seen in 25% to 50% of symptomatic patients. Patients may report bright red blood per rectum, indicating a brisk bleed, or melanotic stools, indicating a slow bleed. Bleeding is usually due to ulceration of the ectopic gastric mucosa. Another common complication is small bowel obstruction, which is associated with the same symptoms described in the previous section.

Physical Exam and Signs Exam findings and signs depend on the type of presenting complication. A patient bleeding from Meckel's diverticulum may present simply with anemia secondary to chronic bleeding or, in more serious cases, with an acute massive hemorrhage.

Differential The differential varies according to the presentation. GI bleeding (see Algorithm 3) or obstructive symptoms change the differential.

Diagnosis In children, the test of choice is nuclear scanning with ^{99m}Tc-pertechnetate. In adult patients, the nuclear scan is not as sensitive; therefore, if the nuclear scan is normal, barium studies are the next best step.

Labs. Findings that reflect the complication, such as ↓Hgb/Hct (in the case of GI bleeding), electrolyte abnormalities (in the case of obstruction).

Imaging. Nuclear scan reveals an area of uptake in the gastric mucosa and the ectopic gastric mucosa in the diverticulum. Barium may demonstrate a single diverticulum arising from the antimesenteric border of the intestine.

Complication(s) GI bleeding and obstruction are the most common complications. Meckel's diverticulitis occurs in 15% to 20% of symptomatic patients, and presentation is clinically indistinguishable from that of appendicitis—diagnosis is made at the time of surgery.

Treatment In cases of acute presentation, surgical resection must be performed in a timely manner. Debate regarding the best approach when Meckel's diverticulum is an incidental finding is ongoing, although current studies support resection as an acceptable option.

SMALL BOWEL TUMORS

Definition Small bowel tumors are benign or malignant tumors of the small intestine.

Etiology Unknown. Risk factors such as Crohn's disease or familial adenomatosis polyposis influence the incidence of malignant tumors. Carcinoid tumors arise from enterochromaffin or **Kulchitsky cells**, also known as **argentaffin cells,** because they are stained by silver compounds. Carcinoid tumors produce biologically active substances, such as serotonin, histamine, dopamine, substance P, and others.

Epidemiology Small intestinal neoplasms are extremely rare, representing only 5% of all gastrointestinal tumors. The most common **benign tumors** are adenomas, gastrointestinal stromal tumors (GISTs) (previously designated **leiomyomas**), and lipomas. The most common **malignant tumor** of the small bowel is adenocarcinoma, which represents 50% of malignant small bowel tumors, followed by carcinoid, malignant GISTs, and lymphoma. Adenocarcinoma is more common in the duodenum and jejunum. Lymphoma is more common in the jejunum. Primary carcinoid, called **apudoma**, has been reported in the small bowel, the stomach, the colon, the appendix, the lungs, the ovaries, the biliary tract, and the pancreas. However, the most common site of carcinoid tumor is the appendix, followed by the terminal ileum. Approximately 40% of carcinoid cases are multiple. Carcinoid tumors smaller than 1 cm in diameter present with metastases in 2% of cases, but if larger than 2 cm in diameter, metastases are present in 80% of cases.

Symptoms Benign tumors are generally asymptomatic and are found incidentally during autopsy or surgery for other reasons. When benign tumors produce symptoms, pain, usually due to obstruction, is the most common complaint. Obstruction, in turn, is most commonly due to intussusception, and a benign tumor is the most common cause of this complication in adults. The second most common symptom is bleeding, usually occult. Malignant tumors usually are symptomatic; the most common symptoms are pain and weight loss. Approximately 10% of those with carcinoid tumor will present with carcinoid syndrome, which consists of cutaneous flushing (caused by kallikrein secretion), diarrhea (caused by serotonin secretion), and bronchoconstriction (uncommon), along with right-sided cardiac valvular disease in 50% of syndrome cases. In general, it can be assumed that a patient who presents with carcinoid syndrome has metastatic disease because hepatic metastases and ovarian or lung carcinoids release vasoactive substances directly into the circulation.

Physical Exam and Signs Findings on physical exam are uncommon. Occasionally, a mass might be palpable in patients with lymphoma or adenocarcinoma.

Differential Depending on the presentation, benign and malignant tumors most commonly require a differential between all neoplasms that can affect the small bowel.

Diagnosis Definitive diagnosis of most small bowel tumors is not made until a biopsy or a surgical resection is performed. The diagnosis of carcinoid tumor may be suspected preoperatively when elevated urinary levels of 5-hydroxyindoleacetic acid (5-HIAA) over 24 hours or elevated levels of serum chromogranin A are detected.

Labs. Patients with carcinoid syndrome excrete >25 mg of 5-HIAA daily, ±↓Hgb/Hct.

Imaging. CT scan may help in the diagnosis of small bowel tumor. In cases of suspected carcinoid tumor, an octreotide scan with ^{111}indium-labeled pentetreotide may be useful in locating the tumor. A small bowel endoscopy can sometimes be of assistance, as can small bowel capsule endoscopy.

Complication(s) Symptomatic manifestations of small bowel tumor are the result of a complication—obstruction, bleeding, or carcinoid syndrome.

Treatment Tumors, benign or malignant, should be removed surgically whenever possible. Carcinoid tumors should be resected, and any metastatic disease should be resected if feasible, because in general carcinoids progress slowly. Carcinoids of the appendix that are 1 cm in diameter or smaller require only an appendectomy; if 2 cm or larger, a right colectomy is appropriate. Octreotide is now used to treat carcinoid because it suppresses tumor growth and controls the symptoms of carcinoid syndrome.

BIBLIOGRAPHY

Lappas JC, Reyes BL, Maglinte DD. Abdominal radiography findings in small-bowel obstruction: relevance to triage for additional diagnostic imaging. *AJR Am J Roentgenol.* 2001;176(1):167-174.

Clinical Keys: Questions and Answers

Question	Answer
What is a closed loop intestinal obstruction?	A presentation in which the bowel is obstructed in 2 places, with neither inflow nor egress of material
What is a significant complication of a closed loop obstruction?	Ischemia
What is the most common cause of small bowel obstruction?	Adhesions
What does a "stack of coins" appearance represent on X-ray?	Air-fluid levels commonly seen in small bowel obstruction
What are common symptoms of small bowel obstruction?	Nausea, vomiting, and abdominal pain
What is the treatment for small bowel obstruction?	Fluid resuscitation, nasogastric tube, surgery
What laboratory test is highly specific for carcinoid?	24-Hour urinary 5-HIAA
Which disease is known as the "disease of 2s"?	Meckel's diverticulum
What is a Meckel's diverticulum?	A congenital diverticulum of the terminal ileum
How is a bleeding Meckel's diverticulum diagnosed?	Nuclear scanning
How many types of ectopic mucosa can be present in Meckel's diverticulum?	2
What is the most common malignant tumor of the small intestine?	Adenocarcinoma

Colon, Rectum, and Anus   14

The colon, or large intestine, is a muscular tube that measures 4.5 to 6 feet.

The appendix is assumed to lie under McBurney's point, located two-thirds of the distance between the umbilicus and the right anterior superior iliac spine.

The sigmoid is the narrowest segment of the colon.

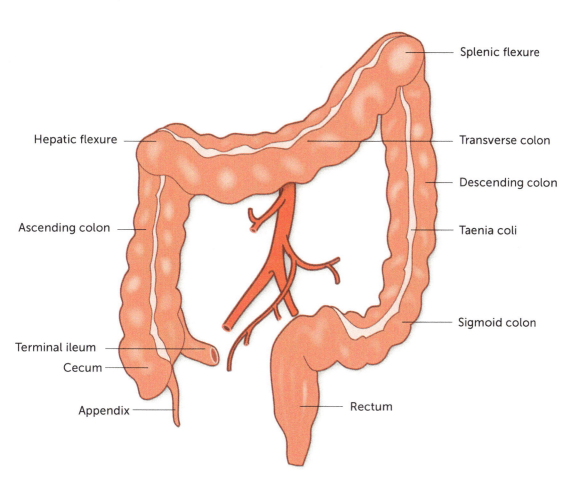

Fig. 14-1. Anatomy of the Colon

The superior mesenteric artery (SMA) and its branches supply the cecum, the ascending colon, and the proximal two-thirds of the transverse colon

The inferior mesenteric artery (IMA) and its branches supply from the distal one-third of the transverse colon to the proximal rectum.

The rectum and the anus receive arterial blood supply mostly from the superior, middle, and inferior rectal arteries.

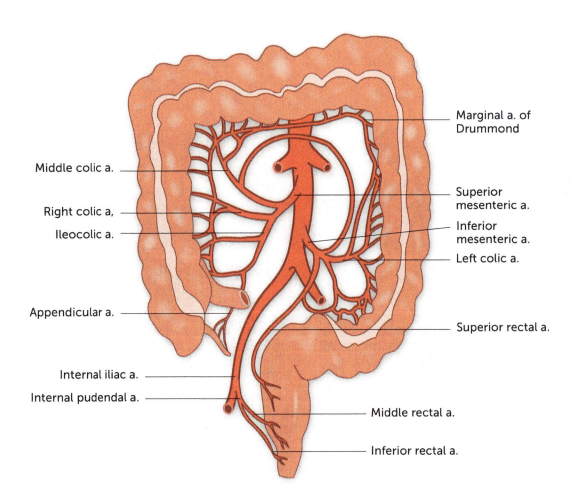

Fig. 14-2. Arterial Blood Supply to the Colon

APPENDICITIS

Definition Appendicitis is an inflammatory process of the appendix.

Etiology It is most commonly due to an obstruction of the appendiceal lumen caused by **hyperplasia of lymphoid tissue (60%)** or a **fecalith (35%).** Obstruction leads to fluid stasis, which promotes bacterial growth and inflammation. Increased pressure within the appendicular lumen compromises blood supply, resulting in ischemia and thrombosis of small vessels. If untreated, necrosis and perforation may ensue, ultimately leading to peritonitis.

Epidemiology Appendicitis is most common in young adults and is slightly more common among young men.

Symptoms The typical presentation includes abdominal pain, anorexia, and sometimes nausea and vomiting. In approximately 50% to 60% of patients, pain starts in the periumbilical region and localizes later to the RLQ. Occasionally, patients report dysuria. Atypical manifestations of appendicitis are more common in children and older patients. Symptoms of atypical presentation may include generalized malaise, diarrhea or constipation, indigestion, and vague, nonlocalized abdominal pain.

Physical Exam and Signs Auscultation of the abdomen may reveal normal to hypoactive bowel sounds. Palpation of McBurney's point typically elicits pain. Coughing may elicit a similar finding. Depending on the degree of the inflammatory process, palpation may be associated with guarding and rebound tenderness (**Blumberg's sign**). *Rebound tenderness* is defined as pain elicited in the abdomen after the examiner's hand is released from deep palpation. This pain does not occur *during* deep palpation. Guarding may be involuntary, in which case the abdomen is firm and the muscles guard involuntarily, or it may be voluntary, in which case the abdominal muscles contract upon palpation of the abdomen. If deep palpation of the LLQ causes referred pain in the RLQ, the patient is said to have a positive **Rovsing's sign.** With the patient lying on the left side, pain with extension of the right leg that is relieved when the leg is flexed is considered a positive **psoas sign.** When the patient is supine, pain in the RLQ with the right thigh flexed and internally rotated is a positive **obturator sign.** Digital rectal exam may elicit pain on the right side, sometimes even when the abdominal exam is inconclusive.

Differential The differential diagnosis varies depending on whether the clinician is approaching an adult, a child, or an elderly patient. **Crohn's disease:** Abdominal pain, weight loss, ±fever, ±gross blood in stool, frequent bowel movements, ±perianal discomfort. **Nephrolithiasis:** Intermittent colicky pain that may radiate from flank to groin, ±hematuria, no bowel alteration, ±n/v. **Meckel's diverticulitis:** Presentation similar to that of appendicitis; diagnosed at time of surgery. **Ectopic pregnancy:** Amenorrhea, ±irregular vaginal bleeding, abdominal pain, occasionally shoulder (referred) pain, elevated human chorionic gonadotropin (hCG) levels.

Diagnosis **CT scan with IV and oral contrast is the test of choice for diagnosis and clear assessment of the inflammatory process.** It has a sensitivity of 98% to 100%.

> *Labs.* Leukocytosis presents in 80% of cases, but it has a low positive predictive value and a better negative predictive value.
>
> *Imaging.* **CT shows an enlarged appendix with wall thickening, fat stranding, and a fecalith in 25% of cases.**

Complication(s) **The most severe complication is perforation with generalized peritonitis.** Pylephlebitis is a suppurative thrombophlebitis of the portal system that is caused by septic emboli resulting from the appendicitis process.

Treatment Appendicitis and its complications is treated surgically. Broad-spectrum antibiotics should be used preoperatively, intraoperatively, and postoperatively. A laparoscopic approach offers the advantages of less discomfort, shorter hospitalization, and earlier return to work. An effort is currently under way to treat some subcategories of patients with appendicitis using antibiotics only. This approach has met with some success.

DIVERTICULAR DISEASE

Definition **Diverticular disease (DD), known as *diverticulosis*, is an *acquired* condition in which the colonic mucosa herniates through areas of weakness in the muscular coat of the colon.** These weak spots are located where the blood vessels (at this level known as vasa recta) pierce the wall to access the submucosal layer. **Not all layers of the colon are present in the wall of each diverticulum.** Instead, only mucosa and submucosa protrude outward as the diverticula are formed. **Thus, colonic diverticula are pseudodiverticula, or false diverticula.** Conversely, congenital diverticula are true diverticula because the protrusion includes all layers of the colon. An example of a true diverticulum is Meckel's diverticulum, which is seen occasionally in the small intestine. **Diverticula are seldom if ever seen in the rectum. They are most prevalent in the sigmoid, although they can be present throughout the colon.**

Etiology The most accepted theory of diverticula formation points to **a deficiency in dietary fiber, which in turn results in low volume stool.** This leads to an alteration in colonic motility, so the colon must compensate by exerting higher pressures to maintain propulsive efficiency. This becomes particularly true in the sigmoid, where local segmenting movements raise the intraluminal pressure above that exerted in other sections of the colon. Increased pressure in the sigmoid leads to hypertrophy of the underlying muscular coats and to an increased prevalence of diverticula.

Epidemiology DD is present worldwide but is highly widespread in industrialized societies such as the United States and Europe. It is interesting to note that although the disease is most commonly seen in the left colon in inhabitants of Western countries, Asian populations frequently exhibit the disease in the right colon. DD is rare among individuals younger than 40 years of age, but its prevalence increases with age, and 65% of Americans will have it by the age of 80.

Symptoms **Uncomplicated DD is asymptomatic in 80% of people,** so it is most commonly an incidental finding, either on barium enema or on colonoscopy. Sometimes episodic abdominal pain, constipation, diarrhea, and bloating are attributed to DD.

Physical Exam and Signs Uncomplicated DD is not associated with physical findings.

Differential The differential diagnosis of uncomplicated DD may include irritable bowel syndrome, which is a diagnosis of exclusion.

Diagnosis **Colonoscopy is the gold standard for diagnosis of DD, although usually asymptomatic DD is an incidental finding.**

There is no reason for any particular type of work-up in cases of asymptomatic, uncomplicated DD.

Labs. No particular abnormality is expected.

Imaging. **Colonoscopy will reveal the typical openings of the diverticula (Fig. 14-3),** which usually are most numerous in the sigmoid colon. Almost invariably, the mucosa will be normal. Barium enema will easily demonstrate diverticula.

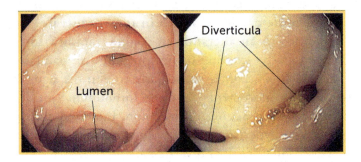

Fig. 14-3. Diverticula Visualized During Colonoscopy

Complication(s) The most common complications of DD are diverticulitis and bleeding (Fig. 14-4). It is estimated that 15% to 25% of patients with DD will develop diverticulitis, and 3% to 5% will develop brisk, significant bleeding.

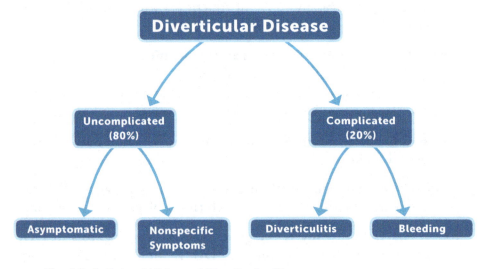

Fig. 14-4. Natural History of Diverticular Disease

1. DIVERTICULITIS is a pericolic inflammatory process resulting from a micro-perforation or macro-perforation of a diverticulum. Usually only one diverticulum perforates, regardless of whether the patient has just a few or many, so the number of diverticula does not predict the rate of perforation. The perforated diverticulum can lead to the formation of a phlegmon, an abscess, or a fistula. A fistula is seen in less than 5% of patients with diverticulitis; more than two-thirds of fistulas are colovesical and are seen in males, because in females, the uterus is positioned between the bladder and the colon. Obstruction can result from an acute attack of diverticulitis, caused by edema and compression of the colon by the inflammatory process surrounding it, or it may be the outcome of chronic recurrent episodes. The severity of the inflammatory process is commonly classified according to the Hinchey categories, on the basis of CT scan findings (Table 14-1).

Table 14-1. Hinchey Stages of Diverticulitis (CT Findings)

Stage I	Pericolic phlegmon or abscess
Stage II	Pelvic, intra-abdominal or retroperitoneal abscess (distant abscess)
Stage III	Generalized, purulent peritonitis (rupture of pericolic or distant abscess)
Stage IV	Generalized, fecal peritonitis (communicating with colonic lumen)

Symptoms. The most common symptom of diverticulitis is acute abdominal pain, which is most prevalent in the LLQ. The pain may be felt in the lower abdomen only, or it may be noted as a generalized abdominal sensation. Nausea and vomiting may occur. Other common symptoms include constipation and diarrhea.

Physical Exam and Signs. Patients with diverticulitis commonly present with fever. The patient may be tachycardic and tachypneic. Auscultation may elicit hypoactive or absent bowel sounds. Asking the patient to cough might elicit pain in the area most affected, usually the LLQ. Palpation may detect a spectrum of findings, from mild discomfort to significant pain in association with guarding and rebound tenderness—signs of peritoneal irritation. Occasionally, a mass is palpable in the LLQ, indicating an inflammatory process that may represent a phlegmon or an abscess.

Differential. Nephrolithiasis: Intermittent colicky pain that may radiate from the flank to the groin, ±hematuria, no bowel alteration, ±n/v. **Colorectal cancer:** Elderly patient, weight loss, ±rectal bleeding, occasionally a palpable mass. **Salpingitis/ pelvic inflammatory disease (PID):** ±Diffuse lower abdominal pain, ±vaginal discharge, ±cervical motion tenderness. **Ectopic pregnancy:** Amenorrhea, ±irregular vaginal bleeding, abdominal pain, occasionally shoulder (referred) pain, elevated hCG levels. **Mesenteric ischemia:** Abdominal pain out of proportion to physical exam findings, ±gross blood in stool, ±heart murmur, ±abdominal bruit(s), ±lactic acidosis, ±ischemic risk factors, such as ↑ cholesterol and ↑ triglycerides.

Diagnosis. CT with IV and water-soluble oral contrast is the test of choice for diagnosing diverticulitis. Free air is seen on CT or with a flat plate of the abdomen in 10% to 15% of diverticulitis cases. This immediately contraindicates the use of barium because it can extravasate, causing further complications. A colonoscopy should be done 6 to 8 weeks after the episode subsides, to assess the colon and to rule out other diagnoses. **Because diverticulitis is a *pericolic* process, the colonic mucosa is usually normal.** A colonoscopy is contraindicated during an acute episode unless there is a specific reason to do so, because this procedure could unseal the perforation that caused the diverticulitis.

Labs. Commonly leukocytosis, ±guaiac, ±hematuria, ±pyuria, ±bacteriuria.

Imaging. Abdominal radiographs may help to rule out or rule in other diagnoses, such as ileus or obstruction. **CT shows** pericolic fat inflammation, fat stranding, diverticula, and bowel wall thickening in 70% to 100% of cases.

2. DIVERTICULAR BLEEDING is the most common cause of lower GI bleeding, accounting for 30% to 40% of cases. Severe bleeding has been reported in 3% to 5% of patients with DD. Bleeding occurs because the vasa recta rupture as they course over the dome of the diverticulum, although the cause of this is unclear. Bleeding from DD ceases spontaneously in 80% of cases, and recurrent bleeding occurs in approximately 30% of patients. For other causes of lower GI bleeding, see Algorithm 3.

Symptoms. **The typical presentation in the adult patient is a sudden and *painless* rectal bleed of maroon or dark red blood called *hematochezia*.** The patient may have diarrhea or constipation and/or may pass maroon or red clots, suggesting that the volume of blood loss is significant. Blood noted on top of or around the stool is suspicious for a lower GI bleed of a more distal origin. Blood mixed with the stool suggests a more proximal source.

Physical Exam and Signs. Diverticular bleeding is frequently unassociated with significant systemic signs. Blood in the intestine may be associated with hyperactive bowel sounds because blood acts as a cathartic. Digital rectal examination (DRE) is mandatory. No stool with the presence of fresh bright blood suggests the possibility of a rapid, significant, and continuing bleed. Stool in the rectum that is guaiac positive but does not present with fresh blood or clots suggests that the bleeding has slowed down or stopped.

Differential. **Vascular ectasia:** Bleeding similar to that seen with DD; diagnostic workup the same as for DD with bleeding. **Mesenteric ischemia:** Abdominal pain out of proportion to physical exam findings, ±gross blood in stool, ±heart murmur, ±abdominal bruit(s), ±lactic acidosis, ±ischemic risk factors such as ↑ cholesterol and ↑ triglycerides. **Upper GI bleeding** (proximal to ligament of Treitz): history of gastroesophageal reflux disease (GERD) and/or nonsteroidal anti-inflammatory drug (NSAID) use, ±bright red blood per rectum (if a brisk upper GI bleed), ±tachycardia, nasogastric (NG) tube + blood aspirate.

Diagnosis. Any pathologic condition distal to the ligament of Treitz may be responsible for hematochezia. History should reveal the nature and duration of the bleeding, any comorbid conditions, and use of medications such as anticoagulants or other agents that might contribute to the bleeding episode. **If the patient's condition is stable, colonoscopy is the next step to find and stop the bleed.** The procedure can be done after a rapid bowel preparation to clear the colon of blood and stool, although it can also be done without this preparation. If the patient's condition remains unstable after initial resuscitation, an angiogram is the next step.

Labs. ±↓Hgb/Hct. If bleeding is rapid, the Hgb/Hct may not have adjusted yet, so serial checks every 4 to 8 hours will reveal the trend. Prothrombin time (PT), activated partial thromboplastin time (aPTT), and platelet count may be altered.

Imaging. Colonoscopy might reveal blood in one area of the colon, but usually the blood is noted throughout the large intestine. Occasionally, a diverticulum may be seen with clots or bleeding; the same is true of an angiodysplastic lesion. Bleeding that persists or recurs may be assessed with a nuclear scan performed with an IV injection of ^{99m}technetium-labeled red blood cells. This scan helps determine whether or not an angiogram is necessary. The angiogram will reveal bleeding only at a certain rate.

Treatment

Asymptomatic DD: The recommended treatment is to encourage the patient to increase fiber intake. This results in a measurable decrease in the incidence of inflammatory complications of DD.

Diverticulitis: Broad-spectrum antibiotics and progression from clear liquids to a soft, nonresidue diet plus the use of bulking agents are the initial treatment modalities. These regimens may be instituted on an inpatient or outpatient basis, depending on the severity of the presentation. A colonoscopy should be scheduled 6 to 8 weeks after resolution of the episode. Twenty-five percent of hospitalized patients require surgery. Of all patients treated medically, approximately 30% will have recurrent episodes of diverticulitis.

Diverticular bleeding: Resuscitation takes precedence over everything else, particularly when treatment is provided for the unstable patient. The source of bleeding may be identified on colonoscopy, and the patient treated with a heater, a bipolar probe, or a laser. An angiographic approach may be needed to stop the bleeding in some cases. If all of these methods fail, surgery is the next step.

Polyps

Definition A polyp is simply a morphologic classification that refers to an accumulation of tissue protruding into the colonic lumen. Polyps may be **pedunculated**, meaning they have a stalk, or **sessile**, meaning they do not have a stalk (Fig. 14-5).

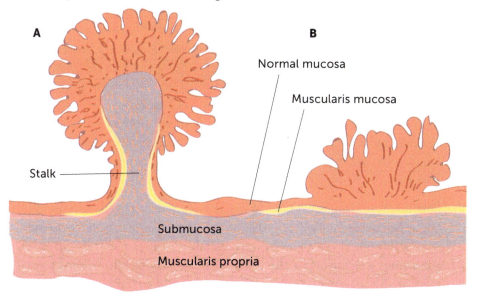

Fig. 14-5. A: Pedunculated Polyp with a Stalk **B:** Sessile Polyp

Polyps may be further classified according to their histologic features (Table 14-2).

Table 14-2. Histologic Classification of Polyps

Cell Types	Histologic Types	Features	Malignant Potential
Inflammatory	Pseudopolyp	Seen in chronic ulcerative colitis	No, except for that of the underlying disease
Non-neoplastic (normal cells)	Hyperplastic polyp	Proliferation of normal cells	No
Non-neoplastic (normal cells)	Hamartoma (juvenile polyp ie, Peutz-Jeghers)	Faulty focal development with disorganization	No (occasionally reported)
Neoplastic (genetically abnormal cells)	Serrated adenoma	Sessile, hyperplastic with adenomatous features	Yes
Neoplastic (genetically abnormal cells)	Tubular adenoma	Most common, usually pedunculated	Yes
Neoplastic (genetically abnormal cells)	Tubulovillous adenoma	Usually pedunculated	Yes/More
Neoplastic (genetically abnormal cells)	Villous adenoma	Usually sessile	Yes/Most

Etiology Other than inflammatory polyps, such as those resulting from ulcerative colitis, the causes of nonhereditary polyp formation are unclear, although the same risk factors influencing the development of the adenoma-carcinoma sequence are connected with polyp formation.

Epidemiology The prevalence of adenoma increases with age; by age 60, approximately 30% to 40% of the population may have adenomas, although these estimates are variable. **Approximately 50% of adenomas are found in the left colon, mostly in the sigmoid and rectum.** About 50% of patients who are found to have one adenoma will have others. **Serrated adenomas are more common in the right colon**, and evidence linking them with colon cancer is fairly clear. Size and epithelial atypia are closely connected with the malignant potential of a polyp, although this might not be true for the small, flat serrated adenomas most often seen in the right colon. **Sessile lesions are more likely to become malignant than pedunculated ones. Pure villous adenomas are usually sessile, and as many as 30% may harbor carcinoma.** The incidence rises to 50% if the villous andenoma is larger than 2 cm. Removal of polyps decreases the incidence of cancer, but the lifetime risk of cancer is higher if the individual has had polyps.

Symptoms Most polyps are asymptomatic. Large polyps are more likely to cause symptoms, the most common of which is rectal bleeding, usually intermittent. Large villous adenomas of the rectum may produce a fair amount of mucus that is visible with bowel movements.

Physical Exam and Signs During a DRE, it is possible to palpate a polyp, although such an occurrence is rare. Occasionally, blood-tinged mucus is seen on digital exam.

Differential The differential diagnosis of asymptomatic polyps focuses on the various polyposis syndromes. **Familial adenomatous polyposis (FAP)**: Rare, but 100% lifetime colon cancer risk. Genetic mutation of the *APC* gene. Associated with ↑ risk of periampullary, thyroid, and adrenocortical cancers and extracolonic manifestations, both benign and malignant. Patients present with hundreds to thousands of polyps of different sizes. **Attenuated FAP**: Fewer than 100 polyps; untreated patients develop colon cancer later in life. **Gardner's syndrome**: *APC* gene mutation, polyps, desmoids tumors, osteomas, sebaceous cysts, ↑ colon cancer risk. **Cowden's disease**: Juvenile polyps, mucocutaneous lesions, ±thyroid cancer ±breast, renal, or endometrial cancer. **Peutz-Jeghers syndrome**: Hamartomas in small and large intestine, +melanotic pigmentation, most often of the lips and gums.

Diagnosis **Colonoscopy is the test of choice for finding polyps in the colon.**

Labs. No specific findings.

Imaging. Air-contrast barium enema (BE) may show a filling defect.

Complication(s) Occasionally, polyps cause bleeding. Rarely, a juvenile polyp protrudes through the anus. Carcinoma develops in untreated multiple polyposis syndromes. Local recurrence is most common for villous adenomas.

Treatment **Polyps are removed by endoscopic snare removal.** If the polyp contains cancer, the clinician applies the Haggit criteria in deciding whether therapy by polypectomy alone is sufficient. Some of the multiple polyposis syndromes are treated with a total colectomy.

ANGIODYSPLASIA

Definition Angiodysplasia, or *arteriovenous malformations* (AVMs), are believed to be acquired degenerative lesions of the large and small intestine. **They are the second most common cause of severe lower GI bleeding after DD.**

Etiology AVMs result from progressive dilatation of submucosal blood vessels.

Epidemiology AVMs occur most often in patients older than 50 years of age. They are found most commonly in the cecum and ascending colon. AVMs are associated with aortic stenosis and renal failure, and occasionally with von Willebrand's disease. Multiple lesions are present in 25% of cases.

Symptoms **Most symptomatic patients present with intermittent, chronic bleeding.** Approximately 10% to 15% present with massive bleeding; in most of these cases, the bleeding ceases spontaneously.

Physical Exam and Signs None.

Differential Severe acute bleeding requires a differential diagnosis similar to that described for DD with bleeding. Chronic intermittent bleeding requires the work-up to include carcinoma, polyps, and hemorrhoids, all which are investigated by colonoscopy/anoscopy.

Diagnosis **Colonoscopy is the test of choice for the diagnosis of angiodysplasia.**

Labs. None specific.

Imaging. **AVMs appear as a red-stellate lesion surrounded by pale mucosa.** Angiography may show the lesion as an early-filling vein, a delayed-emptying vein, or a vascular tuft.

Complication(s) The most common complication is **massive rectal bleeding**.

Treatment If discovered incidentally, no treatment is needed. If the patient is bleeding severely, endoscopic coagulation or injection with sclerosing agents is the initial treatment approach. Angiographic treatment might be otherwise necessary, and vasopressin infusion or foam embolization may be successful. If these methods are ineffective, surgical resection is the next step.

INFLAMMATORY BOWEL DISEASE (IBD): ULCERATIVE COLITIS

Definition **Ulcerative colitis (UC) is an inflammatory disease of the colon**. It is part of a complex presentation that consists of 2 diseases with overlapping characteristics: ulcerative colitis and Crohn's disease (CD) (Table 14-3).

Etiology Although the causes are unknown, those under speculation include infection, environmental factors, and an abnormal immune response resulting from increased exposure to dietary antigens in the presence of a defective mucosal barrier. Some information suggests that smoking may have some beneficial effect on patients with UC.

Epidemiology **UC and CD have a bimodal age distribution**, with a peak incidence between 15 and 30 years and a smaller presentation of cases among people between 55 and 80 years of age. The distinction between UC and CD cannot be made in 5% to 10% of cases. Both UC and CD increase the risk of malignant transformation. UC is more prevalent in industrial societies, and its incidence has remained mostly unchanged for many years.

Symptoms **The most common symptoms of UC are hematochezia and diarrhea, frequently associated with excessive mucus**. Rectal urgency and tenesmus are common in chronic UC, perhaps because of the rectal involvement seen with the disease. Abdominal discomfort is common with acute presentations of the disease, but it is less significant than the same symptom in CD. Fever, anorexia, and weight loss may be noted in severe cases.

Physical Exam and Signs The most telling signs of UC include the presence of rectal involvement and bleeding. In fact, the diagnosis of UC may be called into question if the patient does not have rectal involvement. Segments of the involved colon are affected in a **continuous**

Table 14-3. Ulcerative Colitis versus Crohn's Disease

	Ulcerative Colitis	Crohn's Disease
Disease Location	Colon Terminal ileum (backwash ileitis): 10%	Mouth to anus Terminal ileum most common Both SI and colon: 40% Perianal only: 8% to 10%
Perianal Involvement	No	When TI involved: 30% When colon involved: 50%
Rectal Involvement	Involved 95% of cases	Involved 50% of cases
Symptoms	Hematochezia, diarrhea with mucus/pus, tenesmus, rectal urgency	Crampy abdominal pain, hematochezia (30%), weight loss, less diarrhea, symptoms of complications (eg, obstruction)
Endoscopic Findings	Continuous involvement, friable hyperemic mucosa, shallow ulcers, pseudopolyps (chronic)	Cobblestoning (late), skip lesions, edema, deep linear ulcers, granularity, fissures
Radiology	Barium enema (BE) with shortening and loss of haustra (chronic stage) TI dilated 10% of cases (backwash ileitis)	Colon does not shorten When TI involved, constricted ("string sign")
Gross Findings	Mesentery not thickened, normal serosa unless toxic megacolon	Thickened mesentery, "fat wrapping," enlarged nodes, serositis
Histology	Mucosa and submucosa only +++crypt abscesses	Transmural +crypt abscesses, lymphoid aggregates, fibrosis, granulomas (50%)
Surgery	Usually curative	For complications
Risk for Colorectal Cancer	↑↑↑↑	↑↑

pattern. Histologically, **UC involves the mucosa and the submucosa only**, whereas **CD is a transmural process.** Extracolonic manifestations are possible and are similar for both types of IBD. Arthritis in the knees, ankles, hips, and shoulders is present in 20% of patients. Erythema nodosum appears in 10% to 15% of patients with UC. Other IBD-associated presentations include ankylosing spondylitis, pyoderma gangrenosum, and primary sclerosing cholangitis (PSC); this last one is a progressive and often fatal disease. Bile duct carcinoma may develop, and patients with PSC are at higher risk for developing colon cancer than are patients with UC alone.

Differential The differential may include any of the known causes of lower GI bleeding, but a narrower differential is listed here. *Clostridium difficile* **(pseudomembranous enterocolitis):** History of antibiotic use, diarrhea, ±fever, ±electrolyte abnormalities, +stool toxins. Endoscopy shows inflamed mucosa with yellowish, plaque-like membranes (pseudomembranes). **Chrohn's disease:** Diarrhea, crampy abdominal pain, ±weight loss, ±perianal disease, ±abdominal mass, ±hematochezia. **Infectious colitides**: Various pathogens (eg, *Salmonella, Shigella, Yersinia, Campylobacter, Escherichia coli*), n/v, abdominal cramping, diarrhea, +stool cultures.

Diagnosis **Colonoscopy is the test of choice for the diagnosis of UC.**

Labs. ±Anemia, ±↑perinuclear antineutrophil cytoplasm (pANCA; antibody with 97% specificity, 57% sensitivity), leukocytosis during exacerbations and with steroid use.

Imaging. Colonoscopy/sigmoidoscopy shows **erythema, friability, and continuous involvement starting at the rectum**. Despite its name, UC does not always exhibit ulcerations, particularly in early presentations. When ulcers are present, they may be simply erosions or frank irregular ulcers that appear rather superficial. In the chronic form of the disease, accumulations of inflammatory tissue may occur and are described as *pseudopolyps*. BE in chronic UC may show colonic shortening and loss of haustrations as the result of submucosal fibrosis affecting the colonic wall in continuity. This is not the case in CD, where the inflammation is transmural and the affected colon has normal segments intermingled with diseased ones. When the terminal ileum is involved in UC, it is dilated; this is called *backwash ileitis*.

Complication(s) **Acute dilatation, or toxic megacolon,** is a life-threatening complication reported in 4% to 10% of patients with UC, less commonly in those with CD. The colon becomes severely dilated, mostly in the transverse segment. The patient invariably presents with fever, tachycardia, hypotension, and abdominal distention. The patient with **fulminant colitis** presents with symptoms and signs of toxicity similar to those of megacolon, but without colonic dilatation. Other complications include **obstruction** and **fistula** (more common in CD), hemorrhage, and malignant transformation.

Treatment

Chronic disease: Anti-inflammatory drugs such as the 5-aminosalicylic acid compounds **sulfasalazine** and **mesalamine** are initial treatment approaches. Steroids are used to induce remission, and afterward they are decreased to maintenance doses until they can be discontinued. Immunosuppressors such as **azathioprine** are used when anti-inflammatories alone are ineffective. Antidiarrheals and iron and vitamin supplements are often given. Surgery is necessary when the disease is intractable, manifesting as lack of response to medical therapy, malnutrition, inability to work, or growth retardation in young patients, or when there is danger of malignant transformation. Some patients with severe extracolonic manifestations of IBD will respond well to a total colectomy.

Complicated UC: Toxic megacolon and fulminant colitis require aggressive medical therapy first, with fluid resuscitation, antibiotics, and steroids. Lack of improvement is an indication for surgery. Perforation and mechanical complications such as obstruction and internal fistulas require surgery.

INFLAMMATORY BOWEL DISEASE: CROHN'S DISEASE

Definition Crohn's disease (CD), originally described as regional ileitis, is a form of IBD that **may affect the entire GI tract from mouth to anus but most commonly affects the terminal ileum. CD is a transmural inflammation of the GI tract,** whereas UC involves only the mucosa and the submucosa.

Etiology CD is associated with the same risk factors described for UC. Smoking increases risk, as might the use of oral contraceptives. CD is more prevalent in patients of Jewish ancestry.

Epidemiology **Similar to UC, CD has a bimodal age distribution.** The disease affects the large bowel and the small bowel in 40% of patients, and only the colon in approximately 15% to 30% of patients. CD, unlike UC, has been associated with a slow increase in incidence.

Symptoms The most common symptoms of CD are the **triad of hematochezia, diarrhea with crampy abdominal pain, and weight loss**. Fever is also common. Rectal bleeding is less common in CD, but diarrhea is just as prevalent as in UC. Abdominal pain is more prevalent and significant in patients with CD than in those with UC.

Physical Exam and Signs Rectal involvement is seen in only 50% of patients with colonic CD. Anal and perianal disease is present in 50% of patients with CD and may be seen even if the patient has disease involvement of the terminal ileum only. With colonic CD, anal and perianal manifestations such as pain, skin tags, or fissures should suggest the presumptive diagnosis of CD. Extracolonic manifestations are similar for both types of IBD, although primary sclerosing cholangitis is more prevalent in patients with UC.

Differential *C difficile*, **UC, and infectious colitides** are part of the work-up.

Diagnosis Colonoscopy is the test of choice for both types of IBD, although the combination of clinical, endoscopic, and radiologic findings is more often necessary to reach a conclusion with CD than with UC. **The definitive diagnosis of CD is made when biopsies reveal noncaseating granulomas.**

Labs. ±Anemia, leukocytosis during exacerbations, ±↑anti-Saccharomyces cerevisiae antibody (ASCA; antibody with 97% specificity, 49% sensitivity).

Imaging. Colonoscopy (with ileoscopy when feasible) will show a patchy distribution of normal segments interrupted by abnormal, edematous mucosa. When ulcers are present, they may be superficial early on, or deep and linear late in the disease. The edema separating deep fibrotic, linear ulcers confers onto the mucosa a **cobblestone** appearance, which is recogizable on BE. During colonoscopy, biopsy specimens should be taken from normal-appearing areas, in addition to those taken from affected segments. **When the terminal ileum is involved in CD, it is narrowed and is seen in barium studies as a "string sign."** Strictures seen by endoscopy or BE are more common in colonic CD than in UC.

Complication(s) Colonic CD is associated with the complications described in UC, but toxic megacolon is a less common occurrence. Frequent recurrences are common, and **obstruction and fistula formation are frequently seen in patients with CD.**

Treatment

Chronic disease: Treatment is similar to that for UC. Immunomodulation is similar as well, with the exception that an anti-tumor necrosis factor drug, **infliximab,** is sometimes used in patients with severe CD who do not respond to or tolerate other therapies. Antibiotics such as ciproflaxin and metronidazole are used in CD with mixed results.

Complicated CD: As with UC, severe complications such as perforation, obstruction, and internal fistulas require surgery, as do intractability, growth retardation, and the development of a malignancy.

ISCHEMIC COLITIS (MESENTERIC ISCHEMIA)

Definition Ischemic colitis occurs when there is **decreased perfusion** to sections of or to the entire colon.

Etiology The interruption of blood flow may be due to vascular occlusion or to nonocclusive processes. Common causes include embolic phenomena (30%–50%), atherosclerotic disease, aortic surgery, and conditions causing hypotension. Drug abuse, bacterial and viral pathogens, and even long-distance running have been suspected of triggering this condition.

Epidemiology The disease usually affects the colon in segments at a time. **It most commonly presents in older patients with diseases that may cause emboli formation** (eg, atrial fibrillation), and it affects the sigmoid colon in 40% of cases, followed by the transverse and the ascending. A fairly large number of patients have a transient episode that frequently resolves unrecognized. The disease may present in a variety of ways, from a temporary episode to a chronic condition, to frank colonic gangrene.

Symptoms A typical presentation is manifested by **sudden abdominal pain**, in association with hematochezia and sometimes diarrhea.

Physical Exam and Signs The abdominal exam might reveal **diffuse or localized abdominal pain disproportionate to the actual physical findings**, seldom associated with guarding unless frank gangrene or a perforation has already taken place. Fever is common.

Differential The differential for ischemic colitis may include any of the known causes of lower GI bleeding. *C difficile*, **CD**, **UC**, and infectious colitides are possible etiologies.

Diagnosis Clues to the definitive diagnosis may be found in clinical, endoscopic, and sometimes radiologic information.

Labs. Leukocytosis common, ±lactic acidosis.

Imaging. The first test that should be ordered is a plain abdominal film, which is nonspecific but may show an ileus. Occasionally, sequential depressions may be seen at the colonic edge, resembling "**thumbprinting**," which is caused by edema and sometimes hemorrhage of the colonic wall. This sign is visible on BE as well. However, performing BE is too risky when ischemia is suspected. A flexible sigmoidoscopy done with extreme caution is the next best test to perform, and it may show areas of whitish-pale mucosa surrounded by erythema. In extreme cases, the mucosa might appear gray. There is no way to determine via endoscopy if the ischemia is affecting only the mucosa, or if it is a transmural process.

Complication(s) Milder, reversible episodes may heal with stricture formation. Severe forms may result in perforation and peritonitis.

Treatment Initial treatment consists of IV fluids, antibiotics, and bowel rest. If no improvement is seen, or if the presentation is or becomes severe, surgery is required.

Colorectal Cancer

Definition The most common form of colorectal cancer (CRC) is the sporadic type, meaning that the genetic mutations that took place to cause the malignancy are acquired. If the patient inherits a mutated gene, the CRC is hereditary. Familial cancer may involve both mechanisms.

Etiology CRC results from genetic mutations that are fairly well mapped out. In this manner, a genetic mutation of the *APC* gene turns normal epithelium into a dysplastic one, which progresses to an adenoma and, finally, to carcinoma. CRC usually follows a pattern of metastasis that involves lymphatic and hematogenous spread, not necessarily in sequence. **The liver is the most common site of hematogeneous metastasis.**

Epidemiology CRC is the third most common type of cancer in the United States among both genders. It increases in incidence with age, starting at age 40 and peaking around 70 to 80 years. Its overall incidence and mortality have been decreasing steadily since the mid-90s. In the United States, the lifetime probability of developing CRC is 6%; this risk is greater in individuals with a family history of CRC, adenomatous polyps, or IBD. Over the past few decades, CRC has become more frequent in the right colon, but a slight majority of cases of CRC still present in the left colon and rectum. This is significant because more than 50% of CRCs are no longer within reach of the flexible sigmoidoscope. Synchronous CRC is present in about 3% of patients.

Symptoms CRC presents with varied and nonspecific symptoms, which are related in part to location, size, and lumen involvement by the tumor. CRC is often asymptomatic and is detected only when a routine checkup reveals anemia. However, the most common symptom of CRC is hematochezia. Patients with right-sided CRC may present with melena and postprandial discomfort. The lumen of the left colon is narrower, so cancer of the left colon is more often associated with changes in bowel habits and obstructive symptoms, as compared with right-sided tumors. Left-sided CRC may present with bright red blood per rectum (PR), constipation, colicky pain, nausea, and vomiting. Patients may also experience malaise, anorexia, and weight loss. Occasionally, patients with rectal cancer may exhibit tenesmus.

Physical Exam and Signs The exam must include a DRE, which may detect a mass. The abdomen should be percussed to check for ascites, and the liver should be assessed to check for signs of metastasis. The supraclavicular regions should be examined as well, checking for lymphadenopathies that might also suggest metastatic spread. Occasionally, a mobile mass may be palpated in the cecum if the tumor is large. Rarely, a patient with advanced carcinomatosis will exhibit a nodule palpable in the umbilicus. Although bleeding is the most common sign of CRC, 30% of patients have a normal hemoglobin, and approximately 98% will have a negative guaiac.

Differential The differential includes all of the various polyposis syndromes as possible causes. See the differential on "Polyps." **Hereditary nonpolyposis colorectal cancer (HNCC/Lynch syndrome):** Hereditary form of CRC, with family history as the diagnostic clue. Amsterdam-Bethesda criteria are used to aid in diagnosis. Lifetime risk of CRC is 85%; ↑ risk of brain, gastric, pancreaticobiliary, genitourinary, and endometrial cancers. Hemorrhoids and the presumption of other benign diseases in patients presenting with hematochezia must be carefully studied by colonoscopy/anoscopy. These exams are mandatory even when hemorrhoids are clearly demonstrated.

Diagnosis Colonoscopy is the gold standard and is indicated even if the patient was diagnosed with a BE. In this case, the endoscopy will serve to assess the characteristics of the tumor and to perform a biopsy and inspect for the possibility of associated polyps (a fairly common occurrence) or other lesions. Screening by colonoscopy is an accepted and effective method used to prevent and detect CRC.

Labs. ±↓Hgb/Hct. The tumor marker **carcinoembryonic antigen (CEA)** may be elevated in the presence of CRC, but it is nonspecific and is more useful when used to assess the possibility of recurrence and response to therapy.

Imaging. Colonoscopy can allow visualization of the tumor and can help the clinician determine the best therapeutic approach. **BE may show the typical appearance of an "apple core"** (Fig. 14-6). CT can detect metastatic lesions. For rectal cancer, endorectal ultrasonography can accurately assess the depth of invasion into the rectal wall. It might also detect enlarged pararectal lymph nodes. A chest film should be obtained routinely.

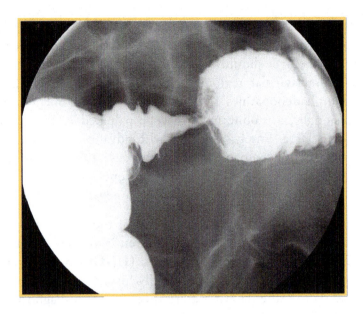

Fig. 14-6. Barium Enema Demonstrating Colorectal Cancer with "Apple Core" Appearance

Complication(s) The most common complication is large bowel obstruction followed rarely by perforation.

Treatment The treatment of patients with uncomplicated CRC depends on the location of the tumor and its stage, which is based on the tumor-node-metastasis (TNM) staging system. The mainstay of therapy is surgical resection, which is possible in approximately 70% of patients: 10% are unresectable at the time of diagnosis, and 20% present with metastatic disease. When the disease has invaded adjacent organs, en bloc resection of the involved tissues is conducted if possible. Some patients in more advanced stages benefit from adjuvant chemotherapy (after surgical treatment). Radiation therapy is most often employed in rectal cancer, in a neoadjuvant (prior to surgery) or adjuvant mode, in combination with or without chemotherapy. In the presence of metastatic disease, the primary tumor may be resected to avoid the complications of obstruction and bleeding; current evidence suggests that this might result in decreased mortality. Liver and/or lung metastases may be resected in selected patients, with similar mortality benefits. A resection requires clear proximal and distal margins, so removing very distal lesions of the rectum may require resection followed by stoma formation (Fig. 14-7).

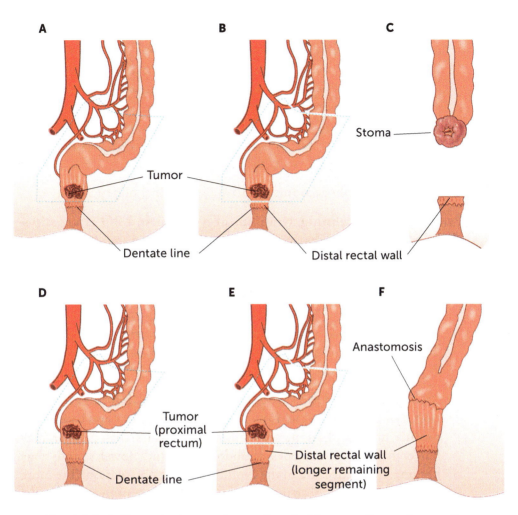

Fig. 14-7. A: Tumor is close to dentate line. **B**: After resection, only a small segment of distal rectal wall remains, so an anastomosis cannot be made. **C**: A stoma is created. If the remaining rectum and anus are also removed, the operation is called an *abdomino-perineal resection*. **D**: Tumor is in the proximal rectum. **E**: After resection there is sufficient room for an anastomosis. **F**: An anastomosis is created.

LARGE BOWEL OBSTRUCTION

Definition A large bowel obstruction (LBO) is an emergency condition in which any segment of the colon is partially or totally occluded.

Etiology The most common cause of LBO is carcinoma of the colon, followed by diverticulitis and volvulus. The obstruction may be due to intrinsic causes (eg, CRC, Crohn's disease) or extrinsic causes (eg, compression from a tumor outside of the colon, inflammation). A closed loop obstruction occurs when both proximal and distal lumina of the colon are obstructed, as would be the case with a volvulus or a strangulated segment of intestine. A closed loop LBO is most commonly seen when the obstructed segment is associated with a competent ileocecal valve. Rarely, if ever, should the clinician assume that a fecal impaction is the cause of LBO.

Epidemiology LBO accounts for 15% of intestinal obstructions.

Symptoms **The defining symptom of a complete LBO is constipation or complete absence of flatus or stool passage**. Patients may have cramping abdominal pain. Nausea is common and vomiting is a late manifestation. The symptoms may be insidious, relatively long-standing, as is possible with CRC, or acute, as is seen with a volvulus. Before the stage of complete obstruction, the patient may have had bleeding per rectum, a change in the characteristics of the stool, or diarrhea. The more proximally the LBO is located, the greater is the likelihood of nausea and vomiting.

Physical Exam and Signs Common signs include **abdominal distention, tympany to percussion**, and **high-pitched hyperactive bowel sounds** on auscultation, sometimes with rushes that may or may not coincide with episodes of abdominal pain. Bowel sounds may become hypoactive late in the evolution of the obstruction. The more distally the colonic obstruction is found, the more pronounced is the distention. Blood on DRE suggests CRC.

Differential **Ogilvie's syndrome (pseudo-obstruction)**: Significant medical comorbidities (renal, respiratory, cardiovascular), trauma (vertebral fractures), ±medications that affect colonic motility, +abdominal distention and tympany, bowel sounds normal or hypoactive, plain abdominal films with mostly distended right and transverse colon, BE diagnostic. **Small bowel obstruction**: ±Vomiting, +air-fluid levels with "stacked coin" appearance.

Diagnosis **The most significant diagnostic test is a water-soluble BE, which will show the level of the obstruction, or will show no obstruction if the patient has Ogilvie's syndrome**. Oral barium should not be administered if the clinician suspects a mechanical obstruction.

Labs. Findings vary according to the duration of presentation, and are mostly nonspecific. Hgb/Hct may be decreased but may be normal if the patient is dehydrated.

Imaging. A plain abdominal radiograph will show a "frame" of gas in a distended colon around the abdomen, with haustrations and a point where the gas column is no longer visible (Fig. 14-8). If the obstruction occurs at the level of the ileocecal junction, the plain films may look like those of a small bowel obstruction. BE will show stoppage of the barium column, and will confirm or rule out the diagnosis. CT is helpful in determining the cause of the obstruction.

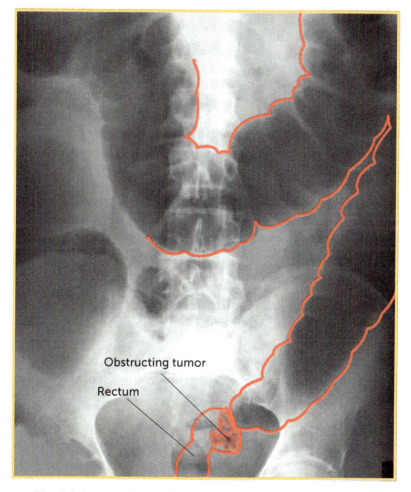

Fig. 14-8. Large Bowel Obstruction on X-ray

Complication(s) Gangrene of the obstructed segments may occur as the LBO progresses. Perforation is a potentially lethal complication. The cecum has the largest colonic diameter, so the **law of LaPlace**—which states that the larger the radius of a cylindrical-shaped structure (eg, a lumen), the greater the wall tension becomes—is quite relevant, and cecal perforation may occur first if the LBO is not treated in a timely fashion.

Treatment Initial therapy must include fluid resuscitation and placement of a nasogastric tube. If ischemia is suspected, antibiotics are indicated. Surgery, the mainstay of treatment for LBO, may consist of a diverting ostomy or a resection. Pseudo-obstruction frequently responds to medical therapy with an anticholinergic agent like neostigmine, which is contraindicated in a mechanical obstruction. Colonoscopy is the initial treatment of choice for pseudo-obstruction if the patient does not respond to medical therapy.

Volvulus

Definition A volvulus is the rotation of a segment of large or small intestine on its mesenteric axis, causing a partial or complete obstruction.

Etiology This presentation is promoted by an elongated and mobile segment of intestine with a narrow attachment of the mesentery to the posterior abdominal wall. Associated risk factors include age over 70 and use of psychotropic drugs; reports have suggested a predisposition to volvulus if large amounts of fiber are ingested.

Epidemiology Sigmoid volvulus represents two-thirds of all cases of colonic volvulus. Approximately 30% of the time, the volvulus involves the cecum and the terminal ileum. Sometimes the cecum alone is involved on account of a cecal bascule, in which the cecum is freely mobile in a caudad-to-cephalad direction. **Volvulus is responsible for 5% of all cases of LBO.**

Symptoms The symptoms are the same as those of a closed loop obstruction. Intermittent colicky pain is seen initially; it eventually becomes continuous and severe if ischemia develops. No stool or gas is passed. Vomiting is almost always present.

Physical Exam and Signs The abdomen is distended and firm, sometimes with associated tachycardia.

Differential Cecal volvulus often requires differentiation from a small bowel obstruction. A sigmoid volvulus requires a differential diagnosis of all possible sources of LBO, including pseudo-obstruction.

Diagnosis A volvulus is diagnosed on the basis of radiologic findings. An abdominal radiograph should be ordered first. This can be followed by a low-pressure barium enema.

Labs. Lab values are nonspecific and correlate with the timing and type of presentation. With ischemia, +leukocytosis, +lactic acidosis. Electrolytes will be altered in relationship to the time elapsed from initial presentation.

Imaging. A plain abdominal radiograph, supine and erect, typically shows a hugely distended loop of bowel that has lost its haustral markings, reaching the diaphragm with a "coffee bean" shape that points toward the left or left lower quadrant (in the case of a sigmoid volvulus). **The radiographic appearance has also been described as that of a bent inner tube, with its apex in the right upper quadrant (Fig. 14-9).** Barium enema shows the

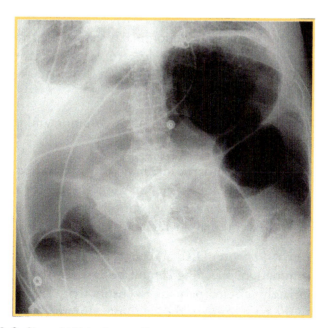

Fig. 14-9. Sigmoid Volvulus on X-ray

characteristic "bird's beak" of the upper end of the lower segment of the torsion. This confirms the diagnosis.

Complication(s) The most common complications include ischemia and perforation.

Treatment Initially, the patient should undergo fluid resuscitation and attempts at nonoperative decompression if no signs of bowel ischemia are noted. Reduction of the volvulus may be attempted with a flexible sigmoidoscope or colonoscope. When this is successful, a sudden gush of gas and fluid is followed by a decrease in abdominal distention. A rectal tube is usually left in place to maintain the decompression until an elective resection is done, which is indicated because the recurrence rate is as high as 50%.

HEMORRHOIDS

Definition Hemorrhoids are anal canal vascular "cushions" consisting of blood vessels, smooth muscle, and elastic and connective tissue, which is present normally to aid in anal continence. These cushions are called *hemorrhoids* when they become symptomatic. They are not varicose veins.

Etiology The causes are unclear, but gravity, straining with bowel movements, and increased intra-abdominal pressure contribute to their formation. All of these elements lead to vascular engorgement and dilatation and rupture of supporting tissues, and are associated with no or varying degrees of prolapse.

Epidemiology Hemorrhoids are extremely common and may be internal (proximal to the dentate line) or external.

Symptoms Internal hemorrhoids may cause painless bright red bleeding per rectum and, depending on the degree of associated prolapse, mucus, fecal leakage, or pruritus. Internal hemorrhoids are insensate, whereas external hemorrhoids may cause pain.

Physical Exam and Signs DRE and anoscopy are mandatory elements of the examination. Bleeding should be investigated via endoscopy in appropriately selected patients to ensure that clearly seen hemorrhoids are the only cause of the symptom. Internal hemorrhoids are classified according to the degree of prolapse:

Grade I: bleeding, no prolapse

Grade II: bleeding, prolapse with spontaneous reduction

Grade III: bleeding, prolapse requiring manual reduction

Grade IV: prolapse, nonreducible/strangulated/thrombosed

Differential Painless bleeding should be followed by a work-up to rule out **CRC**, **DD**, **IBD**, **or polyps**. Painful bleeding is usually associated with a fissure. A nonreducible hemorrhoidal prolapse must be differentiated from a **rectal prolapse**, in which the visible folds of the prolapse are circumferential.

Diagnosis Anoscopy is the test of choice for the diagnosis of hemorrhoids.

Labs. Chronic significant bleeding may lead to anemia.

Imaging. Direct inspection with an anoscope will reveal the hemorrhoids and their associated degree of prolapse.

Complication(s) Complete thromboses with strangulation are an uncommon presentation requiring urgent surgical therapy.

Treatment Initially, medical therapy is appropriate in uncomplicated cases. This includes encouraging patients to increase fiber and water intake. Stool softeners may be used. Topical therapies are seldom helpful. When it becomes necessary, treatment for internal hemorrhoids includes rubber band ligation or infrared coagulation, which is possible because internal hemorrhoids are insensate. Surgical hemorrhoidectomy is reserved for patients for whom other measures fail and is used to treat those with complications such as complete thrombosis, strangulation, or intractable prolapse.

ANAL FISSURE

Definition An anal fissure is an acute or chronic tear of the anoderm distal to the dentate line. A fissure is usually the acute form, whereas the chronic or mature presentation is best described as an ulcer.

Etiology It is likely caused by a hypertensive internal anal sphincter, and the initial insult may be a tear caused by forceful dilatation during a difficult bowel movement.

Epidemiology Fissures are most common at the midline, with approximately 70% of posterior and the rest anterior.

Symptoms Pain during and after defecation is common. Fresh bright bleeding, not mixed with stool, occurs in some patients.

Physical Exam and Signs Inspection is the most important part of the examination. A fissure will be visible in 95% of cases. An ulcer is usually associated with a proximal hypertrophic papilla.

Differential An abscess must be ruled out during an acute presenting episode. It presents with swelling and tenderness and possibly fever. If an anal ulcer is not found at one of the midlines, or if more than one coexist, other causes should be ruled out, such as IBD (Crohn's disease), sexually transmitted disease (STD), or malignancy.

Diagnosis Inspection with visualization of the fissure is the definitive diagnostic maneuver. After the acute episode has resolved, the patient should undergo anoscopy or colonoscopy, depending on associated risk factors.

Complication(s) No significant complications are associated with an anal fissure other than the persistence of the disease and its associated pain.

Treatment The initial medical treatment includes stool softeners, bulking agents, and sitz baths. When conservative measures fail, nitroglycerin or nifedipine ointment might work, although results are variable. Botulinum toxin injection into the internal sphincter has had reasonable results. The surgical procedure of choice is a lateral internal sphincterotomy, which is associated with a low incidence of recurrence.

BIBLIOGRAPHY

Haggitt RC, Glotzbach RE, Soffer EE, Wruble LD. Prognostic factors in colorectal carcinoma arising in adenomas: implications for lesions removed by endoscopic polypectomy. *Gastroenterology*. 1985;89(2):328-336.

Heise CP. Epidemiology and pathogenesis of diverticular disease. *J Gastrointest Surg*. 2008;12(8):1309–1311.

Clinical Keys: Questions And Answers

Where is McBurney's point?	Two-thirds of the distance between the umbilicus and the right inferior iliac spine
Which is the narrowest section of the colon?	The sigmoid
Which anal sphincter is voluntary?	The external anal sphincter
Which artery supplies the cecum and the ascending and proximal two-thirds of the transverse colon?	The SMA. The IMA supplies the distal one-third of the transverse colon to the proximal rectum.
How does the patient with appendicitis typically present?	Pain starts in the periumbilical region and later localizes to the RLQ
What is Rovsing's sign?	Deep palpation to the LLQ causes referred pain in the RLQ
What is the obturator sign?	Pain elicited in the RLQ when the patient is supine and the right thigh is flexed and internally rotated
What is the psoas sign?	Pain with extension of the right leg that is relieved when the leg is flexed while the patient is lying on the left side
What is rebound tenderness?	Abdominal pain that follows the release of the examiner's hand from deep palpation
What is voluntary guarding?	Abdominal muscles contract upon palpation of the abdomen
What is the test of choice to diagnose appendicitis?	CT scan with IV and oral contrast
What is diverticulosis?	An acquired condition in which the colonic mucosa herniates through the muscular coat of the colon
What are the most common complications of diverticulosis?	Diverticulitis and GI bleeding
What is diverticulits?	A pericolic inflammatory process resulting from a micro-perforation or macro-perforation of a diverticulum
What is the most common symptom of diverticulitis?	Acute abdominal pain most prevalent in the LLQ
What is the most common cause of lower GI bleeding?	Diverticular bleeding

What is hematochezia?	A rectal bleed of maroon or dark red blood
What does free air on a flat plate of the abdomen signify?	That a hollow viscous organ has perforated
What are the initial treatment steps for diverticulitis?	Broad-spectrum antibiotics, IV fluids and bowel rest if the patient requires admission
How are polyps classified anatomically?	Sessile or flat, and pedunculated (with a stalk)
Which type of polyp has the most malignant potential?	A villous adenoma
What are arteriovenous malformations?	Dilatations of submucosal blood vessels in the large or small intestine
What is mesenteric ischemia?	Decreased perfusion to sections of the large or small intestine
What is a significant finding on abdominal exam of patients with mesenteric ischemia?	Pain out of proportion to physical findings
What BE finding may indicate mesenteric ischemia?	Thumbprinting
What are the most common symptoms of UC?	Hematochezia and diarrhea, associated with excessive mucus
What are the initial treatment approaches for chronic UC?	Sulfasalazine and mesalamine
Which type of IBD involves the mucosa and the submucosa of the colon only?	UC. Crohn's disease is a transmural process of the bowel wall.
Which IBD may affect the entire GI tract from mouth to anus?	Crohn's disease
What is the meaning of cobblestone appearance?	Elevation of the mucosa between ulcers seen in CD as a result of underlying edema
Which distinctive pathologic characteristic establishes with certainty the diagnosis of CD?	Granulomas
Which anti-tumor necrosis factor drug can be used in severe cases of CD?	Infliximab
What is the most common symptom of CRC?	Hematochezia
What symptoms are associated with left-sided CRC?	Alterations in bowel habits and hematochezia. Nausea, vomiting, and colicky pain are seen when some degree of obstruction is present
What is the lifetime probability of developing CRC?	6%

Liver And Portal System

The liver (Fig. 15-1) is a large solid organ with a major metabolic role—it is responsible for glucose, lipid, and protein metabolism. It encompasses a wide range of other functions as well, such as detoxification, plasma protein synthesis, red blood cell destruction, glycogen storage, immunologic modulation, and regulation of blood clotting.

The liver receives a dual blood supply from the portal vein (75%) and the hepatic artery (25%), and each of these provides roughly 50% of the oxygen to the liver. The portal vein is formed by the confluence of the superior mesenteric and splenic veins. The main portal vein, the hepatic artery, and the bile duct at the hilar region of the liver are collectively referred to as the *porta hepatis*.

Blood from the portal vein and the hepatic artery flows through the sinusoids to reach the central venule of the hepatic lobe, and is then carried in progressively larger branches of the hepatic veins to finally reach the general circulation as these vessels drain into the IVC.

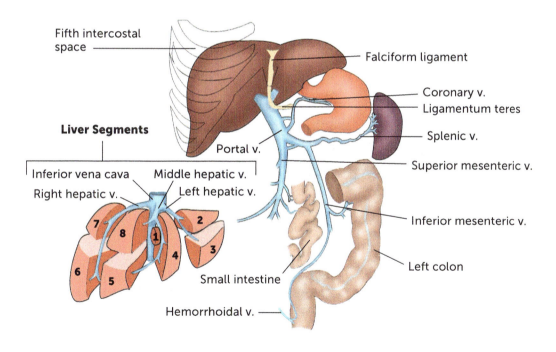

Fig. 15-1 Anatomy of the Liver and Hepatic Veins

Portal Hypertension

Definition Portal hypertension (PH) is an **increase in portal venous pressure.**

Etiology PH is due to resistance in portal venous flow caused by an obstruction or, more rarely, to increased portal venous flow, as is seen in an arteriovenous portal fistula. Resistance to portal venous flow may be prehepatic, intrahepatic, or posthepatic. The most common cause of PH is **intrahepatic obstruction** of portal venous flow from cirrhosis, and in the United States, cirrhosis is most commonly due to consumption of **alcohol.** Other causes of hepatic PH include hepatic fibrosis, hepatitis C, and Wilson's disease, among others. Hepatic resistance to flow, in turn, may be presinusoidal, sinusoidal, or postsinusoidal. Cirrhosis most often causes a **postsinusoidal obstruction.** Less commonly, PH is caused by **prehepatic portal venous obstruction** due to a portal vein thrombosis. **Posthepatic PH** results from increased resistance through the hepatic veins (Fig. 15-1), as is seen in **Budd-Chiari syndrome,** which is a thrombosis of the hepatic veins. This mechanism is also seen in right-sided heart failure and in constrictive pericarditis. Other causes of prehepatic, intrahepatic, and posthepatic PH are presented in Table 15-1.

Table 15-1. Causes of Portal Hypertension

Types of Portal Hypertension	Causes	
Prehepatic	Portal vein thrombosis Congenital abnormalities Extrinsic compression (tumors)	
Intrahepatic	Cirrhosis Hepatitis C Fibrosis (congenital) Hemochromatosis	Wilson's disease (congenital) Schistosomiasis Metastatic disease Vitamin A toxicity
Posthepatic	Hepatic vein thrombosis Inferior vena cava obstruction Cardiac disease (right-sided heart failure, constrictive pericarditis)	Budd-Chiari syndrome Arteriovenous fistula (traumatic, congenital)

Differential The differential diagnoses of PH centers around the various causes of the syndrome (Table 15-1).

Epidemiology The precise prevalence of PH is not known. The prevalence of portal vein thrombosis is also unknown, but it is seen in 30% of patients with hepatocellular carcinoma and in 5% of patients with cirrhosis and PH.

Symptoms PH exhibits nonspecific symptoms, such as anorexia, weight loss, and fatigue.

Physical Exam and Signs A constellation of physical signs suggest PH due to liver disease at different stages in the evolution of the illness. The patient may exhibit scleral icterus, spider nevi, palmar erythema, gynecomastia, splenomegaly, asterixis, caput medusae (distended and tortuous veins radiating from the umbilicus), and hemorrhoids. The liver may be enlarged and easily palpable early on, or it may be shrunken in late stages of the disease.

Differential The differential diagnosis of PH centers around the various causes of the syndrome (see Table 15-1).

Diagnosis A combination of laboratory and imaging tests is needed to determine the presence and causes(s) of PH. This condition is diagnosed when the hepatic venous pressure gradient (HVPG) is **8 mm Hg or greater** (normal is between 1 mm Hg and 5 mm Hg). Varices develop when the HVPG reaches between 10 and 12 mm Hg.

Labs. Commonly, patients with cirrhosis may reveal anemia, thrombocytopenia, ↑PT, ↑aPTT, ↑INR, ↑AST, ↑ALT, ±↑ALP, ↓Na⁺, and ↓K⁺. Chronic disease is associated with ↓albumin. Hepatitis serologies must be obtained because cirrhosis is a common sequela of hepatitis B and C that may also lead to hepatocellular carcinoma. An alpha-fetoprotein (AFP) level can be used to detect carcinoma in 50% to 60% of patients with the disease. α_1-Antitrypsin deficiency has also been associated with hepatocellular cancer. The functional reserve of the liver, also used as a traditional measure of surgical risk for patients with cirrhosis and PH, is derived by calculating the Child-Pugh score (Table 15-2), which is used to classify the liver disease by severity, according to the Child-Pugh classes (Table 15-3). The Model for End-Stage Liver Disease (MELD), which is based on serum bilirubin, creatinine levels, and international normalized ratio (INR), and on the etiology of the liver disease, has been found to be an accurate method of predicting surgical mortality in cirrhotic patients when used in conjunction with the Child-Pugh classification. Hepatic transplantation is considered in Child-Pugh class C patients, and has been performed with good results.

Imaging. The safest and simplest method of screening for PH is **duplex** ultrasonography, which, despite its limitations, can demonstrate portal and splenic vein thromboses, features of cirrhosis, and portal flow. A more invasive method for determining PH is performed indirectly by advancing a catheter into one of the hepatic veins via the jugular or femoral vein and obtaining a **hepatic wedge pressure**. The HVPG can then be calculated. This is not commonly used because ultrasonography is preferred. A computed tomography angiography scan (CTA) may show the portal vasculature. An angiogram of the superior mesenteric artery (SMA) with a venous return phase may demonstrate occlusion of the portal vein.

Table 15-2. Calculating Child-Pugh Score

Clinical Findings	1 Point	2 Points	3 Points
Hepatic encephalopathy	None	Grade I–II: controlled medically	Grade III–IV: refractory to medication
Ascites	None	Mild	Moderate to severe
Total bilirubin, mg/dL	1–2	2.1-3	≥3.1
Serum albumin, g/dL	≥3.5	2.8-3.4	≤2.7
PT (↑ in seconds)	<4	4–6	>6
INR (↑ in seconds)	<1.8	1.8-2.2	>2.2

Table 15-3. Child-Pugh Classification of Liver Disease

Class	Points	Perioperative Mortatlity	1-Year Survival	2-Year Survival
A	5–6	10%	100%	85%
B	7–9	30%	81%	57%
C	10–15	70%–80%	45%	35%

Complication(s) The most common complications of PH are **variceal bleeding, ascites,** and **hepatic encephalopathy.**

1. **Variceal bleeding.** Because of the connections between the portal system and the systemic venous circulation (Fig. 15-1), PH may lead to portosystemic shunting. This increased blood flow through the portal vein leads to increased flow through the collateral, systemic circulation—most clinically important is the shunting between the left gastric portal vein and the esophageal vein (systemic) at the level of the gastroesophageal junction. Increased pressure here can lead to variceal dilatation of thin-walled vessels, namely, the submucosal venous plexuses in the esophagus and stomach, resulting in variceal bleeding. (See later section, "Esophagogastric Variceal Bleeding," for more information on this topic.) Portosystemic shunting may also cause the development of collaterals with the umbilical, retroperitoneal, and hemorrhoidal network of veins, which explains the many physical signs seen in patients with cirrhosis. All patients with cirrhosis should undergo a screening upper GI endoscopy to assess their risk of bleeding.

2. **Ascites.** This condition is caused by salt and water retention by the kidneys, which detect a decrease in circulating blood volume and attempt to compensate for this. It is also caused by a decrease in plasma oncotic pressure and increased lymphatic flow.

3. **Hepatic encephalopathy.** This condition results from an accumulation of neurotoxins normally cleared by the liver, such as ammonia and γ-aminobutyric acid. Clinically, it can manifest with hyperreflexia and asterixis.

Treatment

Variceal bleeding: For patients at **high risk** of variceal bleeding (large varices and small ones with red color signs), the **gold standard** is the prophylactic use of **nonselective beta-blockers,** such as **propranolol.** Prophylactic endoscopic variceal ligation can be used in patients with contraindications or intolerance to beta-blockade, or to prevent recurrent bleeding in patients who have had an episode of bleeding. (See later section, "Esophagogastric Variceal Bleeding," for more information on the treatment of active variceal bleeding.)

Ascites: Treatment consists of salt restriction (<1000 mg/day) and administration of diuretics. **Spironolactone** is the diuretic of choice, and **furosemide** may be added if spironolactone is minimally effective. **Large-volume paracentesis** (up to 10 L) is used for symptomatic relief. Refractory ascites is sometimes treated with a jugular-peritoneal shunt known as a *LeVeen shunt.*

Hepatic encephalopathy: This condition is most commonly acute and requires identification and elimination of precipitating factors. Spontaneous development of this complication is seen in less than 10% of patients with PH. The first step in treating encephalopathy is to **limit dietary protein.** If ineffective, the oral agent **lactulose** may be used, which decreases the amount of intestinal ammonia and inhibits its absorption. Lactulose is also used to produce 2 to 3 stools daily. Lactulose may be given with the antibiotic **neomycin** to suppress urease-producing bacteria. **Metronidazole** may be added.

ESOPHAGOGASTRIC VARICEAL BLEEDING

Definition Upper GI (UGI) bleeding caused by **ruptured varices** of the **distal esophagus** and the **proximal stomach.**

Etiology Portal hypertension.

Epidemiology Variceal bleeding is the most life-threatening complication of PH, and it is responsible for 30% of all deaths in patients with cirrhosis. The risk of death is closely related to the degree of liver disease, and it is highest in patients with Child-Pugh class C disease. Patients with PH due to extrahepatic disease rarely die from variceal bleeding. The risk of bleeding becomes greater as varices enlarge. Eighty percent of patients bleed from esophageal varices, and 20% bleed from gastric ones. Approximately 40% of patients will have recurrent bleeding within 6 weeks of the presenting episode, and 80% of untreated patients will have a recurrent bleed within 2 years.

Symptoms The severity of the bleeding determines symptoms. Patients with acute, significant bleeding may present with weakness, pallor, and mental status changes.

Physical Exam and Signs Most patients with bleeding varices have alcoholic cirrhosis (the signs and stigmata of cirrhosis have been described in the previous section). Jaundice, hepatosplenomegaly, and ascites may be present. Signs of bleeding may include hemodynamic alterations, such as tachycardia, hypotension, and even shock. Patients may have melena and even bright red blood per rectum if the bleeding is severe.

Differential The workup of an UGI bleed should include a rapid assessment of the various causes of this presentation (see Algorithm 3).

Diagnosis The first test for the diagnosis of variceal bleeding is an **upper GI endoscopy,** which can also serve as a therapeutic maneuver if varices are confirmed.

Labs. The possibility of coagulopathies needs to be investigated, so a PT/INR and an aPTT are required. Serial hemoglobin measurements help in assessing the clinical evolution of the patient. Other lab tests may be performed to determine the underlying cause of the PH.

Imaging. CTA has replaced the need for an angiogram, but it is seldom used in acute situations.

Complication(s) Severe hemodynamic instability, exacerbation of liver failure, and shock may occur. Mortality is higher with progressive degrees of liver failure.

Treatment The first and most important step is to provide **resuscitation** with restoration of vascular compartment volume, usually with **isotonic crystalloid solutions.** Patients must be admitted to an intensive care unit, blood should be typed and crossmatched, and prophylactic antibiotics must be administered. Endotracheal intubation is indicated to allow an upper GI endoscopy (and other procedures) once the patient is stable, and either **variceal ligation with rubber bands**—the preferred, more successful method—or **sclerotherapy** may be used to control bleeding. Hemostasis is achieved through endoscopic therapy in 80% of cases. **Octreotide**—a synthetic analogue of somatostatin, which decreases the blood flow to the portal system through vasoconstriction—is administered intravenously. In cases of massive bleeding, a temporizing treatment is the use of a balloon tamponade, usually a Sengstaken-Blakemore tube, which requires tracheal intubation. This tube should not be in place longer than 24 hours; another definitive therapy must be provided after this time. When all else fails, a surgical procedure must be considered, and an effective and preferred approach is the **transjugular intrahepatic portosystemic shunt** (TIPS) procedure, which is performed by an interventional radiologist under fluoroscopic control. It is done by placing a stent between the hepatic and portal venous circulation. The TIPS procedure also serves as a bridge to liver transplantation. If TIPS is not feasible, a more traditional surgical approach may be needed (eg, portosystemic shunt).

SOLID BENIGN LIVER TUMORS

Definition A variety of benign tumors of the liver that include hemangiomas, focal nodular hyperplasia (FNH), and hepatic adenoma (HA).

Etiology The etiology of hemangiomas is not well understood. It is thought that they are outgrowths of endothelium. FNH is believed to be related to a developmental vascular malformation. HAs are the result of benign proliferation of hepatocytes and are strongly associated with **oral contraceptive use.**

Epidemiology Approximately 15% to 20% of the population has benign localized liver masses. The most common benign tumor of the liver is a **hemangioma** (3%–20% of cases). The second most common benign liver tumor is FNH (8%), followed by HAs. All 3 benign tumors are more common in women, and FNH and HA are predominantly seen in **young women.**

Symptoms FNH is asymptomatic and is usually discovered incidentally, at the time of a laparotomy or during imaging studies. The same is true of hemangiomas, although sometimes large masses can produce vague symptoms. HAs become symptomatic approximately 75% of the time, frequently with upper abdominal pain caused by hemorrhage into the tumor.

Physical Exam and Signs Exam is almost always negative, even in cases of a ruptured HA, unless the hemorrhage is severe.

Differential A finding through imaging (or laparotomy) frequently triggers an investigation to establish whether the tumor is benign or malignant. With modern imaging, the distinction is usually reasonably easy to make, but occasionally it might be necessary to obtain tissue for histopathologic confirmation. Tumor markers are helpful in separating these tumors from hepatocellular carcinomas.

Diagnosis All 3 of these tumors may be investigated by **CT scan** and **MRI.**

Labs. Liver function tests and tumor markers are normal.

Imaging. The imaging of choice for the diagnosis of a hemangioma is MRI, with a specificity of 85% and a sensitivity of 95%. Hemangiomas can be seen on CT as well, and on both imaging studies they appear as bright lesions with **peripheral enhancement.** Hemangiomas are usually single, and they seldom measure greater than 5 cm in largest diameter. When they are larger, they are called *giant hemangiomas.* FNH is best diagnosed via CT scan, on which it appears as a **homogeneous mass,** characterized by a **central scar with radiating septa.** However, in 15% of patients, this is not the case, making radiologic differentiation between a benign tumor and a malignant tumor not possible. FNH usually presents as a mass measuring less than 5 cm. A HA appears as a well-circumscribed **heterogeneous mass** with early enhancement on CT scanning, but it can be difficult to distinguish from FNH, in which case an MRI is indicated.

Complication(s) HAs have a 25% chance of rupturing and hemorrhaging, and they rarely undergo malignant transformation. Complications of FNH are exceedingly rare, and the possibility of rupture of a hemangioma is just as unlikely.

Treatment If asymptomatic, hemangiomas and FNH are managed by observation. HAs must be evaluated according to their risk of rupture.

Serial imaging and expectant management are indicated when these tumors measure less than 4 cm, and those that are greater than 4 cm should be resected. Oral contraceptives should be discontinued.

MALIGNANT LIVER TUMORS

Definition Malignant tumors of the liver can be primary, such as **hepatocellular carcinoma** (HCC)—also known as *hepatoma*—or secondary.

Etiology HCC is strongly linked to chronic hepatitis B, hepatitis C, and cirrhosis. HCC may be present in patients with hepatitis B in the absence of cirrhosis, whereas HCC in patients with chronic hepatitis C is commonly associated with cirrhosis. However, cirrhosis is not a prerequisite for the development of HCC, nor is it a predictable consequence. Among patients with cirrhosis, the incidence of HCC is estimated to be 1% to 6%. An association has been noted with hemochromatosis, α_1-antitrypsin deficiency, and nonalcoholic fatty liver disease, also known as *nonalcoholic steatohepatitis*, or NASH, which is a possible sequela of obesity. Other risk factors include alcohol, tobacco, and hepatotoxins.

Epidemiology HCC is the most common **primary malignancy** of the liver, and although it is rare in the United States, it is quite common in Asia and Africa. HCC is more common in men, and its incidence increases with age. In the United States, its incidence has been steadily increasing, and it is becoming one of the most common cancer types responsible for a growing cancer mortality. The most common secondary malignant liver tumor is due to **metastatic cancer.**

Symptoms Patients report **weight loss** and **weakness.** Right upper quadrant pain or epigastric pain is common. This presentation is usually seen at an advanced stage because early on, symptoms are vague or nonexistent. If the patient has underlying cirrhosis, the symptoms may be due to hepatic decompensation. Occasionally, patients may present with symptoms due to distant metastases.

Physical Exam and Signs Hepatomegaly and a **palpable mass** are common findings.

Differential The differential is primarily focused on whether the tumor is benign or malignant, and if malignancy is suspected, it is necessary to determine whether the lesion is primary or metastatic.

Diagnosis The best imaging method is a matter of debate, but **CT** and **MRI** are more accurate than ultrasonography, which nevertheless is a reasonable screening modality if AFP levels are also elevated.

Labs. Besides the lab findings expected with cirrhosis, the patient should be tested for viral infections. AFP level greater than 400 ng/mL may be considered diagnostic if associated imaging studies are confirmatory. AFP levels are helpful in monitoring the results of treatment and in screening for recurrence. An α_1-antitrypsin level should be obtained.

Imaging. Ultrasound is only 60% sensitive, and images are difficult to interpret with a background of cirrhosis. Contrast-enhanced CT findings and MRI reveal a **hypervascular pattern** in the arterial phase. However, MRI is more accurate than CT. Sometimes the tumor is associated with a capsule and a variable internal structure. Small lesions might be missed. Controversy regarding biopsy of the lesion is ongoing, because of the risks of bleeding and seeding the tumor. In general, small lesions (<1 cm) can be observed, and a biopsy is reasonable if the mass measures between 1 and 2 cm in diameter.

Complication(s) Possible complications include hemorrhage, progression of the disease, and liver failure. Metastases are most commonly seen in the peritoneal cavity, bones, and lungs.

Treatment Liver function is a vital element when treatment options are considered. Resection or complete hepatectomy and transplantation is the treatment of choice for noncirrhotic patients; this disease is resectable in only 10% to 20% of patients. Early-stage HCC may be ablated with percutaneous ethanol injection. Cryotherapy (freezing) and radiofrequency ablation (high-frequency alternating current) have been used with variable results.

BIBLIOGRAPHY

Biecker E. Portal hypertension and gastrointestinal bleeding: diagnosis, prevention and management. *World J Gastroenterol.* 2013;19(31):5035-5050.

Chiche L, Adam JP. Diagnosis and management of benign liver tumors. *Semin Liver Dis.* 2013;33(3):236-247.

CLINICAL KEYS: QUESTIONS AND ANSWERS

What is portal hypertension?	An increase in portal venous pressure
What is the most common cause of portal hypertension in the United States?	Alcohol use
What are the signs of portal hypertension?	Scleral icterus up to frank jaundice; stigmata such as spider nevi, palmar erythema, and gynecomastia; splenomegaly, asterixis, caput medusae, and hemorrhoids
What are the most common complications of portal hypertension?	Variceal bleeding, ascites, and hepatic encephalopathy
What is the first-line prophylactic measure used to prevent variceal bleeding?	A beta-blocker, such as propranolol
What is the first step in managing ascites?	Limiting salt intake
What is the first step in managing hepatic encephalopathy?	Limiting dietary protein
What is the Child-Pugh classification system used for?	To determine the functional reserve of the liver

What is the most common cause of variceal bleeding?	Uncontrolled portal hypertension
How is variceal bleeding treated?	Variceal ligation with rubber bands or sclerotherapy
How is a transjugular intrahepatic portosystemic shunt (TIPS) procedure performed?	By placing a stent between the hepatic and portal venous circulation
What is the most common benign liver tumor?	Hemangioma
How is hemangioma diagnosed?	MRI
How do hemangiomas appear on imaging?	Bright lesions with peripheral enhancement
How does focal nodular hyperplasia appear on CT scan?	Homogeneous mass, characterized by a central scar with radiating septa
What is the most common primary malignant liver tumor?	Hepatocellular carcinoma

Biliary System

16

When hepatocytes secrete bile, the bile flows through a network of biliary canaliculi that become confluent to form the **right and left hepatic ducts** (Fig. 16-1).

The right and left hepatic ducts join to form the **common hepatic duct,** which becomes known as the **common bile duct** (CBD) at the point where the **cystic duct** of the gallbladder enters it.

The CBD enters the pancreatic parenchyma for a short trajectory and empties into the second portion of the duodenum at the **ampulla of Vater.** The **sphincter of Oddi** surrounds the CBD at its distal end and is independent of the duodenal musculature.

An anatomic landmark of significance is **the triangle of Calot,** bound by the **cystic duct, the common hepatic duct, and the inferior border of the liver.** Within this triangle lies the **cystic artery.**

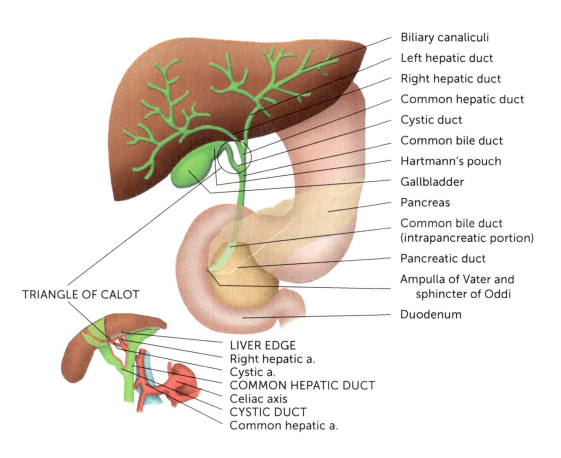

Fig. 16-1. Gallbladder and Triangle of Calot

Surgery 251

Cholelithiasis

Definition Cholelithiasis is the **presence of gallstones in the gallbladder.** The stones are crystalline bodies with varying composition.

Etiology Approximately 70% to 90% of gallstones are composed of **cholesterol.** These stones form when bile is supersaturated with cholesterol (lithogenic bile), which precipitates into crystals and subsequently macroscopic stones. About 15% of patients have **pigment stones**—either brown or black. Black stones are hard and composed of calcium bilirubinate, calcium phosphate, and calcium carbonate. Brown stones are soft, and the presence of both bacteria (*Escherichia coli, Klebsiella*) and ductal stasis is commonly a prerequisite for their development. Most patients have mixed stones.

Epidemiology The disease affects more than 20 million people in the United States. **Native Americans** have the highest incidence of cholesterol stones. Women have a higher incidence of gallstones, with a ratio of 2:1. Other risk factors include increasing age, obesity, rapid weight loss, Crohn's disease, terminal ileal resection, pregnancy, prolonged fasting (eg, patients on total parenteral nutrition), and sickle cell disease.

Symptoms Sixty percent to 80% of patients with cholelithiasis are **asymptomatic.** Approximately 1% to 2% of asymptomatic patients become symptomatic yearly. **Biliary colic** is classically described as **episodic epigastric or right upper quadrant (RUQ) pain,** which may radiate to the back and right shoulder. Pain is commonly **postprandial** and may last from 30 minutes to a few hours. The pain is usually steady, as opposed to the intermittent presentation of intestinal colic, and is not relieved by antacids. The pain is caused by contraction of the gallbladder against a stone that is **transiently** obstructing the gallbladder neck, the cystic duct, or the CBD. Episodes may be associated with nausea and vomiting.

Physical Exam and Signs Asymptomatic cholelithiasis does not exhibit any specific findings on physical exam, and the same is commonly true of transient biliary colic. Patients may sometimes exhibit mild RUQ tenderness.

Differential Duodenal ulcer: Epigastric pain relieved with antacids, negative RUQ ultrasound. **Hiatal hernia:** Epigastric pain/discomfort,

±reflux, upper GI series reveals hernia. **Myocardial infarction:** ±Chest pain, ±ECG findings, ±cardiac-specific enzymes. **Pancreatitis:** Epigastric pain typically radiating to the back, ±↑amylase, ±↑lipase, ±n/v. **Biliary dyskinesia:** Biliary colic symptoms, no stones/demonstrable organic gallbladder abnormality, cholecystokinin hepatoiminodiacetic acid (CCK HIDA) scan ejection fraction <30%.

Diagnosis The test of choice for diagnosing cholelithiasis is an **abdominal ultrasound,** which has a sensitivity of 95% and a specificity of 99%.

Labs. Asymptomatic gallstones have no associated laboratory abnormality.

Imaging. Ultrasound sometimes will show gallstones with **posterior acoustic shadows** (Fig. 16-2). Fifty percent of pigment stones are radio-opaque and as a result are visible on a plain abdominal radiograph.

Treatment Asymptomatic cholelithiasis does not require treatment. Exceptions may be made when gallstones are large (>2 cm), which increases the chance of obstruction, or when the gallbladder is diffusely calcified, because this increases the risk of carcinoma. For **symptomatic cholelithiasis,** laparoscopic cholecystectomy (LC) is the therapy of choice.

Complication(s) The most common complication of cholelithiasis is **acute cholecystitis.** Other complications include choledocholithiasis, cholangitis, and stone-induced pancreatitis.

CHOLECYSTITIS

Definition Cholecystitis is an **inflammatory response of the gallbladder.**

Etiology Cholecystitis occurs when an **unremitting obstruction of Hartmann's pouch or of the of cystic duct takes place.** In 95% of cases, the obstruction is caused by calculi. Typically this is an acute problem. However, patients may develop chronic cholecystitis, a low-grade inflammatory response associated with repeated episodes of biliary colic, which may lead to fibrosis and contraction of the gallbladder wall and loss of function. About 5% of patients present with **acalculous cholecystitis,** in which no calculi are present.

Acalculous cholecystitis has an unclear etiology, although stasis and ischemic insults have been implicated.

Epidemiology Approximately 2% to 3% of patients with symptomatic cholelithiasis develop cholecystitis. Although cholecystitis is an inflammatory process caused by obstruction, it may become infectious in as many as 50% of cases, most often as a polymicrobial insult. The most commonly cultured bacteria are **gram-negative organisms,** such as *E coli, Pseudomonas,* and *Klebsiella* species. Acalculous cholecystitis is more common in patients hospitalized with critical illness, and after trauma, burns, or major operations. In approximately 85% of patients with acute cholecystitis, symptoms subside within a few days.

Symptoms Patients experience RUQ pain that does not subside, unlike biliary colic, and is exacerbated by movement. The pain is more often associated with nausea, vomiting, and anorexia than the symptoms present in an episode of biliary colic.

Physical Exam and Signs Moderate to severe RUQ tenderness to palpation and guarding are typical exam findings. This commonly prevents the examiner from detecting an enlarged gallbladder, although one might be present 15% to 20% of the time. Also common are fever and **Murphy's sign,** represented by pain and inspiratory arrest while the RUQ is palpated during inspiration. Mild jaundice may be present.

Differential Duodenal ulcer: Epigastric pain relieved with antacids, negative RUQ ultrasound. **Pancreatitis:** Epigastric pain typically radiating to the back, ±↑amylase, ±↑lipase, ±n/v. **Acute pyelonephritis:** Flank and/or back pain, ±dysuria, frequency, hematuria (gross or microscopic), bacteriuria, fever.

Diagnosis The initial diagnostic test for cholecystitis is an **ultrasound,** which in this case has a sensitivity of 90% and a specificity of 80%. Confirmation of cholecystitis may be obtained with HIDA scanning, although it is not as sensitive and specific as ultrasound. A HIDA scan that results in non-visualization of the gallbladder suggests that the cystic duct is obstructed (the most common reason for cholecystitits to occur).

Labs. Mild leukocytosis ($12,000/mm^3$–$15,000/mm^3$) is common, but often the white blood cell count is normal. Elevation in alkaline phosphatase, elevation in bilirubin (up to 3 mg/dL), and occasionally elevation in amylase may occur.

Imaging. **Ultrasound** shows **stones in the gallbladder** (not in the cystic duct), **gallbladder wall thickening** (>4 mm), and typically **pericholecystic fluid** (see Fig. 16-2). A **sonographic Murphy's sign** (tenderness over the gallbladder elicited by the ultrasound probe) may be present. A gallbladder that is not visible constitutes a positive result.

Complication(s) The most common complications of acute cholecystitis include:

1. **Empyema.** This condition occurs in approximately 2% to 3% of patients with acute cholecystitis. The pain becomes severe and unrelenting. Fever spikes higher, and the abdominal exam is associated with significant tenderness and/or guarding. Leukocytosis is greater than 15,000/mm3.

2. **Perforation and gangrene.** Ten percent of patients with acute cholecystitis develop a perforation, and in 1% of cases, a free perforation is associated with peritonitis. High fever, systemic signs of toxicity (eg, tachycardia, increased respiratory rate), increasing abdominal pain with rebound tenderness, and hypoactive bowel sounds are indicators that a perforation has occurred. In 1% to 3% of patients, a perforation develops into a hollow viscus, most often in the duodenum, to form a cholecysto-enteric fistula. This complication may lead to a **gallstone ileus,** in which a large stone obstructs the small intestine. Gangrene occurs more rapidly in patients with acalculous cholecystitis.

3. **Emphysematous cholecystitis.** This acute infection of the gallbladder wall is caused by gas-forming organisms, most commonly *Clostridia*. It is a rare event that is more commonly seen in elderly patients with acalculous cholecystitis or diabetes. Treatment requires high doses of antibiotics and surgery. Emphysematous cholecystitis is associated with mortality rates as high as 20%.

Treatment Initial management of acute cholecystitis involves keeping the patient on a **nothing-by-mouth status** (NPO) while administering parenteral fluids and antibiotics. The next step is a **cholecystectomy,** which may be performed immediately or after the acute episode subsides. However, performing the surgery within 72 hours of the onset of symptoms is advantageous. In the case of acalculous cholecystitis, it is imperative to perform the surgery early in the presentation because of the high probability of significant complications otherwise. This is also true in cases of gangrene and perforation.

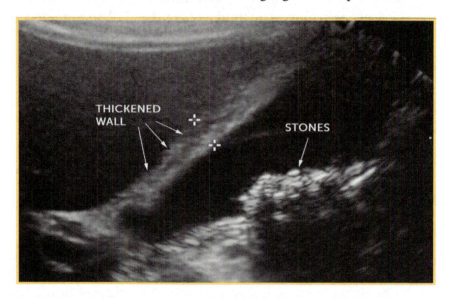

Fig. 16-2. Cholelithiasis with Ultrasonographic Signs of Cholecystitis

CHOLEDOCHOLITHIASIS

Definition Choledocholithiasis is the presence of gallstones in the CBD.

Etiology Gallstones in the CBD are typically the result of them passing from the gallbladder through the cystic duct **(secondary stones)**. Gallstones may also form in the common ducts **(primary stones)**, a phenomenon that applies commonly to brown pigment stones.

Epidemiology Approximately 10% to 15% of patients with cholelithiasis have CBD stones at the time of cholecystectomy. In the United States, 80% to 90% of CBD stones are secondary. Asian populations frequently have primary brown pigment CBD stones, which result from infestation with the parasites *Ascaris lumbricoides* or *Clonorchis sinensis*.

Symptoms Choledocholithiasis is caused by obstruction of a duct in the biliary tree; therefore, it may mimic symptoms of biliary colic that are indistinguishable from those caused by cholelithiasis.

Physical Exam and Signs Exam findings are similar to those seen in cholelithiasis. The most common sign is **jaundice.**

Differential The differential is similar to that of acute cholecystitis, and the workup is related to the presenting symptoms and signs. Jaundice would require investigation of an intrahepatic versus extrahepatic cause.

Diagnosis The initial imaging test is typically an **ultrasound,** although it shows gallstones in the CBD in only 50% of cases. It will, however, reveal stones in the gallbladder and CBD dilatation, a finding expected when the CBD is obstructed.

Labs. An obstructed CBD typically associated with serum bilirubin levels between 3 and 10 mg/dL and an elevation in alkaline phosphatase.

Imaging. After ultrasound, **endoscopic retrograde cholangiopancreatography** (ERCP) may be used to confirm diagnosis and to extract stones (Fig. 16-3). An **intraoperative cholangiogram** (IOC) may confirm choledocholithiasis during LC in some cases.

Complication(s) Cholangitis, jaundice, or biliary pancreatitis may develop.

Treatment Gallstones in the CBD, if less than 1 cm in largest diameter, may pass spontaneously. If they do not pass, the treatment of choice for choledocholithiasis is an **endoscopic sphincterotomy with stone extraction.** In this procedure, the sphincter of Oddi is approached with a side-viewing endoscope and is incised radially to enlarge it (Fig. 16-3). An experienced endoscopist is successful in 85% to 90% of cases. If this is unsuccessful, the patient will require an operative procedure, which may be attempted laparoscopically.

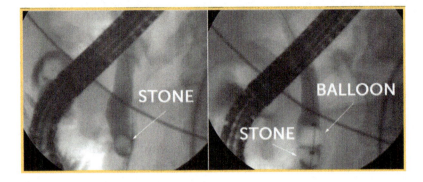

Fig. 16-3. Endoscopic Retrograde Cholangiopancreatography (ERCP) Stone Extraction. *Left panel:* A gallstone is visible in the common bile duct. *Right panel:* A balloon is inserted into the common bile duct to retrieve the gallstone after sphincterotomy.

CHOLANGITIS

Definition Cholangitis is an **ascending bacterial infection** of the biliary ductal system.

Etiology Cholangitis is always due to an obstruction of the biliary ducts, and the most common cause is **choledocholithiasis.** The next most common cause is manipulation of the CBD, usually by ERCP. Other causes include strictures, stents, and carcinoma.

Symptoms The most common symptom is RUQ pain.

Physical Exam and Signs **Charcot's triad,** which includes **fever, RUQ pain, and jaundice,** is seen in 70% to 75% of patients. Of the 3, fever is the most consistent finding and is seen in 90% of cases. A severe form of the disease is **suppurative cholangitis,** which may be associated with **Reynold's pentad** (Charcot's triad with altered mental status and hypotension).

Differential Other diagnostic possibilities are similar to those considered in cases of acute cholecystitis and choledocholithiasis, particularly if the distinction requires separating intrahepatic (eg, acute alcoholic hepatitis, alcoholic cirrhosis) causes of obstruction from extrahepatic ones (eg, carcinoma compressing the CBD).

Diagnosis The test of choice is ERCP, which is both diagnostic and therapeutic. With this test, cholangiography can be performed, as well as a biopsy or stent placement into the common bile duct if necessary.

Labs. Elevated LFTs and leukocytosis commonly >20,000/mm^3. The bilirubin elevation is seldom as high as that seen with a neoplasm, because the obstruction is usually transient, and levels tend to fluctuate.

Imaging. Cholangiography through ERCP shows the level of the obstruction.

Complication(s) Long-standing or repeated bouts of biliary ductal infection may lead to intrahepatic abscess formation.

Treatment Acute ascending cholangitis is a medical emergency. If signs and symptoms of systemic toxicity are not present, initial management consists of correction of fluid and electrolyte imbalances and administration of broad-spectrum antibiotics to cover the most common organisms—*E coli, Klebsiella,* enterococci, and *Bacteroides*. In a toxic patient, an urgent endoscopic decompression with ERCP is mandatory. If unsuccessful, decompression may be accomplished with **percutaneous transhepatic cholangiography** (PTC) and drainage or with traditional operative decompression, which requires T-tube drainage of the CBD.

GALLBLADDER CARCINOMA

Definition Gallbladder carcinoma, as its name suggests, is cancer arising in the gallbladder, most frequently **adenocarcinoma.**

Etiology The risk factor most commonly associated with gallbladder carcinoma is the presence of gallstones (95% of cases). PSC, choledochal cysts, and **porcelain gallbladder** (diffusely calcified) are also associated risk factors.

Epidemiology Gallbladder carcinoma is the most common cancer of the biliary tract and has a poor prognosis unless it is found incidentally during cholecystectomy. More than two-thirds of cases affect individuals older than 70 years, and females are represented by a 3:1 ratio over males. Approximately 1% of cholecystectomy specimens harbor a carcinoma.

Symptoms Abdominal pain is the most common complaint, frequently following the pattern of symptomatic cholelithiasis and/or cholecystitis. Unexplained weight loss is also common.

Physical Exam and Signs Patients may present with a mass in the RUQ, sometimes associated with jaundice.

Differential The workup commonly considers symptomatic cholelithiasis, cholecystitis, obstruction of the CBD, and periampullary tumors if jaundice is associated.

Diagnosis The diagnosis is seldom made preoperatively—one-third of cases are found incidentally during cholecystectomy. Ultrasound is always the first diagnostic test used to diagnose gallbladder carcinoma; it may reveal wall thickening or porcelain gallbladder, or a mass, in which case a CT scan should follow.

Labs. Lab abnormalities depend on presentation and stage of the carcinoma. When it is found incidentally, no abnormalities may be noted. If a tumor obstructs the gallbladder, lab findings may be similar to those of cholecystitis, with an elevated white blood cell count. If surrounding structures are invaded, bilirubin and alkaline phosphatase levels may be elevated.

Imaging. Ultrasound may show a heterogeneous mass within the lumen. CT will also reveal a mass and provide information regarding invasion of adjacent structures.

Complication(s) Obstruction of the CBD or liver abscesses may develop.

Treatment Surgery is the only treatment approach if the tumor is diagnosed at an early stage. Invasion beyond the gallbladder wall makes it unlikely that surgery will be curative.

CHOLANGICARCINOMA

Definition Cholangiocarcinoma (CC) is a rare primary malignancy of the biliary ductal system arising from the bile duct epithelium.

Etiology Unknown. Gallstones, hepatitis, and cirrhosis are not believed to increase risk. PSC, ulcerative colitis, and male gender are commonly associated with CC.

Epidemiology CC is less common than gallbladder carcinoma, with an incidence of approximately 5000 new cases per year in the United States. The average age of onset is 65 years. CC is classified according to its anatomic location and growth pattern. Forty percent of

CC tumors are found in the extrahepatic upper duct region, where the common hepatic duct bifurcates. These are known as Klatskin or *hilar tumors*. Forty percent of tumors are found in the extrahepatic lower duct region, and the remaining 20% are intrahepatic. A great majority are adenocarcinomas, and a small percentage present as squamous cell carcinoma.

Symptoms In advanced stages, pain in the RUQ and weight loss are common. Pruritus may be present if the patient is jaundiced.

Physical Exam and Signs Jaundice is the most common sign. If the obstruction is distal, the gallbladder is frequently distended, and it can be palpated without eliciting pain. This is known as **Courvoisier's sign (painless jaundice),** which is frequently seen in patients with periampullary tumors.

Differential The workup centers around the differential diagnosis of jaundice and its variety of causes (see Algorithm 1).

Diagnosis As is commonly the case with diseases of the biliary tract, ultrasonography is usually the first test used in diagnosis. However, the diagnostic test of choice is **cholangiography** performed via ERCP or PTC. A CT scan eventually needs to be obtained to delineate the extent of the disease. Magnetic resonance cholangiopancreatography (MRCP) may be useful as well.

Labs. Elevated bilirubin and alkaline phosphatase levels are common lab findings.

Imaging. Ultrasound may reveal dilatation of the intrahepatic ductal system, and sometimes may show a mass. ERCP is extremely useful in detecting tumors through cholangiography and offers the added benefit of allowing cells to be obtained for cytologic/histologic analysis. PTC may delineate the level and degree of the obstruction, particularly when ERCP cannot show proximal (hilar) lesions.

Complication(s) Obstruction may lead to severe jaundice, pruritus, and cholangitis.

Treatment The primary treatment is resection, but frequently this is only palliative. ERCP may be used for therapeutic decompression when surgery is not possible.

Bibliography

Boutros C, Gary M, Baldwin K, Somasundar P. Gallbladder cancer: past, present and an uncertain future. *Surg Oncol.* 2012;21(4):e183-191.

Duncan CB, Riall TS. Evidence-based current surgical practice: calculous gallbladder disease. *J Gastrointest Surg.* 2012;16(11):2011-2025.

Clinical Keys: Questions and Answers

What are the borders of the triangle of Calot?	The cystic duct, the common hepatic duct, and the inferior border of the liver
What are the majority of gallstones composed of?	Cholesterol
What are some of the risk factors for developing gallstones?	Increasing age, obesity, pregnancy, terminal ileal resection, Crohn's disease
What is the test of choice to diagnose cholelithiasis?	Ultrasound
How does symptomatic cholelithiasis present?	Episodic epigastric and right upper quadrant pain, typically postprandial
What is the treatment of choice for symptomatic cholelithiasis?	Cholecystectomy
What is cholecystitis?	Inflammation of the gallbladder due to an obstruction of the cystic duct
What are the symptoms of cholecystitis?	Right upper quadrant pain and low-grade fever; nausea and vomiting common
What is a positive Murphy's sign?	Pain and inspiratory arrest while the right upper quadrant is palpated, signaling cholecystitis

What are the ultrasonographic findings of cholecystitis?	Gallstones in the gallbladder, thickened gallbladder wall, pericholecystic fluid
What is the treatment of choice for cholecystitis?	Cholecystectomy
What is cholangitis?	An ascending bacterial infection of the biliary ductal system
What is Charcot's triad?	Fever, right upper quadrant pain, and jaundice, a manifestation of cholangitis
What is Reynold's pentad?	Charcot's triad with altered mental status and hypotension (associated with cholangitis)
What is the treatment of choice for cholangitis?	IV antibiotics and ERCP with decompression of the common bile duct
What is Courvoisier's sign?	Painless jaundice with a palpable distended gallbladder, signaling a periampullary tumor
What organisms are most commonly associated with cholangitis?	*Escherichia coli, Klebsiella,* enterococci, *Bacteroides*

Pancreas 17

The pancreas is an entirely retroperitoneal structure that is divided into 4 anatomic segments—the head, the neck, the body, and the tail (Fig. 17-1).

The pancreatic duct exits into the duodenum via the **duct of Wirsung,** which fuses with the distal common bile duct. This exit point in the second portion of the duodenum is called the **ampulla of Vater,** or *major papilla.*

The complex muscle mechanism that controls the outflow of pancreatic secretions and bile into the duodenum is called the **sphincter of Oddi.** An accessory pancreatic duct, the **duct of Santorini** (present in ~40% of individuals), drains through a lesser papilla that is more proximal than the ampulla of Vater within the duodenum.

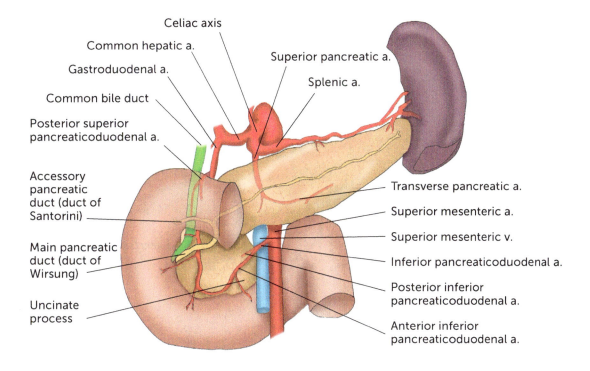

Fig. 17-1. Anatomy of the Pancreas

Acute Pancreatitis

Definition Pancreatitis is an **inflammatory process of the pancreas** of variable severity.

Etiology In the vast majority (~80%) of cases, pancreatitis is caused by **gallstones or chronic alcohol use.** In another 5% of cases, it is induced by **endoscopic retrograde cholangiopancreatography (ERCP).** In the remaining cases, it results from medications, hypertriglyceridemia, hypercalcemia, obstructing neoplasms, heredity, trauma, and pancreatic divisum. Gallstones cause a temporary obstruction (Fig. 17-2) as they flow into the distal common bile duct. The exact mechanism of how this triggers pancreatitis is not completely understood. Possibly, pancreatitis is caused by reflux of bile into the pancreatic duct or from pancreatic duct hypertension induced by the obstruction.

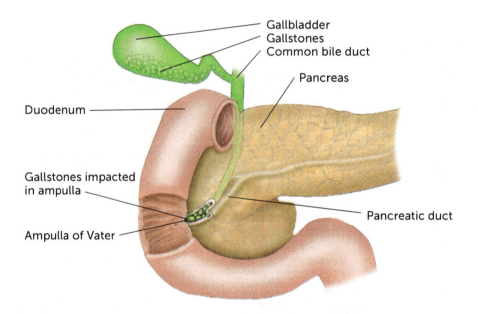

Fig. 17-2. Mechanism of Biliary Pancreatitis

Epidemiology There are various causes of pancreatitis, so there is no specific age range in which the disease is more prevalent.

Symptoms Most patients report severe **epigastric pain** that often **radiates to the back.** Nausea and vomiting is common.

Physical Exam and Signs Patients typically appear ill. **Tachycardia** may be present as can **hypotension secondary to hypovolemia.** Palpation of the abdomen illicits severe pain and possibly guarding. Abdominal distention may be noted. Flank ecchymosis, known as **Grey Turner's sign,** or periumbilical ecchymosis, **known as Cullen's sign,** result from hemorrhage associated with severe pancreatitis. Blood travels through the retroperitoneum and is visible on the abdomen. These signs have been associated with a 40% mortality rate.

Differential Acute cholecystitis: Epigastric/right upper quadrant (RUQ) pain, ±Murphy's sign, fever, fatty food intolerance, nausea/vomiting. **Perforated peptic ulcer:** Epigastric pain, peritonitis, history of ulcer disease, free air on abdominal radiograph. **Ischemic bowel:** Severe abdominal pain, guarding, ±rebound tenderness, recent hypotension, history of vascular or heart disease that may lead to arterial embolus. **Bowel obstruction:** Abdominal distention, nausea/vomiting, history of prior surgery (adhesions), abdominal wall hernias.

Diagnosis The diagnosis is made with a combination of clinical presentation, labs, and imaging, and it is confirmed when serum amylase and lipase levels are elevated. **Ranson's criteria** (Table 17-1) are used to determine degree of severity and predict mortality.

Labs. **Serum amylase** is considered the most useful test—levels rise within 2 to 12 hours of symptoms. **Serum lipase** is more sensitive for pancreatic disease, but specificity ranges from 50% to 95%. The degree of elevation of amylase and lipase levels does not determine severity. Hepatic function panel should be drawn to assess for biliary involvement.

Imaging. **CT** helps to assess the degree of inflammation and pancreatic necrosis; sensitivity and specificity are 90% and 100%, respectively. It can be used to determine whether abscesses, pseudocysts, and neoplasms are present. **MRI** can be performed instead of CT in patients allergic to contrast or in those with renal failure. **MR cholangiopancreatography (MRCP)** is better than CT at detecting cholelithiasis, choledocholithiasis, and pancreatic duct anomalies.

Table 17-1. Ranson's Criteria and Associated Mortality Rates

Admission
Age >55 yr
White blood cell count >16,000 cells/mm^3
Blood glucose >200 mg/dL
Serum lactate dehydrogenase >350 IU/L
Aspartate aminotransferase >250 IU/L
48 hr after Admission
Hematocrit decrease >10%
Blood urea nitrogen elevation >5 mg/dL
Serum calcium <8 mg/dL
Arterial Po$_2$ <60 mm Hg
Base deficit >4 mEq/L
Estimated fluid sequestration >6 L

Number of Ranson's Signs	Approximate Mortality
0–2	0%
3–4	15%
5–6	50%
>6	70%–90%

Complication(s) Severe pancreatitis can lead to multiple organ system dysfunction, including renal failure, pulmonary effusion, and acute respiratory distress syndrome. Necrotizing pancreatitis, infected pancreatic necrosis, pancreatic pseudocysts or abscesses, or venous thrombosis of the splenic, portal, or superior mesenteric vein may develop.

Treatment Mild cases of pancreatitis are usually **self-limited** and require only **supportive care** with **intravenous hydration** and **pain management.** Gallstone-induced pancreatitis requires **cholecystectomy** after the acute episode subsides to prevent further episodes. More severe forms of pancreatitis require intervention to support any organ dysfunction, such as intubation for respiratory failure or dialysis for renal failure. Clinical data do not definitively suggest that antibiotics should be used to treat severe cases. **Pancreatic abscesses** generally require drainage, either percutaneously or surgically. Nutritional support for severe cases is generally accomplished with total parenteral nutrition (TPN) or enteral feeding from a nasojejunal feeding tube.

Pancreatic Pseudocyst

Definition A pancreatic pseudocyst is a collection of pancreatic fluid contained within a wall of fibrous and inflammatory tissue. It is classified as a pseudocyst instead of a true cyst because there is **no epithelial lining** to the pseudocyst wall.

Etiology Disruption of a portion of a pancreatic duct—with or without obstruction—causes fluid collection within a pseudocyst.

Epidemiology Pseudocysts develop in about 10% of patients with acute pancreatitis. Pseudocysts can develop in up to one-third of patients with chronic pancreatitis, which makes this the most common complication in these patients.

Symptoms Pseudocysts typically are discovered at the time of initial workup for pancreatitis. Symptoms are essentially the same as for pancreatitis, which include **upper abdominal pain, nausea,** and **vomiting.** If the pseudocyst is large, it may cause **early satiety, abdominal fullness,** and **jaundice.** Many pseudocysts are **asymptomatic.**

Physical Exam and Signs Large pseudocysts are significant for abdominal tenderness to palpation and may present as a palpable, firm area on abdominal exam.

Differential The differential mostly centers around the different **histologic types** of cystic pancreatic neoplasms (CPNs). **Mucinous**

cystic neoplasm (MCN): Premalignant lesions, usually asymptomatic, more common in women than in men, represent 35% of CPNs. **Serous cystadenoma:** Benign lesions, more common in women than in men, usually asymptomatic, represent 30% of all CPNs. **Intraductal papillary mucinous tumors (IPMTs):** High malignant potential, slightly more common in men than in women, represent 25% of all CPNs. **Pancreatic abscess:** Peripancreatic fluid collection, fever, leukocytosis, ±rim enhancement or air within cavity on CT.

Diagnosis CT is the radiographic study of choice for diagnosing pseudocysts.

Labs. Lab workup is the same as for pancreatitis; serum amylase, serum lipase, and a liver function test should be obtained. The tumor markers **carcinoembryonic antigen (CEA)** and **CA19-9** should be measured.

Imaging. CT reveals the number of pseudocysts and their sizes (Fig. 17-3) and the qualities of the pseudocyst walls. All of these are factors that determine prognosis and guide treatment.

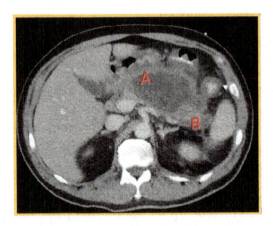

Fig. 17-3. CT Scan. **A:** Large pseudocyst. **B:** Pancreatic tail.

Complication(s) Pseudocysts may become infected and may require percutaneous or surgical drainage. Hemorrhage, obstruction, and rupture may occur.

Treatment Approximately 50% of pseudocysts resolve spontaneously. If no resolution occurs within 6 weeks, **percutaneous drainage** is generally required. The majority of pseudocysts larger than 6 cm require surgery. For pseudocysts that communicate with the pancreatic duct system, drainage alone results in fluid reaccumulation. Therefore, surgically connecting the pseudocyst to the stomach or jejunum, known as a *cystogastrostomy* or *cystojejunostomy,* respectively, keeps the pseudocyst from reforming, because the pancreatic secretions can enter into the GI tract directly.

PANCREATIC NEUROENDOCRINE TUMORS

Definition Pancreatic neuroendocrine tumors are tumors of varying malignant aggressiveness that arise within the islets of Langerhans.

Etiology Most pancreatic neuroendocrine tumors are sporadic without an identifiable cause. However, some are related to known genetic syndromes, such as multiple endocrine neoplasia I (MEN I), von Hippel–Lindau disease (VHL), neurofibromatosis 1, and tuberous sclerosis.

Epidemiology Pancreatic neuroendocrine tumors are rare and represent only about 5% of pancreatic tumors. They are slightly more common in women than in men and are usually discovered in the sixth decade of life. **Insulinomas** are the most common of these types of tumors, followed by **gastrinomas.**

Symptoms The majority of pancreatic neuroendocrine tumors are **asymptomatic** and found incidentally on imaging studies during evaluation for other conditions. Up to 40% cause a characteristic syndrome based on the type of hormone secreted (Table 17-2).

Table 17-2. Hormonally Active Tumors and Associated Clinical Syndromes

Tumor Type	Hormone Produced	Clinical Syndrome
Insulinoma	Insulin	Whipple's triad: (1) hypoglycemic symptoms during fasting, (2) fasting or exertional hypoglycemia with serum glucose levels <45 mg/dL, (3) symptom resolution with glucose administration
Gastrinoma	Gastrin	Abdominal pain, diarrhea, weight loss, multiple peptic ulcers, ~80% with dudodenal ulcers
VIPoma	Vasoactive intestinal peptide	Watery diarrhea, hypokalemia, achlorhydria (WDHA syndrome)
Glucagonoma	Glucagon	Necrolytic migratory erythema (skin rash), hyperglycemia, weight loss, anemia, deep vein thrombosis
Somatostatinoma	Somatostatin	Hyperglycemia, cholelithiasis, steatorrhea

Physical Exam and Signs Findings on exam may vary greatly depending on the type of pancreatic neuroendocrine tumor and its hormone production. The most common finding amongst all of the types of these tumors is **abdominal pain.**

Differential Pancreatic neuroendocrine tumors constitute a small fraction of pancreatic tumors, so the most common types of tumors must be ruled out. **Pancreatic adenocarcinoma:** Usually much more aggressive, commonly presents with jaundice and/or metastatic disease, abdominal pain, weight loss. **Pancreatic cystic neoplasms:** Typically contain cystic component, usually asymptomatic.

Diagnosis CT is the most effective initial imaging modality for detecting the primary lesion and metastatic disease (Fig. 17-4).

Labs. Lab work for functional pancreatic neuroendocrine tumors are specific to the type of tumor and can be tailored based on the clinical syndrome. Obtaining levels of the hormone that is suspected of causing the syndrome is the best initial step. A **chromogranin A** level is generally used as a tumor marker for pancreatic neuroendocrine tumors.

Imaging. Pancreatic neuroendocrine tumors are **hypervascular** and as a result, are **hyperdense** (appear brighter) on CT. If the tumor cannot be localized with CT, an octreotide scan or endoscopic ultrasound may be useful. An added benefit is that endoscopic ultrasound can also be used to obtain a tissue biopsy for pathologic evaluation.

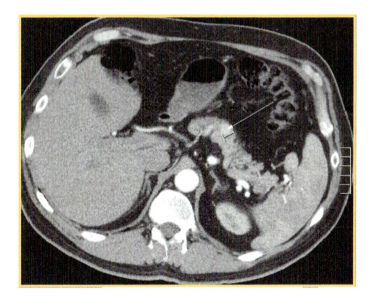

Fig. 17-4. CT with Pancreatic Neuroendocrine Tumor (hyperdense) in Pancreas Body

Complication(s) The complications are directly related to the hormone syndrome that is produced by functional pancreatic neuroendocrine tumors. Untreated tumors may metastasize and ultimately lead to death.

Treatment Surgical resection is the mainstay of treatment, which may require a **distal pancreatectomy** or a Whipple procedure depending on the tumor location. Treatment of metastatic disease must be individualized for each case. Most metastatic lesions are found in the liver. If amenable to resection, the metastatic disease should be resected along with the primary tumor. Systemic chemotherapy is not useful. Chemotherapy techniques directed into the liver have been shown to be beneficial. Somatostatin analogues are helpful in controlling symptoms from hormone secretion and may aid in slowing tumor growth.

Pancreatic Cancer

Definition Pancreatic cancer is a malignancy of the pancreas.

Etiology The exact etiology is unknown; however, hereditary disease, smoking, alcoholism, and chronic pancreatitis may increase the risk of developing pancreatic cancer.

Epidemiology **Pancreatic adenocarcinoma** is the most common type of pancreatic cancer. Pancreatic cancer is the fourth leading cause of cancer deaths in the United States. Patients are usually 65 years of age or older at the time of diagnosis. African Americans have a higher incidence of pancreatic cancer. Most patients present with incurable disease, and the **5-year survival rate is less than 5%.**

Symptoms Typically, symptoms are gradual in onset and nonspecific. Advanced disease may present with dull midepigastric pain and back pain, malaise, weight loss, nausea, and vomiting.

Physical Exam and Signs Scleral icterus, acholic (gray or light-colored) stools, dark-colored urine, and pruritus are signs related to an obstructed bile duct. An obstructed bile duct (Fig. 17-5) can cause a palpable, firm gallbladder with painless jaundice, which is known as **Courvoisier's sign.** Advanced metastatic disease may present with a palpable left supraclavicular lymph node known as **Virchow's node,** or a periumbilical lymph node, known as **Sister Mary Joseph's node.**

Differential Other types of pancreatic neoplasms should be ruled out and so should other causes of obstructing jaundice. **Cholangiocarcinoma (bile duct tumor):** Usually presents in the same manner as pancreatic cancer; treatment is essentially the same. **Pancreatic neuroendocrine tumor:** Less likely to present with jaundice. **Pancreatic lymphoma:** May present with bulky, locally advanced tumors; treatment is chemotherapy. **Benign biliary stricture:** Usually caused by gallstones; may be difficult to rule out malignancy.

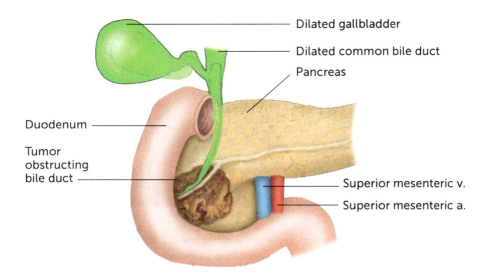

Fig. 17-5. Pancreatic Carcinoma

Diagnosis CT provides the best information for determining the extent of the disease and whether surgical resection is possible.

Labs. The level of tumor marker **CA19-9** is generally elevated with pancreatic adenocarcinoma. If the common bile duct is obstructed, the total bilirubin level remains elevated until the obstruction is alleviated with surgery or stent placement.

Imaging. **Endoscopic ultrasound** can help determine resectability by identifying possible vascular invasion from the tumor and can be used to obtain a biopsy of the tumor.

Complication(s) Pancreatic adenocarcinoma causes **biliary obstruction** and can also cause **gastric outlet obstruction** (Fig. 17-6). Biliary obstruction is treated with **ERCP** and **biliary stent placement.** Gastric outlet obstruction is treated **endoscopically** with stent placement or with **surgical bypass** of the tumor with a **gastrojejunostomy.** Metastatic disease is frequently present and greatly reduces survival.

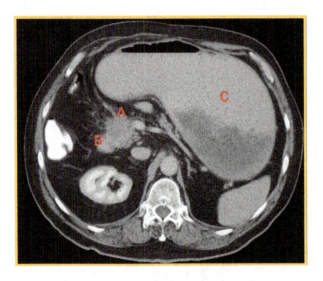

Fig. 17-6. CT Scan. **A:** Large pancreatic head mass. **B:** Duodenum (obstructed by tumor). **C:** Massively dilated stomach.

Treatment **Surgery** is the mainstay of treatment for pancreatic adenocarcinoma. If the tumor is in the pancreatic head, a Whipple procedure, in which an en bloc resection of the head of the pancreas, the entire duodenum, the distal stomach, the distal common bile duct, and the gallbladder is performed (Fig. 17-7). A **distal pancreatectomy** and **splenectomy** are performed for **pancreatic body and tail tumors.** Because pancreatic cancer is aggressive, all patients are offered chemotherapy following surgery. If the tumor is considered unresectable, chemotherapy and radiation may be offered as palliative treatment. Even with the best treatment options, cure is unusual, and lengthening survival may be the only attainable goal.

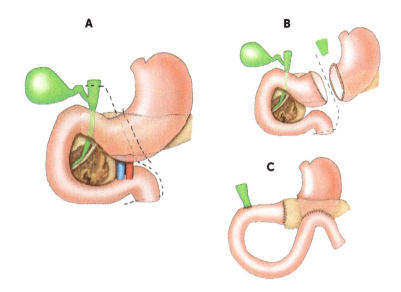

Fig. 17-7. Whipple Procedure. **A:** Tumor in head of pancreas. **B:** Resected specimen. **C:** One type of surgical reconstruction.

BIBLIOGRAPHY

April EW. *NMS Clinical Anatomy*. 3rd ed. Baltimore, MD: Williams & Wilkins; 1997.

Bartlett DL, Thirunavukarasu P, Neal MD. *Surgical Oncology: Fundamentals, Evidence-Based Approaches and New Technology*. New Delhi, India: Jaypee Brothers Medical Publishers; 2011.

Brunicardi FC, Andersen DK, Billiar TR, Dunn DL, Hunter JG, Pollock RE. *Schwartz's Principles of Surgery*. 8th ed. New York, NY: McGraw-Hill Medical Publishing; 2005

Clinical Keys: Questions and Answers

What is pancreatitis?	Inflammation of the pancreas
What are the 2 most common causes of pancreatitis?	Gallstones and alcohol use
What are the symptoms of pancreatitis?	Epigastric pain, nausea, and vomiting are common
What is Grey Turner's sign?	Flank ecchymosis from severe pancreatitis
What is Cullen's sign?	Periumbilical ecchymosis from severe pancreatitis
How is pancreatitis diagnosed?	Elevation of serum amylase and lipase, CT, clinical presentation
What is the initial treatment for pancreatitis?	IV fluids, pain management, nothing by mouth (NPO)
What is a pancreatic pseudocyst?	A collection of pancreatic fluid contained within a wall of fibrous and inflammatory tissue (no epithelial lining)
What are the symptoms of a pancreatic pseudocyst?	Similar to pancreatitis: upper abdominal pain, nausea, and vomiting
What is the treatment for a pancreatic pseudocyst?	Percutaneous drainage or surgery
What are the 2 most common types of pancreatic neuroendocrine tumors?	Insulinomas followed by gastrinomas
What clinical syndrome is associated with an insulinoma?	Whipple's triad: (1) hypoglycemic symptoms during fasting, (2) fasting or exertional hypoglycemia with serum glucose levels <45 mg/dL, (3) symptom resolution with glucose administration

What clinical syndrome is associated with a gastrinoma?	Abdominal pain, diarrhea, weight loss, multiple peptic ulcers, ~80% with dudodenal ulcers
What is the treatment of choice for a pancreatic neuroendocrine tumor?	Surgery
What is the most common type of pancreatic cancer?	Adenocarcinoma
What is the 5-year survival rate for pancreatic cancer?	Less than 5%
What is Courvoisier's sign?	Painless jaundice with a palpable gallbladder
Levels of which tumor marker are generally elevated with pancreatic adenocarcinoma?	CA19-9
What is a Whipple procedure?	Resection of the head of the pancreas, the entire duodenum, the distal stomach, the distal common bile duct, and the gallbladder
What is Virchow's node?	A palpable left supraclavicular lymph node
What is Sister Mary Joseph's node?	A periumbilical lymph node

Spleen

The spleen represents the largest single collection of **lymphoid tissue** in the body. It is located in the posterior left upper quadrant of the abdomen between the ninth and eleventh ribs and is protected by the costal cage.

The blood supply to the spleen is derived from the splenic artery, a tortuous branch of the celiac axis that reaches the spleen by traveling along the superior border of the pancreas. The splenic artery branches to form the short gastric arteries, the left gastroepiploic artery, and the terminal splenic arteries. Once these vessels enter the splenic pulp, they further branch within the trabeculae.

Seventy-five percent of the splenic parenchyma is composed of **red pulp;** the rest is **white pulp.** The area where the red pulp and the white pulp meet is called the **marginal zone.** The white pulp is associated with the arterial blood supply, and it is made up mostly of lymphocytes that carry out immune functions. Lymphatic tissue in the white pulp contains T lymphocytes that replace the native adventitia of the distal central arteries to become the periarteriolar lymphoid sheets, or *PALS*.

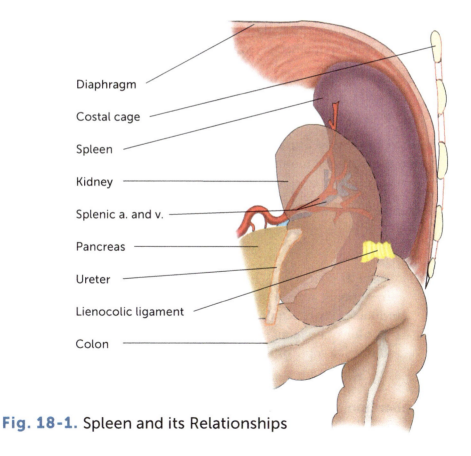

Fig. 18-1. Spleen and its Relationships

Immune Thrombocytopenic Purpura

Definition Immune thrombocytopenic purpura (ITP) is also called *idiopathic thrombocytopenic purpura*. It is characterized mainly by a low platelet count (thrombocytopenia), leading to subcutaneous bleeding.

Etiology ITP is caused by the presence of an antiplatelet IgG, which binds to antigens of circulating platelets. These autoantibody-coated platelets are then destroyed, and they are removed by the reticuloendothelial system of the spleen. Most often, the disease presents in patients who are otherwise healthy. In adults, thrombocytopenia can be caused by systemic lupus erythematosus, leukemia, viral infection, drug hypersensitivity, and HIV. These causes of thrombocytopenia are sometimes mistaken for ITP.

Epidemiology In adults, ITP is more common among women, affecting females in 70% of cases. ITP is the most common cause of thrombocytopenia in children. In this group, both sexes are affected equally, with spontaneous remission occurring in about 80% of cases.

Symptoms Patients often present with epistaxis and gingival bleeding and, rarely, with GI bleeding or hematuria. Occasionally, patients may present with a cerebral hemorrhage.

Physical Exam and Signs The spleen is not palpable on physical exam, and the most common sign is petechiae. Other causes of thrombocytopenia must be ruled out.

Diagnosis Based on the exclusion of other possibilities, the diagnosis of ITP is made in the presence of low platelets and mucocutaneous bleeding.

Labs. Platelet counts are <100,000/mm^3, and large, immature forms may be seen on peripheral smears. Testing for antiplatelet antibodies is not required for diagnosis but may prove helpful. The value of bone marrow aspiration and biopsy is questionable and is still a topic of debate.

Imaging. No specific findings.

Complication(s) Bleeding is the most common complication.

Table 18-1 Indications for Splenectomy (Absolute and Relative)

	Benign Hematologic Conditions	Malignancies	Miscellaneous
Red blood cells	**Congenital Disease** HS Hemoglobin abnormalities Sickle cell anemia Thalassemias **Acquired Disease** Autoimmune Hemolytic anemia Parasitosis		
Platelets	ITP TTP		
White blood cells		Leukemias Lymphomas	
Bone marrow	Polycythemia vera	Chronic myeloid leukemia Acute myeloid leukemia	
Miscellaneous			Abscesses Cysts Storage diseases Splenic artery aneurysm Felty's syndrome Sarcoidosis Wandering spleen

Abbreviations: HS, hereditary spherocytosis; ITP, immune thrombocytopenic purpura; TTP, thrombotic thrombocytopenic purpura.

Treatment For asymptomatic patients with platelet counts greater than 50,000/mm^3, close observation is the only requirement. For symptomatic patients or those with platelet counts between 30,000/mm^3 and 50,000/mm^3, the first line of therapy consists of oral steroids, such as prednisone at a dose of 0.5 to 1 mg/kg per day. If the patient has internal bleeding, or if platelet counts remain low, intravenous immunoglobulin (IVIG) may induce a response, and it commonly does, although transiently. Lack of response to medical therapy, side effects from prolonged use of steroids, and relapse are indications for splenectomy (Table 18-1). In children, observation is the initial approach. Splenectomy is successful in 70% to 80% of cases; therefore, a thorough search for accessory splenic tissue must be performed during surgery. ITP is the most common indication for **elective splenectomy.**

Hereditary Spherocytosis

Definition Hereditary spherocytosis (HS) is an abnormality of the red cell membrane that leads to hemolysis and, as a result, anemia.

Etiology HS is due to a congenital deficiency of one of the red blood cell membrane proteins called *spectrin,* which in turn renders the erythrocytes spherical (spherocytes), small, and stiff (non-deformable), with increased osmotic fragility. As a result, erythrocytes cannot pass through the circulation of the spleen; this leads to their sequestration and destruction within the red pulp.

Epidemiology HS is seen in 1 out of 5000 people, and it is transmitted as an autosomal dominant trait. Is the most common hereditary hemolytic anemia among people of Northern European descent, and it is the most common hemolytic anemia for which splenectomy is indicated. It presents as mild, moderate, or severe disease. A high prevalence of associated pigment gallstones has been noted in patients with HS.

Symptoms Most patients are asymptomatic. Some patients exhibit fatigue. Rarely, a hemolytic crisis may occur in association with infection. Occasionally, right upper quadrant (RUQ) pain or discomfort may signal cholelithiasis.

Physical Exam and Signs With a severe presentation, patients are anemic with splenomegaly and occasionally are jaundiced. Jaundice, however, is most prevalent in infants.

Differential Other anemias associated with hemolysis.

Diagnosis The diagnosis of HS is made by obtaining a **peripheral blood smear.**

Labs. Minimal or no anemia is noted with a mild presentation. Peripheral smear reveals spherocytosis, and lab values reveal reticulocytosis >6%, an increase in the mean corpuscular hemoglobin concentration (MCHC), and an abnormal osmotic fragility test. Coombs test is negative.

Imaging. Ultrasound of the gallbladder is prudent when splenectomy is considered.

Complication(s) In adults, cholelithiasis is present in approximately 85% of cases. Leg ulcers rarely may be seen with severe disease; these respond only to splenectomy.

Treatment Splenectomy is the only treatment, and it is performed if the patient is symptomatic, even if anemia is not present. In children, it is best to wait until age 6 to establish an immunologic record and to reduce the risks posed by infection.

SPLENOMEGALY

Definition Splenic enlargement reaching 400 g may be considered splenomegaly. Commonly, splenomegaly is associated with an exaggeration of splenic function, or **hypersplenism**. In general, hypersplenism is the presence of **pancytopenia** resulting from increased destruction or sequestration of normal or abnormal cells.

Etiology The most common cause of splenomegaly is liver disease, usually cirrhosis, followed by hematologic malignancies. The reasons for splenomegaly can be divided according to the particular function of the spleen that has become hyperactive.

Immune/inflammatory response: eg, endocarditis, mononucleosis, sarcoidosis

Removal of erythrocytes: eg, HS, thalassemia major

Obstructive: eg, portal hypertension, splenic vein thrombosis, congestive heart failure

Neoplastic: eg, lymphomas, leukemias

Myeloproliferative disorders: eg, myelofibrosis, polycythemia vera

Miscellaneous disorders: eg, Gaucher's disease, Niemann-Pick disease, amyloidosis

Epidemiology Varies with the cause of the splenomegaly.

Symptoms The most common symptom is vague abdominal pain, sometimes referred to the left shoulder. In general, symptoms are those of the underlying disease: weight loss (malignancy), pallor (anemia), fever (infection), and so on.

Physical Exam and Signs A palpable spleen is not always abnormal—approximately 2% of spleens are palpable. To detect splenomegaly, it is best to examine patients in right lateral decubitus position, with the left knee and hip flexed. Hematologic malignancies and myelofibrosis may cause massive splenomegaly, in which case the lower pole of the spleen reaches the pelvis and crosses the midline.

Differential The differential includes all causes of splenomegaly, as mentioned in "Etiology."

Diagnosis The diagnosis aims to determine the underlying cause of splenomegaly, which is often suggested by the clinical history.

Labs. Anemia, leukopenia, and thrombocytopenia define hypersplenism, a functional result of splenomegaly in many cases.

Imaging. CT scan is the test of choice in most cases of splenomegaly.

Complication(s) Splenic rupture and bleeding, splenic infarct.

Treatment Splenectomy is used to control symptoms and to prevent complications of the underlying disease. Whenever a splenectomy is considered, patients must be immunized before surgery with a pneumococcal vaccine. Prophylaxis against *Haemophilus influenzae* and *Neisseria meningitidis* is a prudent choice.

OVERWHELMING POSTSPLENECTOMY INFECTION

Definition Overwhelming postsplenectomy infection (OPSI) is a severe complication of asplenia.

Etiology Splenectomy renders patients vulnerable to infection, in particular from *Streptococcus pneumoniae*, *H influenzae*, and *N meningitidis*. Other organisms identified in OPSIs include *Streptococcus* and *Salmonella* species.

Epidemiology OPSI is the most common fatal late complication of splenectomy. It occurs more frequently after splenectomy performed to treat a malignancy or a hematologic disease than after splenectomy performed to treat splenic trauma. The risk is higher in children younger than 4 years of age. Infection is more common 2 years after splenectomy, but it may occur up to 5 years postsurgery. The mortality rate ranges from 50% to 70% despite administration of antibiotics and intensive supportive care.

Symptoms Fever, chills, sore throat, myalgias, altered mental status, and vomiting may occur.

Physical Exam and Signs Depending on the progression of the syndrome, hypotension, respiratory distress, and manifestations of disseminated intravascular coagulation (DIC) may be present. Pneumonia and meningitis may occur.

Differential Other sources of infection must be considered.

Diagnosis The diagnosis of OPSI is made on the basis of clinical and laboratory evidence of sepsis.

Labs. ±Hypoglycemia, ±electrolyte abnormalities, ±acidosis, ±hematologic evidence of disseminated intravascular coagulation.

Imaging. No specific findings.

Complication(s) OPSI is associated with a high mortality rate. Patients may progress to coma and death within 24 to 48 hours.

Treatment IV fluids, frequently steroids, antibiotics, and aggressive supportive therapy are treatments for OPSI. Prevention for patients at increased risk for pneumococcal infection is best achieved by administering the polysaccharide-based pneumococcal vaccine. It is recommended for the asplenic adult patient, with revaccination every 6 years, as suggested by the Centers for Disease Control and Prevention. The vaccine should be given 2 weeks before elective splenectomy is performed.

BIBLIOGRAPHY

Lakin RO, Bena JF, Sarac TP, et al. The contemporary management of splenic artery aneurysms. *J Vasc Surg.* 2011;53:958-965.

Perrotta S, Gallagher PG, Mohandas N. Hereditary spherocytosis. *Lancet.* 2008;372:1411-1426.

Clinical Keys: Questions and Answers

Question	Answer
What is immune thrombocytopenic purpura (ITP)?	The presence of an antiplatelet IgG, which binds to antigens of circulating platelets, leading to thrombocytopenia
Which vaccine should be given to patients undergoing splenectomy?	Polyvalent vaccine against *H influenzae* type B, *Meningococcus*, and *Pneumococcus*
What are 3 symptoms of immune thrombocytopenic purpura (ITP)?	Purpura, gingival bleeding, and epistaxis
What is the most common cause of splenomegaly	Liver disease
What is hypersplenism?	Splenomegaly and a decrease in the number of one or more types of blood cells
What is hereditary spherocytosis (HS)?	A congenital deficiency of spectrin, a red blood cell membrane protein, resulting in the formation of spherocytes
What can be seen in the peripheral smear after splenectomy?	Target cells (immature cells), Howell-Jolly bodies (nuclear remnants), Heinz bodies (denatured hemoglobin), and iron granules (Pappenheimer bodies)
What is an overwhelming postsplenectomy infection (OPSI)?	A severe infection that is a complication of asplenia
What is the first-line treatment for symptomatic patients with ITP or for those with platelet counts between 30,000/mm^3 and 50,000/mm^3?	Oral steroids
What is the treatment for HS?	Splenectomy
What is the most common indication for elective splenectomy?	ITP

Abdominal Wall Hernias   19

The abdominal wall is composed of a series of muscular and aponeurotic layers under the skin and subcutaneous tissue, which vary in structure slightly at different levels (Fig. 19-1). At the midline, these layers fuse to form an aponeurotic structure called the **linea alba,** or *midline*, which is wider in the supraumbilical section of the abdomen.

The muscular structures immediately lateral to the midline are the paired **anterior rectus abdominis muscles,** which insert into the costal cage superiorly and into the pubic bone inferiorly. They are transversely divided into 4 segments by fibrous bands at variable intervals and are surrounded by a fascial envelope called the **rectus sheath.**

Lateral to the anterior rectus muscle are 3 layers of flat muscles, with fibers in each running in different directions: (1) the **external oblique muscle,** the most superficial layer; (2) the **internal oblique muscle,** the middle layer; and (3) the **transversus abdominis muscle,** the deepest layer.

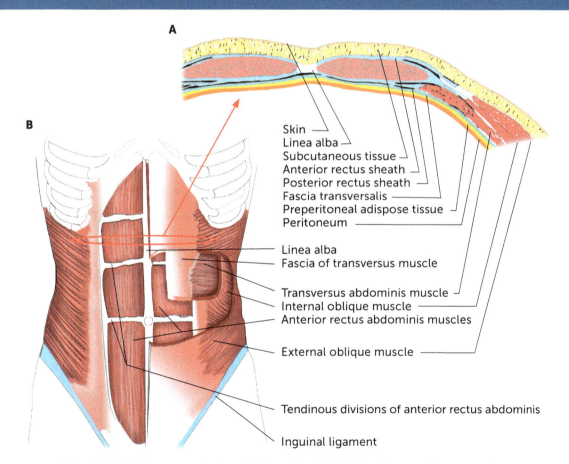

Fig. 19-1. Layers of the Abdominal Wall **A.** Cross-Sectional View **B.** Anterior View

The inguinal canal is a tunnel that traverses all layers of the lower abdominal wall, and it is a counduit through which an indirect hernia protrudes.

In the inguinal region, an anatomic landmark known as **Hesselbach's triangle** is bound medially by the **anterior rectus muscle,** superolaterally by the **inferior epigastric vessels,** and inferolaterally by the **inguinal ligament** (Fig. 19-2).

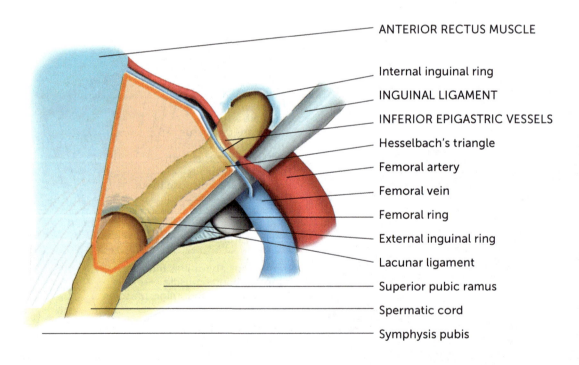

Fig. 19-2. Hesselbach's Triangle

The inguinal ligament, also known as *Poupart's ligament*, is the lower, thickened edge of the external oblique aponeurosis. It arises at the anterior superior iliac spine laterally, and inserts onto the pubic tubercle medially.

The **internal inguinal ring** is an evagination, or outpouching, in the transversalis fascia—much like the finger of a glove—that extends into the spermatic cord.

The **external inguinal ring**, or the *superficial inguinal ring*, is an ovoid opening in the lower, medial portion of the external oblique aponeurosis, close to the pubic tubercle (Fig. 19-3). The spermatic cord passes through the external inguinal ring before entering the scrotum to reach the testicle.

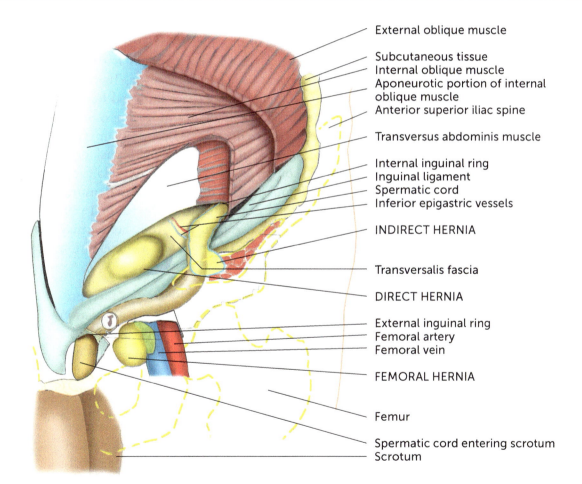

Fig. 19-3. Anatomy of the Inguinal Region and Three Types of Hernias (Anterior View)

Inguinal Hernia

Definition An **inguinal hernia** is an externally detectable bulge of tissue that protrudes into the groin through a defect in the abdominal wall. An inguinal hernia can be classified as **indirect, direct,** or **femoral** (Fig. 19-3).

Etiology An **indirect hernia** extrudes through the **internal inguinal ring lateral to the inferior epigastric vessels;** it follows the spermatic cord in men and the round ligament in women. An indirect hernia may enlarge and extend all the way into the scrotum, although such a situation is more common in hernias that have been present for a long time. An indirect hernia is the result of a **patent processus vaginalis,** which is a tube-like peritoneal extension that accompanies the testicle when it descends into the scrotum. After the testis is in place, the processus vaginalis should occlude. When this does not occur, an open peritoneal sac persists and a hernia may form. Therefore, indirect hernias are considered congenital. **Direct inguinal hernias** protrude through Hesselbach's triangle in an area of weakness of the transversalis fascia and are considered an acquired problem (Fig. 19-2). Conditions that persistently increase intra-abdominal pressure, such as obesity, chronic cough, prostatism, and habitual lifting, may contribute to the development of a direct hernia. A **femoral hernia** protrudes into the femoral canal medial to the femoral vein and below the inguinal ligament. Ocasionally, a groin hernia may have simultaneous direct and indirect components, a presentation called a *pantaloon* ("trousers") hernia.

Epidemiology Inguinal hernias are a common problem, but their precise incidence is unknown. It is estimated that 5% of the population has a hernia, and 75% to 80% of these are inguinal hernias. Of these, approximately **75%** are **indirect inguinal hernias,** the most common type by far in men and women. Lifetime prevalence of inguinal hernias is 25% in men and 2% in women. **Femoral hernias** are common in women (~70%) and rare in men. They comprise approximately 25% of groin hernias in women and 2% of groin hernias in men. In 10% of women and in 50% of men, femoral hernias are associated with an inguinal hernia , either simultaneously or sequentially. The prevalence of hernias and the incidence of strangulation increases with age. **Strangulation** is the most serious complication of hernias, most commonly seen with indirect hernias. This complication occurs in 1% to 3% of patients, usually in children or older adults. However, femoral hernias have the highest rate of strangulation (~20%).

Symptoms Most inguinal hernias are asymptomatic. Occasionally, patients may experience aching or some other form of discomfort. Occasionally, pain may radiate to the scrotum.

Physical Exam and Signs A hernia manifests with an intermittent bulge in the groin that is more apparent with straining. Patients should be examined in both supine and standing positions while performing a Valsalva maneuver (such as coughing) to increase intra-abdominal pressure and reproduce symptoms. The hernia sac is detected against an examining finger by invaginating the scrotum of the affected side into the inguinal canal through the external inguinal ring.

Differential Musculoskeletal pain in the groin may be interpreted as a hernia, but if the physical exam is inconclusive, it is best to wait and reexamine the patient sequentially. Differentials to consider include a hydrocele of the spermatic cord, lymphadenopathy, and ectopic testes.

Diagnosis Physical exam findings are the mainstay of the diagnosis.

Labs. No specific findings.

Imaging. In some cases, ultrasound may help diagnose or differentiate a hernia from a hydrocele. However, imaging is rarely indicated.

Complication(s) An **incarcerated hernia** (Fig. 19-4) is one that is trapped in its location after it protrudes, and it cannot be manually reduced into the abdominal cavity. An incarcerated hernia will remain in its detectable position whether the patient is standing or supine. A **strangulated hernia** (Fig. 19-4) is an incarcerated hernia associated with compromised blood supply. Incarceration and strangulation occurs in approximately 25% of femoral hernias. A **recurrent hernia** is one that reappears after surgical repair.

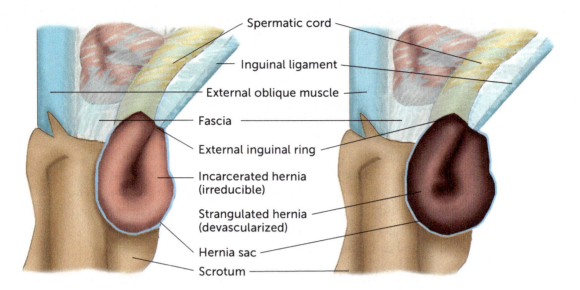

Fig. 19-4. *Left:* Incarcerated hernia. *Right:* Strangulated hernia.

Treatment Small, asymptomatic inguinal hernias may be observed depending on the circumstances calling for this conservative approach. In general, however, hernias usually enlarge, and it is best to surgically repair them when they are diagnosed. The majority of hernias are treated with synthetic mesh repair, which has been shown to substantially reduce recurrence rates. Surgery can be performed by an anterior open approach or laparoscopically. There are pros and cons to each of these methods, but a laparoscopic approach is probably better suited for bilateral and recurrent hernias. The fundamental principle of hernia correction with an open surgical approach is to make sure that the repair creates no tension in the tissues approximated to close or reinforce the underlying defect.

OTHER TYPES OF HERNIAS

An **umbilical hernia** protrudes through the umbilicus. This type of hernia is common in infants, and it may close spontaneously by age 2 years. If it does not close, surgical repair is required. In adults, umbilical hernias are acquired and should be surgically repaired.

An **epigastric hernia** presents at the linea alba, between the xyphoid process and the umbilicus. It is more common in men than in women. Epigastric hernias are multiple in 20% of cases and are commonly located just off the midline. Epigastric hernias usually contain preperitoneal fat, which is difficult to reduce; therefore, it is best to surgically repair this type of hernia once it is diagnosed.

A **Richter hernia** occurs when a portion of the antimesenteric wall of the bowel is trapped through the hernia defect. This type of hernia may reduce with a necrotic portion of the bowel wall, which may later perforate.

A **Littré's hernia** contains a Meckel's diverticulum in the sac. It is most commonly found in inguinal hernias in men.

A **spigelian hernia** pushes through the semilunar line, usually at the level where it crosses the linea semicircularis. It may require CT or ultrasound for diagnosis.

A **sliding hernia** is an indirect inguinal hernia in which an intra-abdominal viscus (such as the colon or bladder) forms a portion of the wall of the hernia sac. They are most common on the left side, and the sigmoid colon is usually the involved viscus.

BIBLIOGRAPHY

Connor K, Brady RR, de Beaux A, Tulloh B. Contemporary hernia smartphone applications (apps). *Hernia*. 2013 Jun 26. [Epub ahead of print]

Henry CR, Bradburn E, Moyer KE. Complex abdominal wall reconstruction: an outcomes review. *Ann Plast Surg*. 2013;71(3):266-268.

Clinical Keys: Questions and Answers

What are the boundaries of Hesselbach's triangle?	The anterior rectus muscle, the inferior epigastric vessels, and the inguinal ligament
What anatomic landmark can be used during surgery to help determine whether a hernia is direct or indirect?	The inferior epigastric vessels—if the hernia is lateral to them, then it is indirect; if the hernia is medial to them, then it is direct
Through what anatomic landmark do direct hernias protrude?	Hesselbach's triangle
What is a strangulated hernia?	A hernia with compromised blood supply
What is an incarcerated hernia?	A hernia that cannot be reduced into the abdominal cavity
What is a Richter hernia?	A hernia with a trapped (incarcerated) portion of the antimesenteric wall of the bowel
What is a Grynfeltt hernia?	A hernia protruding through the back via the superior lumbar triangle
What is a sliding hernia?	An indirect inguinal hernia in which an intra-abdominal viscus (such as the colon or bladder) forms a portion of the wall of the hernia sac
Why do hernias require repair?	To prevent obstruction, strangulation, and pain
What is a Bochdalek's hernia?	A hernia that protrudes through the diaphragm posteriorly
Which is the most common type of inguinal hernia?	Indirect inguinal hernia
What type of hernia has the highest risk of strangulation?	A femoral hernia

Where does an indirect hernia protrude in a woman?	Into the round ligament
Is a femoral hernia lateral or medial to the femoral vessels?	Medial
Is a femoral hernia more frequent in men or women?	Women

Topic VII

Urology

Common Urologic Problems

20

The kidneys are paired solid retroperitoneal organs that border the psoas muscles. The primary microscopic functional unit of the kidney is the **nephron,** which is responsible for regulating serum electrolytes, maintaining red blood cell mass, regulating blood pressure and blood pH, and ridding the body of metabolites through urine.

The core of the nephron is the **glomerulus,** a tuft of capillaries that allows substances to pass into **Bowman's capsule,** followed by the **proximal convoluted tubule,** the **loop of Henle,** and the **distal convoluted tubule** before joining other nephrons in the **collecting tubules.**

Nephrons reside in the **renal cortex,** except for the long loops of Henle and the collecting ducts, which pass through the higher osmotic environment of the **renal medulla.**

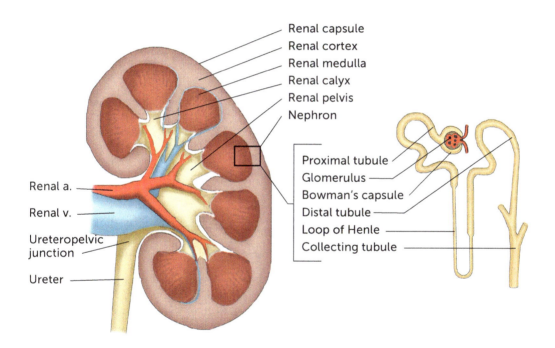

Fig. 20-1. Anatomy of the Kidney

Surgery 301

Through the ureters, urine enters the **urinary bladder** (Fig. 20-2), which is a hollow, muscular organ that stores urine. The bladder mucosa is lined by a transitional epithelial layer of cells.

In men, the **testis**, or *testicle;* the **epididymis;** and the **vas deferens** join the **seminal vesicle** at the level of the **ejaculatory duct** in the **prostatic urethra,** which runs through the **prostate gland.** From there, the male urinary and genital tracts form a single conduit through the ventral aspect of the **penis.**

The 2 **spermatic cords** extend from the internal inguinal rings and traverse the inguinal canals to reach the testes. Each cord contains the vas deferens, the spermatic arteries, the spermatic vein, artery of the vas deferens, nerves, and lymphatics, all of which supply and drain the testicles. As it reaches the testicle, the vas deferens becomes the epididymis. The **tunica vaginalis** covers the anterior two-thirds of the testicle and forms a serous membrane pouch; inadequate fixation of the testes to the tunica vaginalis can result in testicular torsion.

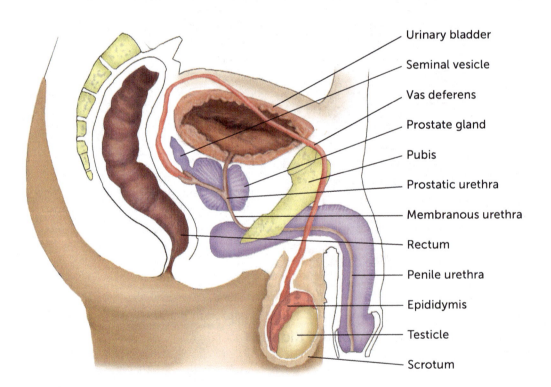

Fig. 20-2. Anatomy of the Male Genitourinary System

Nephrolithiasis

Definition Concretions arising in the urinary tract at any point along its course are called **nephroliths,** or *stones*.

Etiology **Calcium oxalate** stones are thought to form when material that is normally soluble (eg, calcium) **supersaturates** the urine leading to **crystal formation.** The risk factors for developing calcium oxalate stones include hypercalciuria, hyperparathyroidism, high sodium intake, high animal protein intake, or low fluid intake. **Uric acid stones** form in an acidic environment (pH <6.0) and can be associated with gout. **Struvite stones** may form when there is an upper urinary tract infection caused by a **urease-producing organism,** such as *Proteus* or *Klebsiella*. Struvite stones can grow large enough to form a cast of the renal pelvis and the renal calyces, which is known as a **staghorn calculus. Cystine stones** are typically the result of a genetic mutation that causes decreased tubular reabsorption of cystine, resulting in **cystinuria.**

Epidemiology The majority of stones are **calcium based** (80%) and usually composed of **calcium oxalate; calcium phosphate stones occur** less frequently. More rare stone types include **uric acid stones** (10%), **cystine stones** (4%), and **magnesium ammonium phosphate,** or *struvite,* stones. Approximately 15% of the population will develop a kidney stone, typically between the third and fifth decades of life, so the sporadic occurrence of nephrolithiasis in an otherwise healthy person is not pathologic. Stone formation has a **male predominance**.

Symptoms The most common symptom of ureteral obstruction from nephrolithiasis is acute, severe, intermittent **flank pain** (renal colic) resulting from hydronephrosis and distention of the renal capsule. Lower ureteral obstruction may cause pain that radiates to the testicle or labium. Pain may be associated with **nausea and vomiting.** Chronic obstruction may present more subtly. Many such patients describe a persistent backache that does not subside. Stones that traverse the UVJ may cause bladder irritation and resultant urinary **frequency** and/or **urgency**. Typically, only large stones (>1 cm) cause ongoing discomfort once they pass into the bladder, as stones smaller than this may be voided without great difficulty.

Physical Exam and Signs Patients with renal colic usually cannot stop moving as a result of severe discomfort. **Tenderness to palpation** over the affected kidney or retroperitoneum may be noted.

Differential Acute renovascular occlusion (eg, renal artery embolism), retroperitoneal bleed, pyelonephritis, and testicular torsion may be considered.

Diagnosis The diagnosis is made from a combination of clinical presentation, urinalysis, and imaging.

Labs. Urinalysis typically reveals microscopic or gross **hematuria,** although 15% of patients may not have hematuria. Urine pH is usually 5.0. The hallmark of **cystinuria** is hexagonal crystals seen on microscopic examination of urine sediment.

Imaging. **Noncontrast CT** is currently the imaging study of choice, although there still is a role for **intravenous pyelography** (IVP) to assess degree of obstruction.

Complication(s) Persistent obstruction may lead to permanent renal damage if untreated. Nephrolithiasis may lead to septic shock if associated with fever or immunocompromised status. Renal forniceal rupture with leakage of urine into the perinephric space as a result of acute distal ureteral obstruction is an uncommon complication.

Treatment Many patients can be managed with **oral nonsteroidal anti-inflammatory drugs (NSAIDs), opioids,** and **hydration.** Small stones (<5 mm) typically pass spontaneously—the use of oral **alpha-blocker therapy** (eg, tamsulosin or terazosin) may aid this process by relaxing ureteral smooth muscle. Larger stones may cause obstruction at any point in the ureter, but they are most commonly found at the UPJ, the iliac crossing, or the UVJ (Fig. 20-3). In these cases, a variety of treatments are currently available, including extracorporeal shock wave lithotripsy, endoscopy, and, rarely, open surgery.

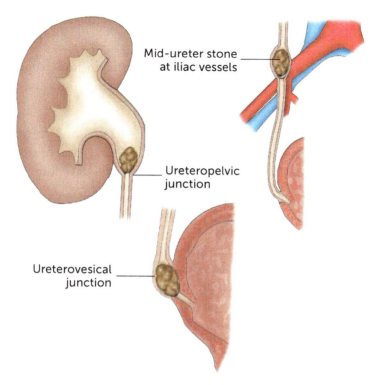

Fig 20-3. Common Locations of Kidney Stones

RENAL CANCER

Definition Renal cancer is a malignant tumor of the kidney that is either a primary renal tumor or a metastasis.

Etiology Cause is currently unknown. Risk factors include smoking and exposure to chemical carcinogens.

Epidemiology **Renal cell carcinoma** (RCC) represents 85% to 90% of all primary renal cancers. Oncocytomas and renal carcinomas are uncommon. In the United States, there are approximately 30,000 cases of renal cancer every year. In children, **Wilms' tumor** is the most common type of renal cancer. Certain syndromes (eg, tuberous sclerosis, von Hippel–Lindau disease) are associated with multiple renal cell carcinomas; however, the vast majority of cases are sporadic (no familial tendency).

Symptoms Most patients are asymptomatic until the disease is advanced. Patients may describe flank pain.

Physical Exam and Signs The triad of hypernephroma (palpable upper abdominal renal mass), flank pain, and hematuria may be noted but is uncommon.

Differential The differential includes benign renal tumor (eg, oncocytoma, angiomyolipoma), lobar nephronia (renal mass caused by acute focal infection), complex renal cyst, and dromedary hump.

Diagnosis The diagnosis of renal cancer is made with CT. Many tumors are diagnosed incidentally.

Labs. There is no serum marker for RCC. Patients with advanced RCC may have normal or decreased hemoglobin levels. Lab abnormalities may include an elevation in a variety of hormones, such as erythropoietin, parathyroid hormone, renin, glucagon, and insulin.

Imaging. Features characteristic of renal carcinoma on CT include enhancement of the lesion after injection of IV contrast or **thickened, irregular walls.**

Complication(s) RCC typically metastasizes to the lungs, bones, and regional lymph nodes. When this occurs, it is usually incurable. Some tumors grow into the renal vein and/or inferior vena cava, making surgery more challenging.

Treatment **Radical nephrectomy** is the mainstay of initial management of RCC, and it may be recommended for patients who have advanced disease and those who require palliative measures. Chemotherapy and immunotherapy are used in patients with metastatic disease.

BLADDER CANCER

Definition Bladder cancer is a malignancy of the urinary bladder.

Etiology Bladder cancer was one of the first malignancies to be linked to environmental exposures (eg, aluminum, paint, and textile and hair dyes). In fact, exposure to these chemicals accounts for more than 20% of bladder cancer cases. Cigarette smoking increases the risk of developing bladder cancer.

Epidemiology **Transitional cell carcinoma** (TCC) accounts for more than 90% of bladder cancer cases.

Symptoms The most common symptom is **gross or microscopic hematuria.** The presence of gross hematuria in older patients is suspected to be bladder cancer until proven otherwise.

Physical Exam and Signs Exam may be unrevealing. A palpable suprapubic mass may indicate advanced disease.

Differential The differential includes cystitis, prostatitis, overactive bladder, and bladder stones.

Diagnosis The diagnosis of bladder cancer is made with cystoscopy and biopsy, urine cytology, and imaging.

Labs. Urinalysis may show hematuria. Urine should be cytologically evaluated.

Imaging. CT/MR urogram or IVP is useful.

Complication(s) Many patients present with advanced disease.

Treatment If the cancer is confined to the transitional cell layer of the bladder (superficial), it may be treated with **transurethral resection** (TUR) and bladder washings with a variety of immunologic or chemotherapeutic agents. Tumors involving the muscular layers of the bladder usually require **radical cystectomy** with urinary diversion. About half of these patients eventually succumb to metastatic disease.

PROSTATE CANCER

Definition Prostate cancer is a malignancy arising from the prostate gland.

Etiology Risk factors include the natural permissive effect of androgens on the prostate gland, African American race, advanced age, and family history.

Epidemiology Prostate cancer is the **most common noncutaneous cancer** in American men. Men have an approximately 16% lifetime risk of developing prostate cancer, and 20% of men die from the disease. Nearly all cases of prostate cancer are **adenocarcinoma.**

Symptoms Most patients are asymptomatic, although in some cases, men may exhibit sudden onset of **urinary retention** or unexplained bleeding in the urine or ejaculate. Other urinary symptoms include **nocturia, frequency,** and **urgency.** Men who present with advanced disease may have back pain from bony metastases.

Physical Exam and Signs **Digital rectal exam** (DRE) is used to evaluate the prostate gland. Eighty percent of prostate cancer cases are associated with a normal digital rectal exam. Firmness or a palpable nodule may be noted in about 20% of patients.

Differential The differential includes prostatitis, benign prostatic hypertrophy, bladder neck contracture, and chronic pelvic pain syndrome.

Diagnosis DRE, prostate-specific antigen (PSA) levels, and biopsy confirm malignancy. Either an abnormal finding from DRE or elevated PSA levels require evaluation of the prostate with imaging and needle biopsy.

Labs. PSA screening remains controversial. **PSA levels greater than 2.5 ng/mL** are considered suspicious for prostate cancer.

Imaging. Biopsy is the gold standard for evaluation of prostate cancer, which is staged according to the **Gleason scoring system. Transrectal ultrasound** is usually done at the time of biopsy of the prostate; however, the gross tumor is usually difficult to see on images. **CT/MRI** of the abdomen and pelvis and **bone scans** are performed to evaluate patients with advanced disease.

Complication(s) Left untreated, prostate cancer may obstruct the bladder neck and spread to regional lymph nodes in the pelvis, the bones, and various internal organs.

Treatment There are myriad treatment options available for both localized prostate cancer and advanced disease. Those with disease confined to the prostate may undergo **active surveillance** (involves obtaining serial PSA levels and having regular check-ups), **radical prostatectomy,** or **radiation therapy**. Those with advanced disease may undergo a combination of treatments.

TESTICULAR TORSION

Definition Testicular torsion (Fig. 20-4) is a rotation of the testicle on its vascular pedicle within the scrotal compartment, leading to vascular compromise and possible testicular loss if diagnosis and treatment are delayed. It is a true urologic emergency.

Etiology Torsion may occur **at rest** or may result from **blunt trauma** to the scrotum. Testicular torsion may be **extravaginal,** when the spermatic cord and the tunica vaginalis rotate as a unit, or **intravaginal,** when the testicle rotates within its tunica.

Epidemiology Approximately 1 in 4000 men has the anatomic testicular mobility to torse, known as "**bell clapper**" anatomy. Intratunica vaginalis torsion is most common in boys 12 to 18 years of age, although it may occur at any age. Extravaginal torsion occurs in the newborn period and may be present at birth. The presence of torsion of one testicle implies approximately a 25% lifetime risk of contralateral torsion. Cases of simultaneous bilateral torsion have been reported.

Symptoms Testicular torsion may exhibit variable symptoms, which may lead to a delay in diagnosis. Many patients report testicular pain and swelling, whereas others report numbness in the affected testicle. Some patients relate previous episodes, which resolved spontaneously. Some patients may only experience nausea and vomiting and/or abdominal pain.

Physical Exam and Signs Typically, the affected testicle is **high riding** (as a result of shortening of the spermatic cord from twisting) with a **transverse lie, mildly swollen,** and **tender.** Although the **cremasteric reflex** (retraction of the testicle elicited by stroking the ipsilateral inner thigh) is classically absent on the affected side, it is not a reliable indicator of the presence of torsion. Elevation of the scrotum does not provide the pain relief (**Prehn's sign**) that typically occurs with the same motion in cases of epididymitis. Some patients with testicular torsion may not have any gross abnormality on physical exam.

Differential The differential includes torsion of a testicular appendage, incarcerated inguinal hernia, testicular tumor, and epididymitis.

Diagnosis Testicular torsion is a clinical diagnosis made primarily by history and physical examination.

Labs. Urinalysis, urine culture, and complete blood count should be obtained to rule out other causes, such as epididymitis.

Imaging. **Ultrasound** or **nuclear testicular scans** are useful if surgical exploration is not indicated, but these studies should not be performed if they will delay diagnosis.

Complication(s) Irreversible testicular damage may begin as soon as 6 hours after torsion occurs. Testicular salvage is rare after 24 hours of torsion. A nonviable testicle that has been detorsed too late will likely atrophy. A long-term complication of atrophy involves the production of anti-sperm antibodies against the healthy contralateral testicle, with resultant infertility later in life.

Treatment In a cooperative patient, **manual detorsion** of the affected testicle may be attempted. Even if this maneuver is successful, emergency **scrotal exploration** and **bilateral orchiopexy** is required. An ice pack may be placed on the scrotum to help preserve the ischemic testicle until surgical exploration can be performed.

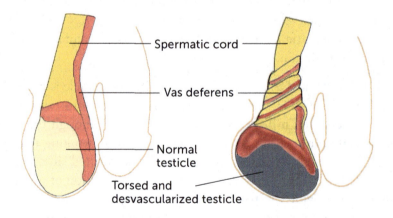

Fig. 20-4. Testicular Torsion

Testicular Cancer

Definition Testicular cancer is a malignancy of the testes.

Etiology Risk factors include cryptorchidism, HIV infection, and gonadal dysgenesis.

Epidemiology Testicular cancer is the most common solid tumor in men aged 15 to 35 years, and the lifetime risk is 1 in 500. It has become one of the most curable solid neoplasms, with an overall 5-year survival rate of 86% for seminomas. **Germ cell tumors** (GCTs) account for 95% of cases and are further classified into 2 categories: **pure seminomas** or **nonseminomatous germ cell tumors.**

Symptoms Typically, patients develop a **painless nodule** or swelling of 1 testicle. About one-third of patients report a dull ache or a sensation of heaviness.

Physical Exam and Signs A palpable mass is often noted.

Differential Epididymo-orchitis, testicular infarct, testicular trauma, testicular hematoma, and tunica albuginea cyst may be considered.

Diagnosis The diagnosis of testicular cancer is made with a combination of lab analyses, imaging, and clinical findings. **Biopsy with histologic evaluation** confirms the diagnosis.

Labs. Serum levels of the tumor marker alpha-fetoprotein (AFP), the beta subunit of human chorionic gonadotropin (beta-HCG), and lactate dehydrogenase (LDH) should be obtained to help identify the tumor and stage disease.

Imaging. **Scrotal ultrasound** is mandatory. Staging is accomplished with **CT scan** of the abdomen and pelvis and a **chest X-ray.**

Complication(s) Chemotherapy may cause infertility. Other complications include loss of seminal emission, which may occur after retroperitoneal lymph node dissection, and metastasis to other sites.

Treatment Initial therapy for all cases of testicular cancer is **radical inguinal orchiectomy.** Further treatment is determined by the stage and type of tumor.

Spermatocele, Hydrocele, and Varicocele

A **spermatocele** is a benign dilatation of the tail of the epididymis or proximal vas deferens.

A **hydrocele** is a fluid collection around the testicle that **transilluminates.** Ultrasound is required for further evaluation.

A **varicocele** consists of tortuous or dilated testicular veins within the spermatic cord. On exam, a varicocele is described as feeling like a "bag of worms."

Bibliography

Resnick MI, Novick AC. *Urology Secrets*. 2nd ed. Philadelphia, PA: Hanley & Belfus; 1999.

Hall PM. Nephrolithiasis: treatment, causes, and prevention. *Cleve Clin J Med*. 2009;76(10):583-591.

Clinical Keys: Questions and Answers

What is nephrolithiasis?	The formation of nephroliths, or stones, along the urinary tract
What are the majority of kidney stones composed of?	Calcium oxalate
What causes the formation of struvite stones?	An upper urinary tract infection caused by a urease-producing organism, such as *Proteus* or *Klebsiella*
What is the most common symptom of nephrolithiasis?	Acute flank pain
How is nephrolithiasis diagnosed?	Clinical presentation, urinalysis, and CT
What is first-line treatment for small kidney stones (<5 mm)?	NSAIDs, opioids, and hydration

Common Urologic Problems

What is the most common type of malignancy of the kidney?	Renal cell carcinoma
What is the most common type of bladder cancer?	Transitional cell carcinoma
What are the screening methods for prostate cancer?	Digital rectal exam and measurement of prostate-specific antigen levels
What is testicular torsion?	The abnormal rotation of a testicle on its vascular pedicle within the scrotal compartment
What are the symptoms of testicular torsion?	Pain or numbness in the affected testicle, sometimes associated with nausea
What is Prehn's sign?	Relief of pain with scrotal elevation, an indication of epididymitis
What is the cremasteric reflex?	Retraction of the testicle elicited by stroking the inner ipsilateral thigh
What is the treatment for testicular torsion?	Surgical exploration and bilateral orchiopexy
What is a spermatocele?	Benign dilatation of the tail of the epididymis or proximal vas deferens
What is a varicocele?	Tortuous or dilated testicular veins within the spermatic cord
What is a hydrocele?	A fluid collection around the testicle that transilluminates
What is the typical symptom of testicular cancer?	Painless mass or swelling of one testicle
What is the most common type of testicular cancer?	Germ cell tumors
What lab tests should be obtained when testicular cancer is suspected?	Serum levels of alpha-fetoprotein (AFP), the beta subunit of human chorionic gonadotropin (beta-HCG), and lactate dehydrogenase (LDH)

Interpreting Common Presentations

Algorithm 1: Managing Obstructive Jaundice

Cholestasis is a condition where there is an absence of bile excretion, which can be the result of decreased bile production or obstructed flow. This algorithm focuses on the adult patient with cholestatic jaundice of obstructive origin.

1. **History:** The history, physical exam, and overall clinical assessment of a patient are approximately 86% to 97% accurate in differentiating hepatic from extrahepatic causes of cholestasis. For instance, a history of alcohol abuse, hepatitis exposure, or drug use increases the suspicion for hepatic cholestasis.

2. **Physical exam:** If jaundice is noted, the patient should be examined in natural light. Occasionally, diet or medication may cause discoloration of the skin but not of the sclerae or mucous membranes. In these rare cases, bilirubin levels are not elevated. Pruritus in patients with cholestasis is associated with high concentration of bile acids, and this symptom can sometimes be unbearable. Stigmata of liver disease such as spider angiomas and caput medusae, and ascites or altered mental status strongly suggest a hepatic cause of jaundice. Right upper quadrant (RUQ) pain and fever suggests cholangitis. Painless jaundice (Courvoisier's sign) associated with an abdominal mass suggests a malignant obstruction. Abdominal pain, fever, and jaundice (Charcot's triad) are diagnostic of cholangitis until proven otherwise. Some patients with advanced cholestasis may develop xanthomas (yellowish fat deposits beneath the surface of the skin) or xanthelasmas (yellowish fat deposits around the eyelids).

3. **Laboratory tests:** For jaundice to become clinically evident, the total bilirubin level must be at least 2 mg/dL. Dark urine due to elevated bilirubin as well as pale stools indicate that the bilirubin is mostly conjugated, or *direct,* and that there is possibly an extrahepatic obstruction. Urine and stool of normal color suggest indirect, or *unconjugated,* hyperbilirubinemia. Unconjugated bilirubin has not yet been combined with glucuronic acid, a step that takes place in the liver. Conjugation

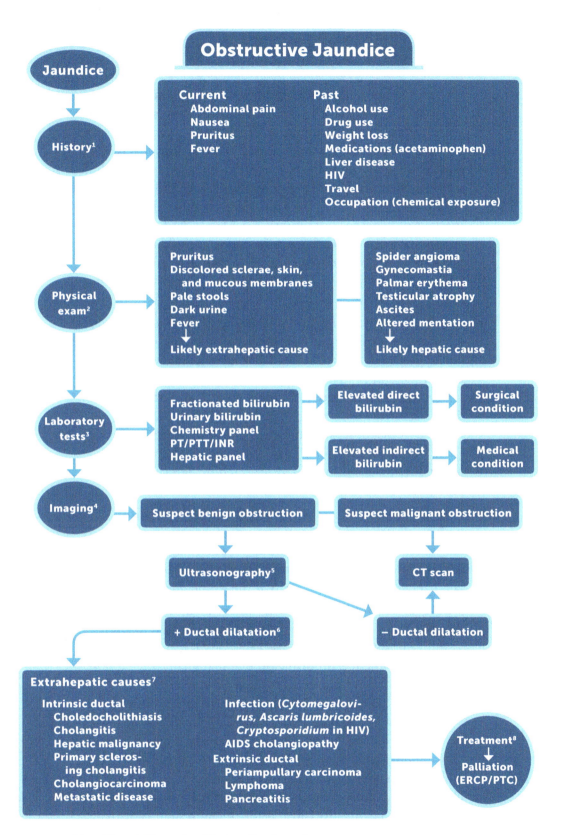

Algorithm 1. Managing Obstructive Jaundice

renders the bilirubin water soluble and it can then be excreted in urine. Unconjugated hyperbilirubinemia is mostly a medical presentation, whereas conjugated hyperbilirubinemia is relevant to the surgical practitioner. Elevated alkaline phosphatase (AP) and elevated γ-glutamyltransferase (GGT) levels suggest a biliary tract obstruction. Alanine aminotransferase (ALT) and aspartate aminotransferase (AST) are liver enzymes commonly used as markers of hepatocellular injury. An AST-to-ALT ratio of 2:1 suggests alcoholic liver disease. An elevated cholesterol level is common in cholestatic jaundice. A chemistry panel and a coagulation profile (PT/PTT/INR) contribute to the assessment of hepatic function.

4. **Imaging:** The gold standard of imaging is direct visualization of the biliary tree, as can be done with an endoscopic retrograde cholangiopancreatogram (ERCP) or a percutaneous transhepatic cholangiogram (PTC), but these tests are invasive and no longer used for the initial diagnosis of patients with jaundice. They are instead increasingly performed as a combined method of diagnosis and therapy in some jaundiced patients. Ultrasonography has become the first choice of imaging techniques for patients with a suspected benign cause of jaundice.

5. **Ultrasonography:** Ultrasound detects ductal dilatation with an accuracy of 95% and may detect hepatic pathology, such as cirrhosis or tumor infiltration. It can also easily detect cholelithiasis, which increases the suspicion for choledocholithiasis, particularly if the gallbladder is distended.

6. **Ductal dilatation:** Occasionally, biliary dilatation has not yet developed into an obstructive process and as a result, is not visible with ultrasound. In these cases, a CT scan may be of value even if there is no suspicion of a malignant obstruction. It is also recommended when there is an indeterminate suspicion of obstruction. In the absence of biliary dilatation, a hepatobiliary iminodiacetic acid (HIDA) scan may also be used to evaluate the biliary tree. Magnetic resonance cholangiopancreatography (MRCP) is useful if ERCP fails, or if an alternative is needed to evaluate a patient for choledocholithiasis. Sensitivity and specificity of MRCP are estimated to be 90% to 100% if the ductal system is dilated.

7. **Extrahepatic causes:** Extrahepatic, or *posthepatic,* causes of obstructive jaundice can be considered in relation to the presenting symptoms. So, in patients with an acute presentation of jaundice, pain, fever, and positive findings from laboratory tests the most common cause to consider is choledocholithiasis. An insidious presentation of painless jaundice suggests a malignant obstruction.
8. **Treatment:** ERCP and PTC are used to diagnose, treat, and palliate a malignant obstruction causing jaundice. ERCP is also used in cases of postoperative jaundice.

Algorithm 2:
Managing Acute Abdominal Pain

In some cases, acute abdominal pain in the adult patient overlaps with overt or subtle symptoms that suggest an underlying, more chronic cause that was previously undetected. Such could be the case, for instance, in a patient with a previously undiagnosed acute episode of inflammatory bowel disease. Another example would be a patient with a past episode of ischemia due to atherosclerosis, whose symptoms subsided, and presents now acutely after a complete occlusion.

1. **Hemodynamic stability:** The first step in management is to assess hemodynamic stability. Many of the diagnostic and therapeutic maneuvers are performed in tandem.

2. **History:** Taking an accurate history that focuses on the characteristics of the pain is essential. A mnemonic to help remember all of the elements of the pain is "old cars," where "o" stands for onset, "l" stands for location, "d" stands for duration, "c" stands for character, "a" stands for alleviating or aggravating factors, "r" stands for radiation, and "s" stands for severity. These elements provide a tentative differential. It is important to note that the majority of patients with presenting symptoms including abdominal pain will not require immediate surgery, and in many patients the cause of the pain will be extraperitoneal.

3. **Physical exam:** The physical exam will give the clinician at least 2 major elements to aid in the diagnosis: the location of the pain and the presence or absence of peritoneal signs, such as involuntary guarding and rebound tenderness. The first objective is to determine whether the patient has signs of an acute abdomen, indicating that an immediate surgical procedure is required. This might be the case, for instance, with a ruptured abdominal aortic aneurysm. Pelvic and rectal exams must be performed routinely.

4. **Labs:** Laboratory work should include a CBC with differential, electrolytes, BUN, creatinine, lactic acid, glucose, amylase and

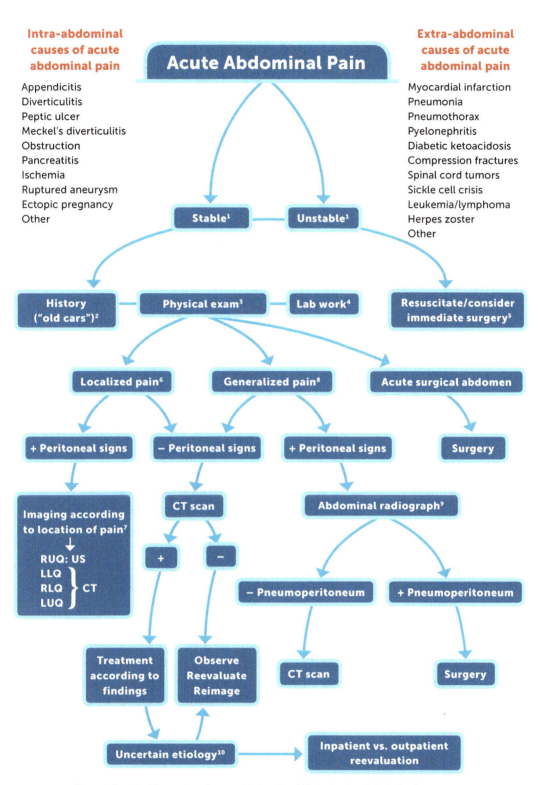

Algorithm 2: Managing Acute Abdominal Pain in the Adult Patient (Excluding Trauma)

lipase levels, liver function tests, and urinalysis. An elevated lactic acid level suggests ischemia. A pregnancy test should be performed on female patients of childbearing age.

5. **Resuscitation:** If the patient is unstable, resuscitation is the highest priority. Inserting central lines and monitoring vital signs and urine output is imperative and performed while making management decisions, specifically considering the need for immediate surgery. Few situations require emergent surgery without first obtaining a reasonably complete workup. Examples of conditions in which this is not the case include a ruptured abdominal aneurysm or a ruptured ectopic pregnancy.

6. **Localized pain:** If peritoneal signs are present in association with localized pain, the need for surgery is more likely, either urgently or after the diagnosis is confirmed. The location of the pain guides the differential diagnosis. Pain in the right upper quadrant (RUQ)/epigastric area may suggest cholecystitis, peptic ulcer disease, or pancreatitis. Pain in the right lower quadrant (RLQ) may suggest appendicitis, salpingitis, ectopic pregnancy, or inflammatory bowel disease. If there is a lack of peritoneal signs, the diagnosis relies more on the findings of the workup.

7. **Imaging according to location of pain:** Initial imaging technique is selected according to location of the abdominal pain. For instance, if the pain is in the RUQ, an ultrasound might be ordered to investigate the possibility of biliary disease. In general, pain localized to any of the other quadrants is investigated with a CT scan. Treatment for positive results is guided by findings. If there are no imaging findings, usually observation or reevaluation and a different type of imaging is required.

8. **Generalized pain:** In the case of generalized pain with peritoneal signs, surgery is typically required. However, such a decision may occasionally apply to a patient without obvious peritoneal signs. An example of this is an elderly patient whose pain is out of proportion to the physical findings (suggestive of bowel ischemia), or a patient with mild or no peritoneal irritation.

9. **Abdominal radiograph:** Symptoms of generalized abdominal pain with peritoneal signs can be studied first

with an abdominal radiograph to investigate the possibility of pneumoperitoneum. If present, a laparotomy (or laparoscopy) is required. In the absence of pneumoperitoneum, a CT scan is most likely indicated.

10. **Uncertain etiology:** In patients without a clear diagnosis, further inpatient observation or outpatient reevaluation may be required.

Algorithm 3: Managing Acute GI Bleeding

Patients with acute GI bleeding may present with an episode of hematemesis, melena, or hematochezia. **An upper GI (UGI) bleed is defined as one that originates proximal to the ligament of Treitz; a lower GI (LGI) bleed originates distal to the ligament of Treitz.** An UGI bleed may present with hematochezia, if it is a brisk bleed.

1. **Hemodynamic stability:** The first management step is to assess the patient's hemodynamic stability. **If the patient is unstable, ICU admission and resuscitation are the highest priorities.** Placing central lines and monitoring vital signs and urine output are imperative and are performed in tandem with transfusions and correction of any existing coagulopathy.
2. **History and physical:** The history may be obtained from the patient or from a relative of the patient. The goal is to elicit whether the patient has peptic ulcer disease and/or hepatic, cardiac, or renal disease. It is also necessary to find out whether the patient takes any medications that affect coagulation, such as warfarin or any nonsteroidal anti-inflammatory drugs (NSAIDs). Recent trauma, previous surgical procedures, and alcohol use are also relevant to the history. The physical exam seldom yields a great deal of information, but aside from determining whether hematemesis, hematochezia, or melena is present, the clinician might find stigmata such as caput medusae, or signs such as jaundice, ascites, bruits, or masses, which can provide clues to the cause of the bleed.
3. **Labs:** Relevant labs include CBC, liver and renal function panel, PTT, and PT/INR. The patient's blood should be typed and screened.
4. **Nasogastric aspirate:** The first step is to place a nasogastric (NG) tube. If it returns bloody fluid, this confirms an UGI bleed. If the aspirate is clear without bile, bleeding of duodenal or hepatic sources remains a possibility, as the bleed could be originating beyond a closed pylorus. If no blood is noted in the

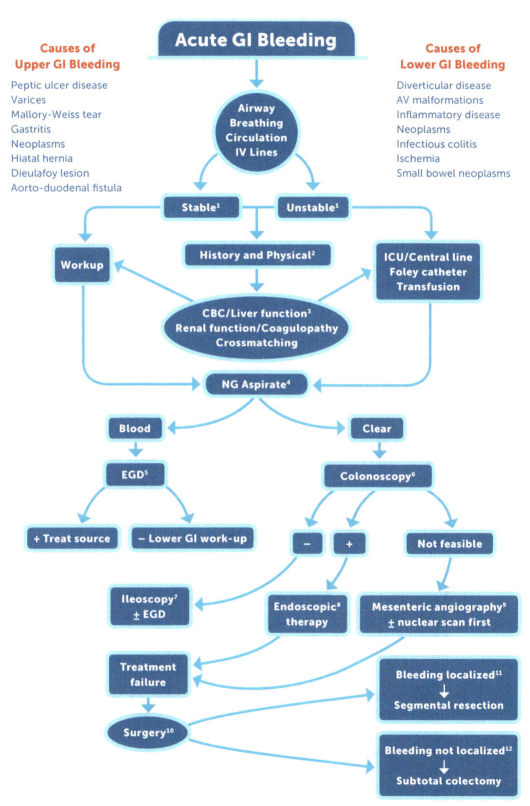

Algorithm 3. Managing Acute GI Bleeding

aspirate, but bile is evident, an upper GI source of bleeding is unlikely, unless the bleeding stopped before the NG tube was inserted.

5. **Esophagogastroduodenoscopy (EGD):** An EGD is the test of choice for diagnosing and locating the source of an UGI bleed. It also provides therapeutic possibilities such as thermal coagulation, injection therapy, argon plasma coagulation, and clip placement.

6. **Colonoscopy:** If bleeding is suspected to arise from a lower GI source, a colonoscopy is the first step in diagnosing and treating it. This procedure can be done even if there is no opportunity to cleanse the bowel.

7. **Ileoscopy:** If no bleeding source is seen during colonoscopy, an attempt should be made to enter the terminal ileum (enteroscopy) with the scope. If colonoscopy and ileoscopy do not reveal a bleed, EGD must be considered to rule out an UGI bleed.

8. **Endoscopic therapy:** If colonoscopy reveals a bleeding source, it can also be used to provide treatment through modalities such as fulguration, injection of vasopressors, or placement of clips.

9. **Mesenteric angiography:** Sometimes the volume of blood is so significant that a colonoscopy is not feasible or helpful. If this is the case, selective angiography is the next step. Angiography can reveal the bleeding source and can be used to treat the patient with infusion of vasopressin or embolization. Before angiography is performed, a bleeding scan may or may not be done to target a bleeding site with greater accuracy, or to assess whether the bleeding persists or has ceased.

10. **Surgery:** If endoscopic or angiographic therapy is not possible, or if it fails, surgery is the next approach.

11. **Segmental resection:** If the colonic lesion has been localized before surgery is performed, a segmental resection is the treatment modality.

12. **Subtotal colectomy:** If the lesion has not been identified before the time of surgery, the surgeon might attempt to do so while the patient is under anesthesia. If the bleeding source still cannot be determined, a subtotal colectomy must be performed.

Algorithm 4:
Managing Acute Limb Ischemia

Acute limb ischemia (ALI) is a sudden loss or reduction of blood flow to an extremity that threatens the viability of the limb. It is distinguished from chronic ischemia when the symptoms have been present for less than 2 weeks.

1. **History and physical exam:** A detailed history frequently suggests the cause of the ischemia. Arterial thrombosis over a preexisting arterial plaque or stenotic segment of a vessel is the most frequent cause of ALI (85%), whereas embolic sources account for most of the remainder. Thrombosis also may occur in a synthetic graft. Symptoms from an embolus usually have a rapid onset and are severe because there is no time for collateral circulation to develop. This could be the case with an already semioccluded vessel that later became fully blocked by a thrombus. Other, less common causes of ALI include dissection and trauma. Chronic causes of limb ischemia include vasculitides (eg, thromboangiitis obliterans), atherosclerosis, and connective tissue disorders. Some conditions may mimic ischemic pain, such as gout, neuropathy, and venous hemorrhage. Patients with presenting symptoms of ALI often have associated comorbidities that may lead to life-threatening conditions. These patients are at risk for coronary artery disease, myocardial infarction, congestive heart failure, and stroke, so they may exhibit severe arrhythmias, acid-base disturbances, respiratory compromise, and cardiovascular collapse.
2. **Resuscitation:** If a patient is hemodynamically unstable, resuscitation with IV fluids and other appropriate measures must be performed immediately in tandem with treatment of the affected limb.
3. **Assess limb:** A careful vascular exam of all limbs must be done, including palpation of all pulses, and the presence of flow must be assessed with a Doppler instrument. If flow can be heard, a blood pressure cuff can be used at the ankle or wrist proximal to the Doppler probe to assess the blood pressure of that limb.

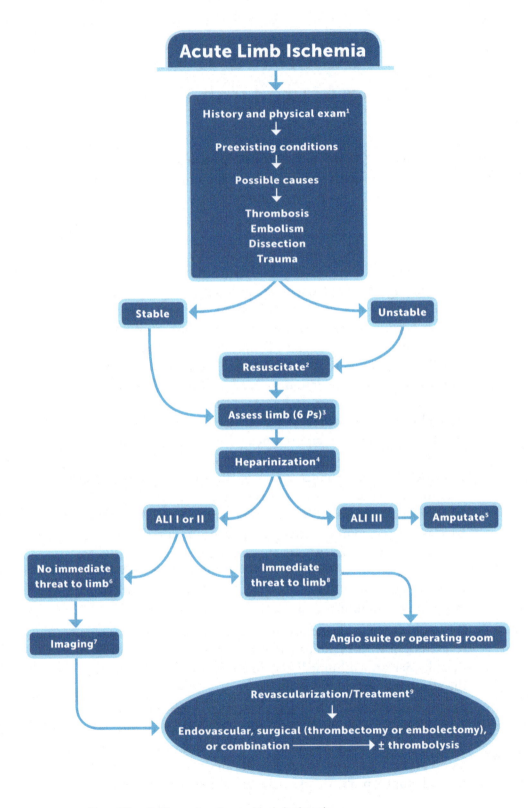

Algorithm 4. Managing Acute Limb Ischemia

A pressure less than 50 mm Hg confirms limb ischemia. The clinical features of acute limb ischemia (commonly referred to as the 6 *P*'s) must be assessed: paresthesia, pain, pallor, pulselessness, paralysis, and poikilothermia (coldness). Paresthesia (loss of nerve function) and paralysis (loss of nerve function and muscular function) indicate severe ischemia. The 6 *P*'s establish the severity of the ischemia and provide a baseline exam that can later serve to gauge the success of therapy. Comparison with the contralateral extremity may also give insight into the severity of disease as well as suggest possible causes. ALI is classified in 3 categories: class I signifies that the limb is viable and not immediately threatened, class IIa and IIb signify that the limb is salvageable if treated promptly or immediately, and class III signifies that the limb is irreversibly damaged.

4. **Heparinization:** Anticoagulation therapy with heparin must be initiated promptly to prevent propagation of the thrombus and to protect and optimize collateral circulation. This frequently results in relief of symptoms and lessening of critical ischemia and may convert an emergent high-risk procedure into an elective one, thereby reducing morbidity. This step should be taken initially in all categories of ALI.

5. **Amputate:** A limb categorized as class III ischemia requires amputation. Amputation of a lower extremity for ischemia is associated with a mortality rate of 5% to 16% as a result of the associated comorbidities typically found in these patients. Attempting revascularization of a nonviable extremity (ALI III) may result in even a higher mortality.

6. **No immediate threat to limb:** For patients who fall into ALI classes I and IIa, and when the limb is not immediately threatened, imaging studies may be performed to obtain information regarding the nature and extent of the occlusion and to plan an appropriate intervention.

7. **Imaging:** Duplex ultrasonography, computed tomography angiography (CTA), or magnetic resonance angiography (MRA) can be used and are over 90% sensitive and specific.

8. **Immediate threat to limb:** In the past, patients with ALI category IIb were taken directly to the operating room. Now, in facilities with the appropriate infrastructure, patients can be treated in a specially designed angio suite.

9. **Revascularization/treatment:** Improved endovascular approaches, such as angioplasty and stenting, allow for simultaneous imaging and revascularization during a single procedure. Surgical approaches, such as thrombectomy and embolectomy, are generally preferred for patients with a limb that is immediately threatened. If the limb is not threatened, thrombolysis can usually be performed through an intraarterial catheter to direct the infusion and restore flow. The decision to infuse a thrombolytic agent must be measured against the risk of bleeding that may complicate its use. Various trials suggest that thrombolysis has the best results in patients with a recent occlusion, thrombosis of a synthetic graft or stent, and at least 1 identifiable distal runoff vessel.

Algorithm 5: Managing Acute Mesenteric Ischemia

Acute mesenteric ischemia (AMI) is defined as a sudden decrease in blood flow through the mesenteric vessels, which can lead to the devastating consequences of bowel ischemia, shock, and frequently death. A high mortality rate of approximately 70% has persisted over the last several decades despite significant advances in diagnosis and therapy. Although mesenteric ischemia may affect the small and the large bowel, the pathophysiology of each differs.

The blood supply to the GI tract is complex and redundant, and it is derived mainly from the celiac axis, superior mesenteric artery (SMA), and inferior mesenteric artery (IMA). This is supplemented by an extensive network of collateral vessels, which provide redundancy.

1. **Causes:** The causes of acute mesenteric ischemia (AMI) include: (1) acute thrombosis of the SMA, typically superimposed on an atherosclerotic plaque at the origin of the vessel; (2) an embolism to the SMA; (3) SMA dissection; (4) mesenteric venous thromboses; and (5) a low-flow state described as nonocclusive mesenteric ischemia (NOMI).

2. **History:** The most important factor in making the diagnosis is maintaining a high index of suspicion. The typical presentation of AMI is acute onset of abdominal pain in an elderly patient, without obvious findings on physical exam, described classically as "pain out of proportion to physical exam findings." The pain is often reported in the periumbilical or epigastric region, and it may be associated with nausea, vomiting, and bloody bowel movements. A careful history will identify predisposing risk factors. Previous symptoms such as postprandial abdominal pain, food fear, and weight loss suggest underlying chronic mesenteric ischemia. It is important to separate an acute from a chronic presentation, especially if the presentation is subacute, because the treatment for chronic mesenteric ischemia is different from the treatment in the acute

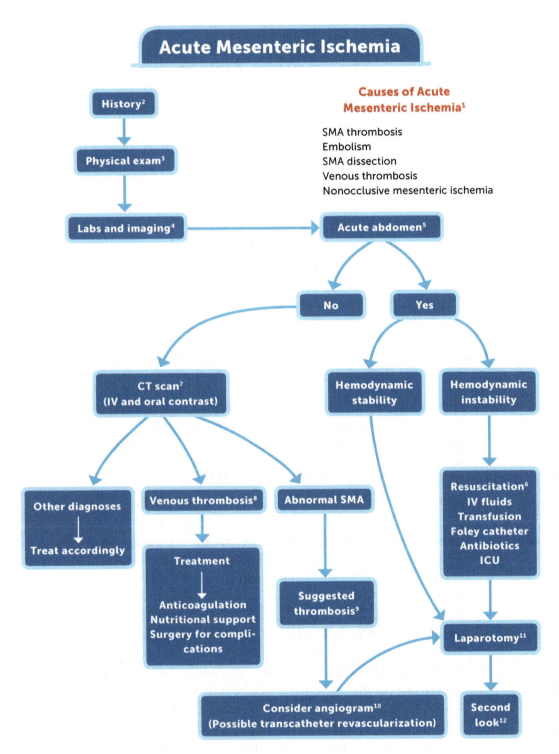

Algorithm 5. Managing Acute Mesenteric Ischemia

situation. Thromboembolism from cardiac sources accounts for the majority of cases of AMI. Cardiac risk factors include arrhythmias, valvular abnormalities, recent heart attack, congestive heart failure, arteriosclerosis, previous embolic phenomenon, and ventricular aneurysms. Other factors that promote the development of arteriosclerosis include a history of smoking, hypertension, hyperlipidemia, and diabetes mellitus. A history of a malignancy has also been associated with AMI. A subacute presentation may elicit suspicion of mesenteric venous thrombosis, and in these cases, it is important to rule out a hypercoagulable condition. NOMI is typically seen with a low perfusion state (eg, decreased cardiac output) resulting in secondary ischemia. Rapid diagnosis remains the key to decreasing the morbidity and mortality associated with AMI.

3. **Physical exam:** Sudden decrease in blood flow to the mesenteric vessels leads to rapid ischemia of the bowel mucosa first, followed over time by full thickness ischemia with eventual necrosis and perforation. An elderly patient with blood in the stool should signal the possibility of AMI. On exam, the presence of an arrhythmia or hypertension may be noted. The presence of peritoneal signs typically indicates later stages of AMI.

4. **Labs and imaging:** Lab work should include a CBC with differential, lactic acid level, chemistry panel, amylase and lipase levels, and hepatic and coagulation panels. An elevated lactic acid level should readily increase the suspicion of ischemia. Blood typing and cross-matching might be necessary. An ECG and a three-view abdominal radiograph should be performed to rule out an obvious perforation. In the late stages of AMI, radiographs may show gas in the portal system or bowel wall.

5. **Acute abdomen:** An acute abdomen is a manifestation of a sudden intra-abdominal process that causes severe pain. It always requires immediate medical judgment and often leads to a surgical intervention. The causes can be inflammatory (eg, appendicitis), mechanical (eg, bowel obstruction),

6. **Resuscitation:** Hemodynamic stability and stabilization should follow established protocols. Airway protection, fluid resuscitation, administration of vasopressors, transfusion (if needed), correction of any coagulopathy, Foley catheter

insertion, and invasive hemodynamic monitoring should be undertaken according to the clinical picture. These steps are intended to prepare the patient for surgical exploration as soon as possible.

7. **CT scan with IV and oral contrast:** This imaging can be obtained rapidly in stable patients to confirm AMI or suggest an alternative diagnosis. The scan can demonstrate lack of filling of the SMA or its branches, and it may show thickening of the bowel wall.
8. **Venous thrombosis:** A "target" sign from a thrombus in the superior mesenteric vein may be noted on CT.
9. **Suggested thrombosis:** Indications of SMA thrombosis may be seen on CT scan. For instance, distal branches might show a "cutoff" sign, where the filling of the vessels with contrast stops abruptly.
10. **Angiogram:** This test can demonstrate mesenteric ischemia, and in the stable patient, it allows for simultaneous therapeutic options such as angioplasty, arterial stenting, or infusion of vasodilators or thrombolytic agents. In the low-flow setting of NOMI, a classic angiographic finding is the presence of a narrowing at the vessel origin with spasm of the distal branches. In these cases, the angiographic catheter permits infusion of vasodilators to improve perfusion.
11. **Laparotomy:** If angiography is not the final therapeutic step, exploration of the abdominal cavity must be performed promptly and systematically. The entire bowel should be assessed, and the distribution of the ischemia should be noted. Thrombosis at the origin of the SMA causes global ischemia. Embolic events typically spare the most proximal jejunal branches and cause an occlusion distal to the take-off of the middle colic artery. Global ischemia is incompatible with life, forcing a decision of comfort care only. If localized necrosis or perforation is present, resection is indicated. In the presence of marginal viability, the status of the vasculature may help determine surgical options. For example, if there appears to be an occlusion of the SMA at its origin, a bypass may be performed. Or if the source of the ischemia is an embolic phenomenon, an embolectomy may be indicated.

12. **Second look:** A "second look" laparotomy is a planned procedure conducted 24 to 48 hours after the initial exploration to assess the viability of the remaining bowel. It is not always a mandatory step, but it is used frequently in patients presenting with AMI.

Appendix

Surgical Signs and Syndromes by Chapter

	Signs and Syndromes	Presentation	Associated Diagnosis
Chapter 4	Chvostek's sign	Twitching of facial muscles after tapping area through which the facial nerve courses	Hypocalcemia
	Trousseau's sign	Carpal spasm after decreased blood flow to forearm, provoked with a blood pressure cuff	Hypocalcemia
Chapter 5	Rule of 10s	10% are malignant; 10% are incidental; 10% occur in children; 10% are bilateral; and 10% are extra-adrenal	Pheochromocytoma
Chapter 6	Boerhaave's syndrome	Vomiting and retching followed by severe and acute pain in the chest, neck, or epigastric area, and dysphagia	Esophageal perforation
	Mackler's triad	Vomiting, pain, and subcutaneous emphysema	Esophageal perforation
Chapter 7	Horner's syndrome	Anhidrosis, miosis, and ptosis	Pancoast's tumor of the lung
Chapter 8	Peau d'orange	Skin erythema and edema	Inflammatory breast cancer

	Signs and Syndromes	Presentation	Associated Diagnosis
Chapter 10	Dressler syndrome	Inflammatory reaction involving the pericardium and pleura caused by an immune response to cardiac tissue damaged from a myocardial infarction; pericardial effusions often accompany the syndrome	Pericarditis
Chapter 11	Beck's triad	Hypotension, distended neck veins, and muffled heart sounds	Cardiac tamponade
	Leriche syndrome	Decreased femoral pulses, impotence, leg pallor, buttock and leg claudication, and leg muscle atrophy	Atherosclerotic occlusive disease involving the bifurcation of the abdominal aorta
	Virchow's triad	Vascular stasis, hypercoagulability, and endothelial damage	Deep venous thrombosis
	Homan's sign	Calf tenderness on dorsiflexion of the foot	Deep venous thrombosis
	Westermark's sign	Decreased vascular markings on chest radiograph, suggesting focal oligemia	Pulmonary embolism

Surgical Signs and Syndromes by Chapter

	Signs and Syndromes	Presentation	Associated Diagnosis
Chapter 12	Mallory-Weiss syndrome	Upper GI bleeding, nausea, and vomiting	Esophageal tear
	Zollinger-Ellison syndrome	Abdominal pain, steatorrhea, and diarrhea, plus multiple gastrointestinal mucosal ulcerations	Gastrinoma
Chapter 13	Rule of 2s	It occurs in 2% of the population; it is 2 inches long and 2 cm wide; it is 2 feet from the ileocecal valve; 2% of patients are symptomatic; it most commonly presents at age 2 y; and 2 types of ectopic tissue—gastric and pancreatic—may be present	Meckel's diverticulum
	Carcinoid syndrome	Diarrhea, flushing, palpitations, wheezing, and secondary restrictive cardiomyopathy (caused by serotonin-induced fibrosis of the valvular endocardium, mostly tricuspid and pulmonic valves)	Carcinoid tumor
Chapter 14	Blumberg's sign	Pain felt upon sudden release of pressure from the abdomen	A symptom of peritoneal inflammation, frequently described with presumptive diagnosis of appendicitis

Signs and Syndromes	Presentation	Associated Diagnosis
Rovsing's sign	Deep palpation of the left lower quadrant causes referred pain in the right lower quadrant	Appendicitis
Psoas sign	Right lower quadrant pain with extension of the right hip or with flexion of the right hip against resistance (suggests appendix might be retrocecal)	Appendicitis
Obturator sign	Right lower quadrant pain with internal and external rotation of the flexed right hip (suggests that the inflamed appendix is located deep in the right hemipelvis)	Appendicitis
Dunphy's sign	Sharp pain in the right lower quadrant elicited by a voluntary cough	Localized peritonitis
Dumping syndrome	Abnormal postoperative gastric motor function and/or pyloric emptying mechanism	A frequent complication after gastric surgical procedures, such as vagotomy, pyloroplasty, gastrojejunostomy, Roux-en-Y

Chapter 14 (continued)

Surgical Signs and Syndromes by Chapter

	Signs and Syndromes	Presentation	Associated Diagnosis
Chapter 14 *(continued)*	Ogilvie's syndrome	Abdominal pain (80%), nausea and vomiting (80%), obstipation (40%), fever (35%), abdominal distention (90%–100%), abdominal tenderness (64%), hypoactive bowel sounds; most commonly in debilitated, hospitalized patients with multiple medical problems	Acute nonobstructive colonic dilatation
	Laplace's law	The larger the radius of a cylindrical structure (eg, a lumen), the greater the wall tension becomes	Risk of cecal perforation
	Peutz-Jeghers syndrome	Benign hamartomatous polyps in the GI tract, dark spots on the gums and lips	15-fold increased risk of developing intestinal cancer compared with the general population, plus increased risk of extraintestinal cancer
	Gardner's syndrome	Colon polyps, sebaceous cysts, osteomas, desmoid tumors	Colon cancer
	String sign	A narrowed terminal ileum seen in a barium study	Crohn's disease

	Signs and Syndromes	Presentation	Associated Diagnosis
Chapter 15	Budd-Chiari syndrome	Thrombosed hepatic veins	Posthepatic portal hypertension
Chapter 16	Murphy's sign	Pain and inspiratory arrest while the right upper quadrant is palpated	Acute cholecystitis
	Charcot's triad	Fever, jaundice, right upper quadrant pain	Ascending cholangitis
	Reynold's pentad	Fever, jaundice, right upper quadrant pain, altered mental status, hypotension	Suppurative cholangitis
Chapter 17	Courvoisier's sign	Palpable, firm gallbladder with painless jaundice	Periampullary tumor
	Whipple's triad	Hypoglycemic symptoms during fasting, fasting or exertional hypoglycemia with serum glucose levels <45 mg/dL, symptom resolution with glucose administration	Insulinoma
	Grey Turner's sign	Flank ecchymosis	Pancreatitis
	Cullen's sign	Periumbilical ecchymosis	Pancreatitis
	WDHA syndrome	Watery diarrhea, hypokalemia, achlorhydria	VIPoma

	Signs and Syndromes	Presentation	Associated Diagnosis
Chapter 20	Prehn's sign	Testicular pain is relieved with elevation of the affected testicle	Epididymitis

Case Study Questions

Case Study Questions

1. A 67-year-old woman presents with an irregular, 3-cm mass in the upper outer quadrant of the right breast. There appears to be a subtle change of the overlying skin, interpreted as possible peau d'orange. The rest of the exam is unremarkable. The patient has not had any imaging done. A core needle biopsy is performed. What is the next step in management?

   A. Await the pathology report
   B. Order a mammogram
   C. Start chemotherapy
   D. Schedule the patient for surgery
   E. Order an ultrasonography

2. A 22-year-old man in good health is involved in a physical altercation and is stabbed in the left chest. He is rushed to the emergency department with no recordable blood pressure. His pulse is fast and difficult to palpate, and his lungs are clear. His heart sounds are muffled and distant. The jugular veins are distended. What should be done next?

   A. Coronary artery bypass graft
   B. Pericardiocentesis
   C. Insertion of a chest tube
   D. Defibrillation to convert to a normal rhythm
   E. Blood transfusion

3. A 75-year old man with diabetes comes to the emergency department because of a nonhealing wound on his foot. He states that he has tried "all kinds of remedies" at home with no improvement. He reports that he has severe peripheral neuropathy from his diabetes, but no pain. He denies wearing ill-fitting shoes. On exam, there is a 3-cm long, deep, necrotic-appearing ulceration on the dorsum of the right foot without evidence of purulence or erythema. There is no discoloration of the right lower extremity, although the skin has a glossy appearance and absence of hair growth below the knee. There

is also pallor of the involved foot followed by dependent rubor after 1 to 2 minutes of elevation of the foot to above heart level. What is the most likely diagnosis?

A. Venous ulcer
B. Ulcer caused by hobo spider bite
C. Arterial ulcer
D. Diabetic ulcer
E. Cellulitis with ulceration

4. On the fifth postoperative day, a patient confined to bed develops a cough and wheezing. Crackles are heard on auscultation. A chest radiograph shows atelectasis of the right pulmonary base. Pulse oximetry reveals an O_2 saturation of 90%. What test should be performed next?

A. Duplex ultrasound of both lower extremities and a CT angiogram (CTA)
B. CT scan of pelvis
C. Cardiac stress test
D. Echocardiogram
E. CT scan of the chest

5. A 58-year old man has had frequent nausea and occasional vomiting for the past 3 years. He has been trying to decrease his intake of alcohol but has not been completely successful. Vital signs and results of lab work are normal. An upper GI endoscopy reveals areas of atrophic gastritis. A biopsy reveals a microscopic, well-differentiated adenocarcinoma. Which of the following is more likely to have played a role in the development of this cancer?

A. Decreased testosterone levels
B. *Helicobacter pylori* infection
C. Mutations in the *BRCA1* or *BRCA2* gene
D. Epstein-Barr virus (EBV) infection
E. Alcohol consumption

6. A 28-year-old man presents complaining of fatigue and pallor. He states that he is having a great deal of difficulty performing

his daily routines. He also has had several episodes of right upper quadrant pain. A workup reveals a hemoglobin level of 11.1 g/dL and a reticulocyte count of 12%. Unconjugated bilirubin levels are 6.3 mg/dL, and results of a Coombs test are negative. Spherocytes are noted on the peripheral smear. What are the likely findings on physical exam?

A. A palpable gallbladder in the right upper quadrant
B. A palpable spleen in the left upper quadrant
C. A palpable pancreas in the left upper quadrant
D. A palpable spleen in the left upper quadrant and no findings in the right upper quadrant
E. Neither a palpable spleen nor a palpable gallbladder

7. A 72-year-old man is found to have a diverticular abscess arising from the sigmoid colon. The surgeon decides to proceed with a Hartmann's procedure. What does this operation consist of?

A. Removing the diseased segment and re-anastomosing the intestine
B. Draining the abscess and doing a transverse loop colostomy
C. Removing the diseased segment and creating an end colostomy and a distal mucous fistula
D. Draining the abscess and creating an ileostomy
E. Removing the diseased segment as part of an abdominoperineal resection (APR)

8. A 46-year-old woman reports finding a lump in the left breast. She has an average risk profile and says she doesn't examine her breasts habitually. She did this time because she had pain in that breast. What must be determined first during the physical exam?

A. Whether the lump is in an outer or inner quadrant
B. Whether the lump is larger or smaller than 1 cm
C. Whether the lump is dominant
D. Whether the lump has irregular or smooth borders
E. Whether the lump is tender

9. A 46-year-old man presents with increasing midabdominal pain, nausea, and vomiting of foul-smelling material of several days duration. He is taken to the operating room with a diagnosis

of bowel obstruction, and during the laparotomy he is found to have a small, yellowish submucosal tumor in the terminal ileum with a significant inflammatory response around it that is causing the obstruction. The immunohistochemical analysis of the tumor is returned 2 days later and shows a strong positive reaction to chromogranin and synaptophysin. Levels of which marker can be expected to be elevated in this patient?

A. Metanephrines
B. Serotonin
C. Insulin
D. Estrogen receptor
E. Calcitonin

10. A 49-year-old woman is diagnosed with celiac sprue. What condition does she have an increased risk of developing?

A. Intestinal lymphoma
B. Inflammatory bowel disease
C. Lactose intolerance
D. Tropical sprue
E. Whipple disease

11. A 52-year-old man has had an abdominal operation. Six days after surgery, he develops a fever (temperature, 38.4°C). Urine output is normal, but a urinalysis reveals 100,000 CFU/mL of *Escherichia coli*. His IV has been discontinued, and he is ambulating. On exam, there is mild tenderness and swelling at one end of the incision, which is erythematous and warm. What is the next step in management?

A. Perform a duplex ultrasound of pelvic veins
B. Obtain a urine culture
C. Order incentive spirometry
D. Open the wound
E. Perform a CT scan of the abdomen

12. A 69-year-old man presents to the emergency department with severe abdominal pain associated with hematemesis. He has had intermittent episodes of abdominal pain in the past, which

he treated with over-the-counter medications. He has a history of gout and has been taking colchicine to manage it. Recently, indomethacin was added to his medication regimen for pain control. Exam reveals abdominal guarding and moderate rebound tenderness. His hemoglobin level is 9.7 g/dL, and his white blood cell count is 14.1/mm^3. A plain abdominal film suggests, but does not confirm, that there is air under the diaphragm. What should be the initial treatment for this patient?

A. Perform an emergency UGI endoscopy
B. Admit him to the ICU, begin administration of IV antibiotics, and perform serial physical exams and lab work
C. Order a CT scan to confirm or rule out whether there is air under the diaphragm
D. Admit the patient for observation and place him on triple therapy for *H. pylori*
E. Perform a laparotomy

13. A 42-year-old woman is diagnosed with triple-negative breast cancer, and she is considering treatment options. She is undecided between a lumpectomy and a mastectomy. Her history indicates that her mother had ovarian cancer at age 48 years, and her uncle on the maternal side had breast cancer. Her maternal grandmother had pancreatic cancer. What should she be advised to undergo as the next step before making a decision regarding the type of surgical procedure to choose?

A. MRI of both breasts
B. Testing for genetic mutations
C. A mirror biopsy of the opposite breast
D. A bilateral mastectomy
E. An oophorectomy

14. A patient is being prepared for a colon resection. Which bacteria should be targeted by prophylactic antibiotics?

A. *Haemophilus influenzae*
B. *Bacteroides fragilis*
C. *Candida albicans*

D. *Pseudomonas aeruginosa*
E. *Staphylococcus aureus*

15. Which of the following can be released by non–small cell lung cancer cells to induce a paraneoplastic syndrome?

    A. Gastrin
    B. Adrenocorticotropic hormone (ACTH)
    C. Parathyroid hormone–related peptide (PTHrP)
    D. Calcitonin
    E. Antidiuretic hormone (ADH)

16. A 49-year-old woman comes in with a lesion on the areola and nipple of the left breast, which is itching and flaky. On exam, the areola and nipple are reddish, with a crusty lesion and mild flattening of the nipple. Expressing the apex of the breast elicits a droplet of clear fluid from the nipple. Exam of the opposite breast is unremarkable. How should this patient be managed?

    A. Order a 10-day course of a steroid-containing ointment
    B. Order a mammogram and an ultrasound
    C. Perform a biopsy
    D. Reexamine in 6 weeks to assess for the possibility of regression
    E. Order a 10-day course of antibiotics

17. A 63-year-old man is about to undergo a colon resection. Which of the following should not be performed?

    A. Mechanical bowel preparation
    B. Chlorhexidine preparation of the skin before incision
    C. Hair clipping the night before surgery
    D. Administration of antibiotics within 1 hour of incision
    E. Intraoperative body temperature control

18. A 17-year-old girl is performing cheerleading exercises and is thrown in the air. She falls upon landing and strikes her head. She experiences a brief loss of consciousness, and after awakening appears to behave normally, as reported by her friends. The school protocol, however, requires evaluation at the local emergency department. She is found to have a

score of 15 on the Glasgow Coma Scale (GCS), but she has amnesia of the event. A CT scan of the head demonstrates a small left occipital subdural hemorrhage. She is admitted for observation. Late in the evening, she becomes agitated and confused. She is emotionally labile, represented by crying, then yelling and impulsively trying to get out of bed. Her GCS score is now 14. Given the change in her mental status, a repeat head CT is performed that demonstrates a new right frontal intraparenchymal hemorrhage. What kind of injury has the patient suffered?

A. Diffuse axonal injury
B. Stagnant hypoxia injury
C. Waddell's triad injury
D. Second impact syndrome
E. Coup-contrecoup injury

19. An 8-year-old girl wrecks her bicycle, hitting her upper abdomen on the handlebars. Vital signs in the emergency department reveal a blood pressure of 100/60 mm Hg, a heart rate of 110 bpm, and a respiratory rate of 14 breaths per minute. Abdominal CT scan reveals a duodenal hematoma. Her GCS score is 15. What is the most appropriate treatment?

A. Immediate laparotomy
B. Discharge and follow up as an outpatient
C. Laparoscopy
D. Endoscopic retrograde cholangiopancreatography (ERCP)
E. Hospital admission, serial exams, and nasogastric tube insertion if vomiting occurs

20. A 3-year-old girl is brought into the emergency department with a 1-hour history of intermittent coughing. Her mother reports that the sputum is blood streaked. She describes the child as otherwising behaving normally. Stridor is noted on auscultation. What is the most likely cause of the hemoptysis?

A. Metastases
B. Bronchitis
C. Pneumonia

D. Asthma
E. Foreign body

21. A 64-year-old man presents as an outpatient complaining of cramping in his buttocks, thighs, and calves with walking and says that it is relieved with rest. He states that his feet generally feel cooler than they did when he was younger. He has difficulty achieving an erection. His medical history includes tobacco use and coronary artery disease. On examination, femoral pulses are diminished and hair is sparse below his knees. What is the most likely diagnosis?

    A. Spinal stenosis
    B. Diabetic neuropathy
    C. Aortoiliac occlusive disease
    D. Varicocele
    E. Bilateral femoral occlusive disease

22. A 61-year-old woman arrives at the emergency department complaining of right calf pain. She was hospitalized 2 weeks ago for an appendectomy complicated by a wound infection. Vital signs reveal a blood pressure of 145/92 mm Hg and a heart rate of 120 bpm. According to the revised validated criteria of the Wells score to diagnose a pulmonary embolism, her score is greater than 6 points. What does this score signify about the probability that she has a pulmonary embolism?

    A. Low Probability
    B. Moderate probability
    C. Intermediate probability
    D. No probability
    E. High probability

23. A 25-year-old diabetic man has suffered blood loss after an episode of trauma. His blood pressure is stabilized after administration of fluids. He has a Foley catheter in place, and his urine output so far is 430 mL (reference range for daily urine output: 750–2000 mL/d). Laboratory studies reveal a hemoglobin A_{1C} of 5.6%, a serum osmolality of 260 mOsm/kg (reference range: 278–298 mOsm/kg), and a serum Na^+ of 143

mEq/L. Results of an arterial blood gas (ABG) are as follows:

Results	Reference Range
pH = 7.38	7.35–7.45
Pao$_2$ = 78 mm Hg	80–100 mm Hg
Paco$_2$ = 48 mm Hg	35–45 mm Hg
Hco$_3^-$ = 25 mEq/L	22–26 mEq/L
Sao$_2$ = 92%	95%–100%

On physical exam, the extremities are warm and breath sounds are normal. Vital signs are within normal limits. He is receiving oxygen through a non-rebreather mask at a rate of 12 L per minute. His non-rebreather mask collapses 75% with each breath. What action should be performed next?

A. Reduce the oxygen flow to a rate of 10 L per minute
B. Increase the oxygen flow to a rate of 15 L per minute
C. Support the patient with continuous positive airway pressure (CPAP)
D. Initiate mechanical ventilation
E. Add albuterol via nebulizer

24. A 17-year-old man presents to the emergency department with 2-hour history of dyspnea and chest pain. He is 6 feet tall and weighs 170 pounds. He exercises regularly and is in excellenct shape. He denies any foreign travel or trauma. His heart rate is 110 bpm. Physical exam demonstrates absent breath sounds of the left lung with hyperresonance to percussion. What is the most likely diagnosis?

A. Acure coronary syndrome
B. Pulmonary embolism
C. Arotic dissection
D. Pneumonia
E. Primary spontaneous pneumothorax (PTX)

25. A 51-year-old woman presents with a mammographic density, reported as BI-RADS 4. A stereotaxic biopsy is performed, and the pathology report reveals the presence of lobular carcinoma in situ, or *LCIS*. What is the next step in management?

    A. Mastectomy
    B. Lumpectomy and radiotherapy
    C. Irradiation
    D. Bilateral mastectomies
    E. Close observation

26. Which is the most common electrolyte abnormality that occurs in the postoperative period?

    A. Hyperchloremia
    B. Hyponatremia
    C. Hyperkalemia
    D. Hypochloremia
    E. Hypernatremia

27. A 56-year-old woman is seen in the emergency department with significant abdominal pain that does not coincide with the mild findings on abdominal exam. She reports nausea, vomiting, and diarrhea. The patient has known factor V Leiden disease, and had been taking warfarin until 1 month ago. The results from the stool guaiac test are positive. What is an appropriate treatment regimen?

    A. IV fluids and observation
    B. IV fluids, CT scan with contrast, and observation
    C. IV fluids, CT scan with contrast, and papaverine infusion
    D. IV fluids, CT scan with contrast, heparin and papaverine infusion through an angiographic catheter
    E. IV fluids, CT scan with contrast, heparin infusion, nutritional support, and serial exams

28. A 14-year-old boy is brought in by his mother because of a mass in his neck. On exam, there is a 2-cm soft, round mass in the anterior midline of the neck, close to the hyoid bone. It is

nontender and moves with deglutition. An ultrasound reveals a hypoechoic lesion without a solid vascular component. What is the most likely diagnosis?

A. Branchial cleft cyst
B. Cystic hygroma
C. Lipoma
D. Thyroglossal duct cyst
E. Enlarged lymph node

29. A 64-year-old man presents with a dominant lump in the left breast, directly underneath the areola. Findings from physical exam of the axilla and supraclavicular areas are normal, and the patient has no comorbid conditions. A biopsy reveals invasive ductal carcinoma. What is the next step in treatment?

A. Lumpectomy
B. Mastectomy and sentinel node biopsy
C. Irradiation
D. Segmental mastectomy
E. Neoadjuvant chemotherapy

30. A patient suffers blunt trauma to the torso. In which one of the following does focused assessment sonography for trauma (FAST) have the greatest detection utility?

A. Mesenteric hematoma
B. Pancreatic transection
C. Free fluid
D. Grading of solid organ injuries
E. Free air

31. An 18-year-old man is seen because of right lower quadrant pain, which began 36 hours ago. The presumptive diagnosis of appendicitis is made. A CT scan is ordered. What will it show if the patient does have appendicitis?

A. The appendix will not be visible because of the inflammatory process
B. The appendix will appear enlarged in diameter, and fat stranding of the mesentery will be noted

C. The appendix will appear shrunken with a radiopaque fecalith in the lumen
D. The appendix will be surrounded by large lymphadenopathy
E. The appendix will not be visible because it will be covered by omentum

32. A 34-year-old man evaluated as American Society of Anesthesia (ASA) Class 1 is seen on postop day 1 after damage control surgery for multiple trauma. He is in the surgical ICU, sedated and receiving ventilatory assistance. Vital signs are stable and urine output is normal. The high-pressure alarm on the ventilator sounds and the bedside capnograph reading is depicted below:

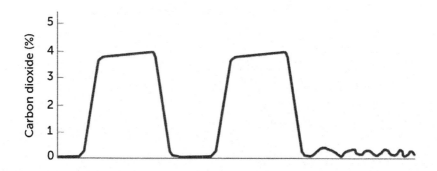

The patient is still breathing. What action is required next?

A. Increase the fraction of inspired oxygen (Fio_2)
B. Increase the tidal volume
C. Extubate the patient and begin manual ventilation
D. Reverse the sedation and reevaluate the patient once he is awake
E. Order a portable chest X-ray

33. A 52-year-old woman presents with epigastric pain, nausea, and vomiting. Lab analyses reveal an amylase level of 2200 IU/L. An ultrasound reveals cholelithiasis. Her symptoms subside after 24 hours, and her amylase level is normal after 48 hours. She wants to go home. What should be done next?

A. Discharge and follow up in 6 weeks

B. Discharge, arrange for an endoscopic retrograde cholangiopancreatography (ERCP), and follow up in 6 weeks
C. Discharge, order a low-fat diet, and follow up in 6 weeks
D. Discharge, arrange for an ERCP, order a low-fat diet, and schedule for cholecystectomy in 6 weeks
E. Perform a cholecystectomy

34. A 60-year-old woman with a history of poorly controlled diabetes presents to the emergency department complaining of significant pain in her right leg at the site of a wound. She does not remember how she first sustained trauma to the area. Vital signs reveal a temperature of 101.8°F and a heart rate of 99 bpm. Systolic blood pressure is 161 mm Hg. The wound appears to be insignificant and looks like a puncture that is almost healed. Her right leg is exquisitely tender to palpation in the area of concern, with significant pain also present in tissue that appears healthy near the wound. The area is warm, with erythema spreading out from the center of the lesion. What is the working diagnosis?

    A. Spider bite
    B. Cellulitis
    C. Necrotizing fasciitis
    D. Deep venous thrombosis
    E. Foreign body

35. A 57-year-old woman presents with a 5-cm mass in her left upper extremity. There are no skin changes, tenderness, or erythema. An MRI demonstrates a soft tissue mass arising from the body of the muscle. What is the next step in management?

    A. Biopsy of the lesion
    B. Radiation
    C. Chemotherapy
    D. Surgical resection with sentinel lymph node biopsy
    E. Surgical resection with axillary node dissection

36. A 65-year-old man is admitted after he is seen in the emergency department because his wife noticed that he appeared "yellow."

He has no specific complaints. The emergency department lab analyses revealed a total bilirubin of 9.6 mg/dL and a direct bilirubin of 7.9 mg/dL. What CT scan finding best explains this presentation?

A. Pancreatic pseudocyst
B. 2.5-cm pancreatic tail mass
C. 3-cm mass in the right lobe of the liver
D. 2-cm pancreatic head mass
E. Inflammatory changes around the pancreas indicative of pancreatitis

37. A 69-year-old man has been having intermittent episodes of pneumaturia and dysuria. He has a history of occasional bouts of lower abdominal pain. A urinalysis reveals bacteria and a small number of red blood cells. What is the most likely cause of this presentation?

A. Colon cancer
B. Bladder cancer
C. Cystitis
D. Diverticular disease
E. Prostatic cancer

38. A 40-year-old woman presents to the emergency department with severe abdominal pain. Lab analyses reveal an amylase level of 1050 U/L and a lipase level of 1200 U/L. She denies drinking alcohol. The working diagnosis is acute pancreatitis. What diagnostic test is the best to identify the most common cause of acute pancreatitis?

A. Right upper quadrant ultrasound
B. Cholesterol panel
C. Drug toxicology screen
D. CT scan
E. Endoscopic retrograde cholangiopancreatography (ERCP)

39. A 25-year-old woman who is 28 weeks pregnant is brought to the emergency department after being involved in a motor vehicle accident (MVA). She has a dilated left pupil and her score on the Glasgow Coma Scale (GCS) is 3. Systolic blood

pressure is 80 mm Hg and heart rate is 130 bpm after infusing 2 L saline solution. A blood transfusion is started, and focused assessment sonography for trauma (FAST) is positive for fluid in the pelvis and right upper quadrant. What is the most appropriate next step?

A. Request obstetrics consultation and wait for their evaluation
B. Obtain CT scan of the head
C. Perform diagnostic peritoneal lavage (DPL)
D. Obtain CT scan of the abdomen
E. Perform exploratory laparotomy

40. A 55-year-old woman is referred for evaluation of chronic abdominal pain. An upper endoscopy reveals ulcers in the stomach and several in the duodenum. Gastrin level is elevated, and a gastrinoma is suspected. What is the best test to order first to identify its location?

A. Endoscopic ultrasound
B. Octreotide scan
C. CT scan
D. Ultrasound
E. ERCP

41. A 65-year-old man presents to the emergency department reporting abdominal and back pain. Vital signs reveal a blood pressure of 90/40 mm Hg, a heart rate of 140 bpm, and a temperature of 36°C. A urinalysis is negative for white blood cells and reveals a small number of red blood cells. Lab work reveals a serum creatinine level of 1.8 mg/dL, an elevated serum lactate level, and a hemoglobin level of 8.2 g/dL. Examination reveals a pulsatile abdominal mass and a decreased pedal pulse in the right foot. What is the most likely diagnosis?

A. Nephrolithiasis
B. Severe peripheral vascular disease
C. Gastrointestinal bleed
D. Ruptured abdominal aortic aneuyrsm (AAA)
E. Mesenteric ischemia

42. A patient presents with a 2-mm superficial spreading melanoma on the right arm with involved lymph nodes proven by biopsy at the time of diagnosis. He is taken to the operating room for a wide local excision with axillary lymph node dissection. Six months after the surgery, he presents complaining of swelling and pain of his right arm, which is significantly larger than the contralateral arm. The swelling involves the fingers and is nonpitting. What is the most likely diagnosis?

   A. Hyperhidrosis
   B. Hydrostatic swelling
   C. Lymphedema
   D. Reflexive sympathetic dystrophy
   E. Deep venous thrombosis (DVT)

43. An 18-month old boy is brought into the emergency department with brisk rectal bleeding that started earlier in the day. Physical exam reveals vital signs within the reference ranges, no fever, and no abdominal tenderness. The umbilicus appears to have a small sinus, but there is no drainage. What study should be ordered next?

   A. Radiographic studies of the upper GI tract
   B. Pertechnetate Tc 99m scan
   C. CT scan
   D. Ultrasonography
   E. Plain abdominal radiograph

44. A 68-year-old man undergoes surgical repair of an abdominal aortic aneurysm. On the third postoperative day, he develops acidosis and his volume requirements increase. Abdominal exam is inconclusive because pain at the incision site makes it difficult to evaluate. The results of the stool guaiac test are positive. What diagnostic maneuver should be done next?

   A. Angiography
   B. Rigid sigmoidoscopy
   C. CT scan with contrast
   D. Colonoscopy
   E. MRI

45. Which of the following tests is not helpful to diagnose nonocclusive mesenteric ischemia?

A. Ultrasonography
B. CT scan with contrast
C. Angiography
D. Magnetic resonance angiography (MRA)
E. CT angiography (CTA)

46. Radioactive iodine I 131 may be a useful adjuvant treatment after resection of which one of the following thyroid carcinomas?

A. Papillary and medullary
B. Follicular and medullary
C. Anaplastic and medullary
D. Papillary and follicular
E. Papillary and anaplastic

47. A 45-year-old trauma patient with a history of well-controlled diabetes is admitted to the SICU with systemic inflammatory response syndrome (SIRS) after sustaining multiple trauma injuries. He is sedated and receiving muscle relaxants to assist with mechanical ventilation. He is receiving synchronized intermittent mandatory ventilation (SIMV) assistance at a rate of 12 breaths per minute (reference range: 8–12 breaths per minute). The tidal volume (VT) is set at 550 mL and the fraction of inspired oxygen (Fio_2) is 40%. Positive end-expiratory pressure (PEEP) is set at 10 cm H_2O and pressure support is set at 5 (normal). The nurse reports that his Pao_2 is 95 mm Hg, $Paco_2$ is 35 mm Hg, and his respiratory rate (RR) is 35 breaths per minute. What should be done next?

A. No action required
B. Increase the SIMV rate
C. Decrease the SIMV rate
D. Increase the Fio_2
E. Decrease the Fio_2

48. A 59-year-old woman is diagnosed with extensive necrotizing fasciitis. Which intervention is the most critical in controlling her infection?

   A. Wound management consisting of frequent dressing changes and topical treatments
   B. Wound irrigation with broad-spectrum antibiotics
   C. Intravenously administered antibiotics
   D. Orally administered antibiotics
   E. Surgical débridement

49. Hexagonal crystals on are found during microscopic examination of the urine of an 8-year-old girl with nephrolithiasis. What is the diagnosis?

   A. Calcium oxalate stones
   B. Uric acid stones
   C. Struvite stones
   D. Calcium phosphate stones
   E. Cystine stones

50. A 34-year-old man presents with a history of rectal expulsion of fresh, bright red blood. A colonoscopy confirms the presence of hundreds of polyps. Which one of the following genes should be checked for the presence of a mutation?

   A. *APC*
   B. *MLH1*
   C. *STK11*
   D. *BRCA2*
   E. *Neurofibromin 1*

Answers and Rationales

Answers and Rationales

1. **B.** A mammogram is not performed to confirm an obvious finding, such as a clearly detectable mass with malignant clinical characteristics as is noted in this patient. Peau d'orange (orange peel skin) indicates invasion of the subdermal lymphatics by tumor. However, the management might change if a mammogram detects any other abnormalities not clinically apparent in the affected breast or in the opposite breast. The decision to initiate chemotherapy or perform surgery is done after the workup is completed. Ultrasonography is used to determine whether a mass is solid or cystic. In this case, it would only confirm the presence of a mass that is already clinically apparent, so it is unnecessary.

2. **B.** This presentation is typical of pericardial tamponade, frequently described as Beck's triad (hypotension, distended neck veins, and muffled heart sounds). Therefore, an immediate pericardiocentesis should be performed to remove the blood collecting in the pericardial sac that is not allowing the heart to expand. A coronary artery bypass is not an option because the clinical presentation is secondary to penetrating trauma and does not suggest pathology of the coronary vessels. A chest tube is not indicated because the patient has normal breath sounds and most likely does not have a pneumothorax. Defibrillation is not needed at this time because he does not have an arrhythmia; instead he exhibits tachycardia with a faint pulse. A transfusion is not needed at this time as there is no indication of acute blood loss.

3. **C.** This patient has classic findings of an arterial insufficiency ulcer. Arterial ulcers are normally painful, although in patients with diabetic neuropathy this may not occur. These ulcers are found on the toes, dorsum, and heel of the foot. Atherosclerosis and peripheral neuropathy occur with increased frequency in persons with diabetes mellitus. Peripheral neuropathy causes loss of protective sensation and loss of coordination of muscle groups in the foot and leg, both of which increase mechanical stress during ambulation. The loss of a limb is a significant risk

in patients with diabetic foot ulcers. Venous ulcers are normally associated with "bronzing" of the skin (caused by hemosiderin deposits), and the ulcers are usually painless and are present over the medial and lateral malleoli. These areas are especially prone to venous hypertension because their drainage largely depends on the competence and patency of the entire great saphenous vein and the perforating veins. Diabetic ulcers are painless and occur on the plantar or lateral aspects of the foot. Hobo spider bites are painful and result in purulent necrotic ulcers. Nonpurulent cellulitis is associated with the 4 typical signs of infection: erythema, pain, swelling and warmth.

4. **A.** The fifth postoperative day coincides with the possible complication of a venous thromboembolism. This patient has symptoms of a pulmonary embolism (PE), which usually arises from a DVT. Therefore, a PE clearly must be ruled out, and a duplex ultrasound of the lower extremities to locate a DVT can be ordered simultaneously with a CTA of the chest. There are no clinical indicators that require a CT scan of the pelvis, and a CT scan of the chest is not as helpful in identifying a PE as a CTA. This patient does not have cardiac symptoms, so a stress test and an echocardiogram are not indicated.

5. **B.** Infection with *Helicobacter pylori* bacteria has been found to be a major cause of stomach cancer. Long-term infection of the stomach with this bacterium may lead to atrophic gastritis and precancerous changes of the gastric mucosa. An increased risk of stomach cancer is associated with a diet consisting of large amounts of smoked foods, salted fish and meat, and pickled vegetables. The nitrates and nitrites found in cured meats can be converted by *H. pylori* into compounds that have been shown to cause stomach cancer in lab animals. Consumption of alcohol and mutations of *BRCA1* or *BRCA2* genes appear to increase the risk of gastric cancer, but not to the degree that *H. pylori* does. EBV has been linked to lymphoma, and it is also found in the cancer cells of about 5% to 10% of people with gastric cancer. Decreased levels of testosterone play no role in the development of gastric cancer.

6. **D.** In hereditary spherocytosis, the spleen is usually enlarged and can be palpated upon careful examination. The gallbladder and the pancreas are not palpable in a presentation like this.

7. **C.** A Hartmann's procedure includes removing the diseased segment, usually the sigmoid colon, and bringing the proximal end out through the abdominal wall as a colostomy. Whenever possible, the distal segment is brought out as a mucous fistula, which is simply a nonfunctioning colostomy because no intestinal contents reach it. Commonly, the distal segment is too short to exteriorize, so it is left closed inside the abdominal cavity. The intestine should not be re-anastomosed in the presence of an infection. Simply draining the abscess and creating a proximal stoma, either as a colostomy or an ileostomy, is seldom done anymore because a diverticular infection is the result of a perforation. Therefore, leaving the diseased segment in place means more intestinal contents may leak out. An APR, a procedure in which the rectum is removed, is not indicated.

8. **C.** The normal breast is "lumpy," so the first step is to decide if the patient actually has a true, or *dominant*, lump. If the presence of a true lump is established, the characteristics of the lump, such as its size, borders, and location, must be determined afterward.

9. **B.** This patient has a carcinoid tumor, which relases serotonin and produces a significant inflammatory and scarring mesenteric response out of proportion to the tumor size. The tumor is responsible for the bowel obstruction and the patient's symptoms. The measurement of chromogranin A is considered the gold standard of chemical tests to confirm the diagnosis of carcinoid and neuroendocrine tumors and is also used to monitor their course. Urinary 5-HIAA is a breakdown product of serotonin, and is usually measured when there is a suspicion of a carcinoid. However, even when 5-HIAA is not elevated, serotonin levels might be. The measurement of metanephrines is used to diagnose pheochromocytoma. Insulin levels are measured to diagnose pancreatic insulinomas, and an elevated calcitonin level is associated with thyroid cancer. Estrogen

receptor status is evaluated with a diagnosis of breast cancer.

10. **A.** Celiac sprue is a disorder of the digestive tract that results in the inability to tolerate gliadin, the alcohol-soluble portion of gluten. It results in the malabsorption of nutrients. Intestinal lymphoma of the small intestine is a recognized complication of celiac sprue, and it can also occur with immunodeficiency syndromes, such as HIV infection. Lactose intolerance is a common genetic deficiency. Like celiac sprue, tropical sprue is a malabsorptive disorder and is believed to be caused by bacterial infection with *Klebsiella* species, *Escherichia coli*, and *Enterobacter* species. It typically occurs after travel to third world countries and is associated with folate, vitamin B_{12}, and iron deficiencies. Whipple disease is a systemic disease that affects the small intestine, the joints, the cardiovascular system, and the central nervous system and is most likely caused by the gram-positive bacterium, *Tropheryma whipplei*. In the small intestine, *T. whipplei* infiltrate the villi, causing a malabsorption syndrome.

11. **D.** Fever on the sixth postoperative day plus rubor (erythema), tumor (swelling), calor (heat), and dolor (pain) in the incision are the result of a wound infection, which requires opening of the incision. This patient also has a urinary tract infection that must be treated. However, a urine culture must be obtained in conjunction with initiating broad-spectrum antibiotics until culture results become available. A duplex ultrasound of the pelvic veins, which might be of help in suspected cases of ileofemoral thrombosis, serves no purpose in this patient. Spirometry is useful to reduce the possibility of atelectasis, but it is not the next step in care for this patient.

12. **E.** This patient has clinically clear signs of peritonitis, and this presentation in conjunction with the suggestion of air under the diaphragm requires surgical exploration. On the basis of these signs and symptoms, the patient most likely has a perforated ulcer. Admission to the ICU and serial exams might constitute a reasonable approach in treating a patient without peritonitis, but in this case the patient needs an urgent laparotomy. A CT scan can confirm the presence of free air in the abdomen, but

this finding would not change the recommended management in this case. Treating this patient for *H. pylori* infection is appropriate but would not change the need to perform a laparotomy as the initial step in treatment.

13. **B.** A young patient with a triple-negative breast carcinoma plus this strong family history of breast and ovarian cancers indicates the possibility of a mutation in one of the *BRCA* genes, so testing for it is not only appropriate but indicated as the next step. If this patient is found to have a harmful mutation (known as a *deleterious mutation*), she would be advised that her lifetime risk of developing breast cancer is 85% to 87%, and the risk of developing ovarian cancer would be increased as well. Commonly, patients in this situation choose to have a bilateral mastectomy, with or without reconstruction. An oophorectomy would also be an appropriate choice for the patient to consider if she is found to have a mutation. An MRI of both breasts is commonly indicated in a case like this, but genetic testing could change management, so that should be the next step. A mirror biopsy is not indicated, because the probability of finding disease without a target (which is the principle behind a mirror biopsy) is minimal. For this reason, mirror biopsies have been abandoned.

14. **B.** Over 99% of the bacteria in the gut are anaerobes, and the most common is *Bacteroides fragilis,* which comprises approximately 30% of colonic bacteria. In the cecum, aerobic bacteria reach high densities. All other bacteria are either less common or infrequently found in the colon.

15. **C.** PTHrP is released by non–small cell lung cancer cells and induces a paraneoplastic syndrome of hypercalcemia. PTHrP resembles PTH, and they both bind to the same type of receptor and induce a similar response in the body. For this reason, hypercalcemia of malignancy resembles hyperparathyroidism. In addition to their normal functions, ACTH and ADH can be released by small cell lung cancer cells. Gastrin stimulates the parietal cells of the stomach to secrete gastric acid, and calcitonin is produced by the C cells of the thyroid to reduce serum calcium levels.

16. **C.** This patient presents with typical symptoms of Paget disease of the breast, which is a malignant disease with clinical characteristics similar to eczema. It is not uncommon to interpret an eczematoid lesion on the nipple or the areola as a dermatologic process. With the described characteristics, eczema is unlikely. Therefore, a biopsy is the first step to rule out Paget disease, and it would be imprudent to wait 6 weeks to reexamine this patient. A mammogram and ultrasound will be needed eventually but would not change the need to obtain a tissue diagnosis. The clinical presentation does not have the characteristics of an infection (erythema, pain, swelling). Therefore, antibiotics are not indicated.

17. **C.** The hair should be clipped immediately before incision. All others are important measures that should be performed to decrease incidence of postoperative infections.

18. **E.** A coup-contrecoup injury is commonly seen in high-energy blunt head trauma, and is frequently noted at nearly 180 degrees from the original injury. This occurs when a head in motion strikes a stationary object, causing a coup injury at the site of impact. The abrupt deceleration causes the brain to collide with the opposite side of the skull, which causes the secondary contusion, or contrecoup injury. Diffuse axonal injury is due to rotational acceleration of the brain that causes shearing and tensile forces. This results in axons tearing at the microscopic level. These patients often have mild findings on CT scan but are completely obtunded. This disturbance in the brain can produce temporary or permanent widespread brain damage, coma, or death. A stagnant hypoxia injury, most commonly called *hypoxic brain injury,* results when the brain does not receive enough oxygen. This can be caused by a variety of factors, such as a decrease in the oxygen supply to the brain (eg, smoke inhalation, tracheal compression, carbon monoxide poisoning) or a decrease in blood flow (eg, severe hypotension, drug overdose, drowning). There is no evidence in this patient's presentation suggesting an ischemic insult is the cause of the brain injury. Waddell's triad is a pattern of injury seen when motor vehicles collide with pedestrian children. The pattern of injury includes first a fractured femoral shaft

followed by intrathoracic or intra-abdominal injuries and a contralateral head injury. Second impact syndrome, also termed *recurrent traumatic brain injury,* occurs when a person sustains a concussion followed by a second traumatic brain injury before the symptoms of the first traumatic brain injury have healed. The second injury may occur from days to weeks following the first. This second impact may cause cerebral edema and herniation, leading to collapse and death within minutes. If the patient survives, long-term effects can include muscle spasms, emotionalal lability, hallucinations, and difficulty thinking and learning.

19. **E.** Initial treatment for duodenal hematomas in the stable patient is close observation and serial exams. Furthermore, this patient's GCS score indicates a fully awake patient. If obstructive symptoms develop, nasogastric (NG) tube decompression is warranted. There is no indication for laparotomy in this patient, and similarly there is no indication for laparoscopy because there are neither clinical nor radiologic indications that there is a surgical emergency. ERCP rarely has a role in trauma, unless there is clear concern regarding the integrity of the common bile duct or pancreatic duct.

20. **E.** The most common cause of hemoptysis (coughing up blood) in children is the aspiration of a foreign body. It is associated with stridor, an abnormal, high-pitched breathing sound that is caused by a blockage of the trachea. The most commonly aspirated foreign bodies are small food items such as nuts, raisins, sunflower seeds, improperly chewed pieces of meat, and small, smooth items such as grapes. Lung metastases is an unlikely diagnosis in a child, and it does not present suddenly with the symptoms described. Bronchitis and pneumonia are infectious processes and are typically accompanied by systemic complaints, such as fever. Furthermore, neither has a sudden onset as described in this case. Asthma is a chronic condition and is associated with wheezing on auscultation.

21. **C.** This patient describes classic Leriche syndrome with decreased femoral pulses, impotence, and buttock claudication (cramping). More proximal claudication (eg, buttock or thigh)

typically signifies severe aortoiliac disease. Muscle cramping is typically relieved with rest when blood flow is restored to the area. Spinal stenosis typically causes leg pain and weakness and can even occur with standing and sitting in certain positions. Diabetic neuropathy generally is described as a burning pain. A varicocele is a dilatation of the internal spermatic vein, which is described as a "bag of worms" on testicular exam. It is a potential cause of infertility, but not of impotence. Location of the symptoms correlates to the anatomic location of the arterial lesions. Bilateral femoral occlusive disease most commonly corresponds to disease of the distal superficial femoral artery (located just above the knee joint), which corresponds to claudication primarily in the calf, the muscle group just distal to the arterial disease.

22. **E.** A Wells score greater than 6 corresponds to a high probability of having a pulmonary embolism (PE). The Wells score is the most commonly used validated criteria, which was modified in 2001. In this case, the patient's Wells score is 7.5 points: 3 points are accrued with the clinical suspicion of a deep vein thrombosis, 3 points are accrued with tachycardia, and 1.5 points are accrued with the history of a surgery within the last 4 weeks.

23. **B.** This patient is starting to show a degree of mixed acidosis, with a low O_2 concentration and an elevated $Paco_2$, most likely secondary to the anemia from blood loss. A non-rebreather mask is used to deliver 100% oxygen with each breath. For this to occur, the bag attached to the mask must not collapse more than 50%, and in this patient the bag collapses 75%. Therefore, increasing the flow rate of oxygen will allow the bag to fill more and provide a greater oxygen supply. CPAP is a treatment that delivers mild air pressure to keep the airways open; it is typically used by spontaneously breathing patients with conditions such as sleep apnea. It is functionally similar to positive end-expiratory pressure (PEEP), except that PEEP is an applied pressure against exhalation (to keep the pulmonary alveoli open) and CPAP delivers a constant flow of pressure. In this patient, CPAP would not help because there is no indication of airway problems. If the bag was functioning properly to deliver

the expected concentration of oxygen and the blood gas still continued to deteriorate, then mechanical ventilation would need to be considered. Albuterol is a short-acting β_2-adrenergic receptor agonist used for the relief of bronchospasm in conditions such as asthma and chronic obstructive pulmonary disease, which is not this patient's clinical problem.

24. **E.** This patient fits the classic presentation of a spontaneous PTX, which is associated with tall, thin males and absent breath sounds. He is young, so acute coronary syndrome is unlikley. He has no risk factors for a pulmonary embolism. Aortic dissection is associated with chronic hypertension and atherosclerotic disease and occurs most commonly in the sixth and seventh decades of life. Patients typically describe a tearing chest pain. The clinical presentation does not suggest pneumonia, which is associated with fever and crackles on auscultation.

25. **E.** LCIS is not cancer, but it is a marker of risk, so close observation is the correct way to manage these patients. However, some patients might choose to undergo a mastectomy when the statistics regarding the risk of developing cancer over time are discussed with them. Patients with LCIS have a 25% to 30% risk of developing cancer over 15 to 20 years. Irradiation, a mastectomy, or a lumpectomy are initial therapeutic choices offered to patients who have been diagnosed with a malignancy.

26. **B.** Hyponatremia is the most common postoperative electrolyte imbalance. It is generally attributed to dilution of the vascular compartment, typically as a result of the administration of IV fluids.

27. **E.** This patient presents with a strong diagnostic possibility of mesenteric vein thrombosis because she has a hypercoagulable condition and has stopped taking the prescribed anticoagulation therapy. Fluids, CT with contrast, and anticoagulation therapy are indicated first, but serial exams are critical to make sure that there is no clinical deterioration, which would require immediate surgical exploration. Papaverine infusion is used for an arterial occlusion. Heparin and papaverine are incompatible, so they should not be used together.

28. **D.** A thyroglossal duct cyst (TGDC) is a cystic remnant along the course of the thyroglossal duct between the foramen cecum of the tongue base and the thyroid bed in the visceral space of the infrahyoid neck. It presents almost always in children or young adults as a midline anterior neck mass close to the hyoid bone, and it has a typical cystic appearance on ultrasonography. A branchial cyst is located laterally on the neck. Cystic hygromas have cystic spaces separated by septa, which makes it easy to differentiate from a TGDC on imaging. Lipomas have a feathery pattern and bright or hyperechoic areas on ultrasonography. Lymph nodes have an echogenic vascular hilus.

29. **B.** A man does not have enough breast tissue to attempt a lumpectomy, so there is no reason to consider such an alternative. Furthermore, a tumor right under the areola would make breast-conserving surgery quite difficult even in a female patient. A lumpectomy and a segmental mastectomy are the same thing, and there is no place for irradiation instead of surgery in this case because local control is best achieved with complete resection. Neoadjuvant chemotherapy, which can shrink the tumor and possibly achieve systemic control, is usually reserved for patients with advanced local disease who might not be candidates for a primary surgical approach. Neoadjuvant chemotherapy may also be recommended for patients with operable breast cancer who desire breast conservation but the extent of the disease makes surgery technically infeasible. Invasive ductal carcinoma is the most common type of breast cancer.

30. **C.** FAST is best used to detect free fluid in the abdomen or pericardium. At least 200 mL must be present for the test to be effective. Grading of solid organ injury and free air is revealed best by CT scan. Pancreatic transection and mesenteric hematomas may have subtle findings, and therefore are best imaged by CT scanning as well.

31. **B.** The appendix may appear edematous and enlarged, with periappendiceal fluid and mesenteric fat stranding suggesting an inflammatory process. It is unlikely that the appendix will be fully hidden, and a radiopaque fecalith is present only in 4%

to 6% of cases. Lymphadenopathy is not usually described, and the appendix may or may not be covered by omentum. But even if it is, it is likely to be identified as part of the inflammatory response.

32. **C.** The capnograph is a measure of effective ventilation. A normal capnograph reading has a waveform that begins at the baseline, raises steeply, plateaus with a gradual upslope, and quickly returns to the baseline. The end-tidal CO_2 reading in this patient is within the normal range of 35 to 45 mm Hg.

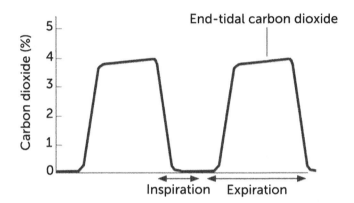

If there is not a defined waveform, the clinician must recognize that there may be an issue with the equipment or that the patient has ceased breathing. Since this is an otherwise healthy patient who continues to breathe, an equipment malfunction or a similar mechanical problem must be assumed. The ventilator high-pressure alarm combined with the loss of the capnograph waveform confirms that the likeliest problem is that the endotracheal tube (ET) has moved out of place. Auscultation can rapidly help to assess the situation. Even if there is a doubt about the patency of the airway, the ET must be removed and the patient's lungs must be ventilated by bag valve mask (BVM), and the airway must be reestablished if indicated. Increasing Fio_2 does not help this situation. Increasing tidal volume could be dangerous because the location of the ET is unknown. Reversing the sedation could be harmful since the airway is not secure. A chest X-ray would show a malpositioned ET, but the priority is to secure the airway and ventilate the patient's lungs.

33. **E.** This patient may develop a recurrent episode of pancreatitis while waiting for surgery, so it is safer to proceed with a cholecystectomy immediately.

34. **C.** The findings of severe pain out of proportion to what is expected for this wound and pain that is also present in uninvolved areas should raise concern for a necrotizing infection. Additionally, given the systemic signs of infection such as fever, necrotizing infection should be highest on the differential. These lesions may be mistaken for necrotizing insect bites, but a high index of suspicion for the possibility of an underlying, severe infection should be maintained. Cellulitis is less likely given the pain to palpation on areas of skin that appears normal. Deep venous thrombosis is not associated with sharp pain and fevers. A foreign body in a wound will have localized symptoms but is seldom associated with the significant systemic response that this patient has.

35. **A.** This finding is suspicious for a muscle sarcoma. A tissue diagnosis obtained from biopsy is important to establish a diagnosis and for multidisciplinary planning. In this situation, given the tumor size, performing a core needle biopsy is more appropriate than attempting surgical excision. If a sarcoma is confirmed, radiation may be considered in an adjuvant or neoadjuvant setting, but it is not appropriate before obtaining a tissue diagnosis. Chemotherapy may also be considered in some circumstances, but it also requires a tissue diagnosis. Surgical resection with sentinel lymph node biopsy is not indicated, because sarcomas do not generally require lymph node sampling, and the same holds true for an axillary node dissection. Common sites of recurrence are local, occurring in the original tissue bed, or distantly in sites such as the lungs.

36. **D.** Obstructive jaundice would most commonly be caused by a pancreatic head mass that was compressing the distal common bile duct. None of the other lesions would usually present with jaundice.

37. **D.** Diverticular disease complicated by a colovesical fistula is the most likely cause of this patient's symptoms. Inflammatory

conditions such as diverticular disease can cause a connection to form between the bowel and the bladder, which allows bacteria and air to enter the bladder. Bladder cancer most commonly presents with hematuria, and cystitis presents with lower abdominal pain with or without hematuria. Neither is associated with a fistula into the bowel. Colon cancer may induce formation of a fistula, but such a presentation is quite uncommon. Prostatic cancer is associated with back pain, hematuria, and urinary retention and is seldom associated with a rectal fistula.

38. **A.** The most common causes of pancreatitis are gallstones and alcohol use. Therefore, in this patient, gallstones are the most likely cause of this episode of acute pancreatitis. An ultrasound of the right upper quadrant is the best imaging study to diagnose cholelithiasis. More than 80% of gallstones are composed of cholesterol, but ordering a cholesterol panel would not change management. This patient has no history of illicit drug use, and furthermore, results of a drug toxicology screen would not change the need for an ultrasound. A CT scan may be used to confirm pancreatitis, but it is not used to diagnose cholelithiasis. An ERCP may visualize gallstones, but it is an invasive test with considerably more risk than an ultrasound. It is performed if there is suspicion of stones in the common bile duct, not to diagnose cholelithiasis.

39. **E.** Although an obstetrician should be consulted, an exploratory laparotomy should not be delayed in a patient like this, who is hemodynamically unstable and has not responded to fluid resuscitation. Optimal care of the fetus involves prompt resuscitation and treatment of the mother. Obtaining imaging studies and performing diagnostic procedures can wait until after this patient has been stabilized.

40. **C.** A CT scan is the best first test to localize a neuroendocrine tumor such as a gastrinoma. Gastrinomas appear hyperdense (brighter) on CT scan compared to surrounding tissue. They are generally found in the pancreatic head or in the duodenum. An endoscopic ultrasound is usually ordered after a CT scan to obtain a biopsy. If the CT scan does not identify the tumor,

an endoscopic ultrasound may be able to locate it. Octreotide scans may also be used if the CT scan is negative. An abdominal ultrasound and ERCP would not be helpful in locating the lesion.

41. **D.** Although the patient has hematuria, in the presence of back pain, hypotension, a low hemoglobin level, and a pulsatile abdominal mass, a ruptured AAA is most likely. Nephrolithiasis is associated with severe back pain, but it is not associated with a low hemoglobin level. Decreased pedal pulses could be attributed to peripheral vascular disease in different circumstances, but in the presence of shock pulses are uniformly decreased. The anemia is most likely not a result of a gastrointestinal bleed, which is associated with blood in the stool. Mesenteric ischemia is seldom associated with a pulsatile abdominal mass, and back pain as a presenting symptom is most uncommon.

42. **C.** Lymphedema is a common postsurgical complication that can occur after lymph node dissection. The incidence can be as high as 30% with complete lymphatic basin resection. Hyperhidrosis is excessive sweating. Although hydrostatic pressures may be involved in the etiology of lymphedema, this is not the proper terminology for this diagnosis. Reflexive sympathetic dystrophy is a rare regional pain syndrome and is not a common side effect of lymphatic resection. This is not the typical presentation of DVT.

43. **B.** Lower GI tract bleeding in children under 2 years originates from a Meckel's diverticulum in 50% of cases, and a nuclear scan is quite specific in localizing the lesion, although it is not highly sensitive. Scan results are positive when the gastric mucosa secretes pertechnetate Tc 99m in the same manner it secretes chloride, which accumulates in the diverticulum and allows detection. An umbilical sinus is an infrequent finding, perhaps seen in 10% of patients with a Meckel's diverticulum. This sinus is usually associated with a tract that must be removed to prevent intestinal obstruction. Radiographic studies of the upper GI tract are not helpful in diagnosing a suspected acute bleeding episode in the lower GI tract, because it is most

unlikely that they will demonstrate a diverticulum, and it obscures visibility of other tests. An ultrasonography and a plain abdominal radiograph are unhelpful as well. A CT scan is rarely used to diagnose Meckel's diverticulum.

44. **D.** This patient might have acute mesenteric ischemia following the aneurysm repair, which is likely to have occluded the inferior mesenteric artery. A colonoscopy might demonstrate areas of mucosal ischemia. An angiography, which would determine if there is an arterial occlusion, is not indicated at this time because the aneurysm repair was performed by placing a graft, and it would be unsafe to run a catheter through the repair this early in the postoperative period. A rigid sigmoidoscope cannot reach proximal affected areas. A CT scan could help if the patient has full bowel necrosis, but at this time the clinical presentation suggests a lesser degree of damage, and a colonoscopy could confirm the diagnosis and guide treatment strategy. An MRI is not indicated.

45. **A.** Ultrasonography does not help in the diagnosis of nonocclusive mesenteric ischemia (NOMI) and is a second-line study in other types of acute mesenteric ischemia. NOMI may be diagnosed with CT scan with contrast, angiography, CTA, and MRA. CTA combines the technology of a conventional CT with angiography.

46. **D.** Papillary and follicular carcinomas are classified as well-differentiated thyroid cancers. Radioactive iodine I 131 is useful in treating well-differentiated cancers of the thyroid. When administered after a total thyroidectomy, iodine I 131 serves 2 purposes. First, it will ablate any small remnants of thyroid tissue left behind during thyroidectomy. More importantly however, it will be taken up by well-differentiated thyroid cancer cells that have retained their ability to take up and process iodine and subsequently destroy them as well. This "targeted therapy" allows treatment of metatstatic disease with minimal toxicity to other tissues, making it an attractive adjuvant treatment for these tumors. Medullary and anaplastic carcinomas are not well differentiated and are not amenable to treatment with radioactive iodine I 131 therapy.

47. **B.** SIMV delivers a minimum number of fully assisted breaths per minute that are synchronized with the patient's respiratory effort. These mandatory breaths are patient-triggered, flow-limited, and volume-cycled. However, any breaths taken between volume-cycled breaths are not assisted, and the volumes of these breaths are determined by the patient's strength, effort, and lung mechanics. Therefore, a patient receiving SIMV assistance may breathe spontaneously as often as they need to. When the RR becomes as high as it is in this patient, breathing may lead to hyperventilation. This is the case in this patient in whom the $Paco_2$ has decreased to 35 mm Hg (reference range: 35–45 mm Hg). To make the breathing more efficient, the SIMV rate must be increased. SIMV allows the patient to exercise their respiratory musculature while on the ventilator by allowing spontaneous breaths and less ventilator support. High respiratory rates on SIMV allow little time for spontaneous breathing, whereas low respiratory rates allow for the opposite. However, this equilibrium must be carefully gauged, because SIMV may increase the work of breathing and cause respiratory muscle fatigue, which would decrease the possibility of future weaning and extubation. Modifying the concentration of delivered oxygen doesn't affect the RR. SIRS is a nonspecific clinical response that can be caused by ischemia, inflammation, trauma, infection, or a combination of insults. It is defined as 2 or more of the following variables: fever greater than 38°C or less than 36°C; heart rate greater than 90 bpm; RR greater than 20 breaths per minute or $Paco_2$ less than 32 mm Hg; white blood cell count greater than $12,000/mm^3$ or less than $4000/mm^3$; or greater than 10% immature forms (bands).

48. **E.** The most important aspect of infection control with necrotizing fasciitis is rapid surgical débridement. Aggressive wound management is inadequate treatment for a necrotizing tissue infection, as is antibiotic irrigation. Intravenously administered antibiotics are an important element of treatment but are not as critical as surgical débridement. Orally administered antibiotics are insufficient in the majority of cases.

49. **E.** Cystinuria is an autosomal-recessive disease. The genetic defect impairs intestinal absorption and renal reabsorption

of cystine, causing elevated urinary levels of cystine and subsequent crystallization and stone formation. Patients with cystinuria usually present with renal colic. Urinalysis may show typical hexagonal or benzene crystals, which are essentially pathognomonic of cystinuria. Microscopic crystalluria is present in 30% to 80% of patients. Cystine is one of the sulfur-containing amino acids; therefore, the urine may have the characteristic odor of rotten eggs. Cystine stones are pale yellow and have a homogeneous or ground-glass appearance on radiographs. Although radiopaque, they are often less dense than calcium-containing stones.

50. **A.** This patient presents with familial adenomatous polyposis, a condition where the *APC* gene mutation can be detected in more than 90% of cases. This patient must have a total colectomy; otherwise colon cancer will develop, most commonly before age 40 years. *MLH1* is mutated in Lynch syndrome, or *hereditary nonpolyposis colorectal cancer*. *STK11* is diagnostic of Peutz-Jeghers syndrome. *BRCA2* is found in hereditary breast cancer, and *Neurofibromin 1* is responsible for neurofibromatosis.

Index

A

Abdominal pain,
  algorithm 320–323
Abdominal wall, anatomy
  and physiology 289–291,
  289f, 290f, 291f
Abscess, pancreatic 269, 270
Achalasia 88–89
Acid-base abnormalities 11,
  15, 15t
Adenomas
  adrenal 66
  intestinal 200, 214
Adhesions 195
Adrenals, anatomy and
  physiology 65, 65f
Adrenal hyperplasia,
  idiopathic 66
Adrenal insufficiency,
  acute 67–68
Adrenal mass, incidental 70–71
Aldosteronism, primary 66–67
Alpha-blockers
  pheochromocytoma 70
  renal stones 304
Alpha-fetoprotein 311
Ampulla of Vater 251, 251f, 265, 266f
Amylase 267
Anal fissure 233–234
Anesthesia 8
  local 8
  general 8–9
  induction 8
  maintenance 8
  physiologic
    monitoring 9–10
  regional 8
Aneurysm
  abdominal aortic 167–170, 168f, 170t
  CTA with contrast 166, 169
  thoracic 165–167, 166f, 167t
  thoracic rupture 167
Angiodysplasia,
  colonic 216–217
Angiography 159, 216
Ankle brachial index
  (ABI) 163, 164t
Anoscopy 233
Antibiotics, prophylactic 10
Antidiuretic hormone 12
Aortic dissection 106, 150–152
  classification 150, 150f
APC gene 215
Apudoma 200
Appendicitis 205–206
Argentaffin cells 200
Arrhythmias 36
ASA physical status 7t
Ascaris lumbricoides 256
Ascites 241, 242
Atelectasis 32, 33
Atherosclerosis 142, 158, 160
Atypical ductal
  hyperplasia 117, 119
Atypical lobular
  hyperplasia 117, 119

B

Bacteria in surgical
  procedures 11t
Bacteroides fragilis 259
Barrett's esophagus 85–86
Basal cell carcinoma 128–129
Beta-blockers
  pheochromocytoma 70
  variceal bleeding 242
Biliary colic 252
Biliary dyskinesia 253
Biliary stent 276
Biliary system,
  anatomy 251, 251f
Billroth I and II
  operations 186
Biopsy
  core 123
  fine needle aspiration
    (FNA) 54, 118
Bladder cancer 306–307
Bladder washings 307
Blumberg's sign 205, 341
Boerhaave's syndrome 89
BRAF gene 32
BRCA genes 119, 120t
Breast
  anatomy and
    physiology 113–116,
    113f, 114f, 115f
  hormonal effects 116f
  milk lines 115, 115f
  lymphatic drainage 114f
  tail of Spence 114f
Breast calcifications 124
Breast cancer 119–125
  adjuvant
    chemotherapy 125
  inflammatory breast
    cancer 123
  invasive ductal breast
    cancer 122
Breast cancer risk 120t, 121t

Breast conserving
   surgery 124
Breast disease, benign 117–119
   cysts 117, 118
   fibrocystic disease (FD) 117
Breast pain 117
Budd-Chiari syndrome 238

C

CA 19–9 270, 275
Calcifications
   breast 124
   thyroid 54
Calcitonin 74
Calot's triangle 251, 251f
Cancer
   basal cell carcinoma 128–129
   bladder 306–307
   breast 119–125
   colorectal 224–227, 226f, 227f
   esophageal 87–88
   gallbladder 259–260
   gastric 189–191
   hepatocellular 246–247
   lung 100–104
   pancreatic 274–277, 275f, 276f, 277f
   prostate 307–308
   renal 305–306
   testicular 311
   thyroid 53–55
Carcinoembryonic antigen 225, 270
Carcinoid tumor 200, 201
   syndrome 200
Cardiac diagnostic testing 141, 142t
Cardiac risk 3t, 5
Carotid artery occlusive disease 158–160
   bruit 158
   duplex scanning 159
   endarterectomy 160
   mortality 159
   neurologic deficits 159, 160
   treatment 159–160
Cerebrovascular accidents (CVA) 158
Charcot's triad 258, 344
Child-Pugh score 239, 240t, 241t
Cholangiocarcinoma 260–262
Cholangitis 258–259
   suppurative 258
Cholecystectomy 253, 269
Cholecystitis 253–256, 256f
   acalculous 253, 254
   emphysematous 255
   empyema 255
   Murphy's sign 254, 255
   perforation 255
   ultrasound 254, 255, 256f
Choledocholithiasis 256–257, 258f
Cholelithiasis 252–253
Chromogranin A 273
Chvostek's sign 14
Cilostazol 164
Cinacalcet 61
Cirrhosis 238
Claudication 162
Clonorchis sinensis 256
Clostridium difficile 219, 221, 223
Colon ischemia 222–223
Colon, rectum and anus, anatomy 203–204, 203f, 204fColonic polyps 213–216, 213f, 214t
Colonic pseudoobstruction (Ogilvie's syndrome) 228, 230
Colonoscopy 215, 219, 221, 225
Complications, perioperative 5
Complications, postoperative 31
   arrhythmias 36
   atelectasis 32–33
   dehiscence 42–43
   fever 32t
   mnemonic 31
   myocardial infarction 35
   pneumonia 33–34
   prevention 10
   procedure specific 43
   pulmonary embolism 40–41
   surgical site infections 41–42
   timing of complications 32t
   urinary 37–38
   venous thromboembolism (VTE) 38–41
Contusion, pulmonary 102
Cooper's ligaments 113f
Coronary arteries 139, 139f, 140f
Coronary artery disease 142–144, 143f
   coronary angioplasty 144
   coronary artery bypass grafting 144
   percutaneous coronary intervention 144
Courvoisier's sign 261
Cowden's disease 215
Crohn's disease 206, 220–222
CTA (Computed Tomography Angiogram) 166
   spiral 172
Cullen's sign 267, 344
Cushing's syndrome 70
Cystectomy 307
Cystic artery 251, 251f
Cystine stones 303
Cystinuria 303, 304

D

Deep vein thrombosis 38–40, 170–175, 173t
   treatment 174
Dehiscence 42–43
Dentate line 233
Dexamethasone suppression test 70
Digital subtraction angiography (DSA) 159
Diverticular disease 206–

213, 208f, 209t
  bleeding 211–212, 213
  complications 208
  diverticulitis, Hinchey
    stages 209–210, 209t
  natural history 208f
Dopamine agonists 72
Ductal carcinoma in situ
  (DCIS) 122, 124f
Dysphagia 86, 87, 88
Dysplasia
  esophageal 86
  endoscopic ablation 86

E

Echocardiography 147
  transesophageal
    (TEE) 141
  transthoracic (TTE) 141
Endarterectomy. *See* carotid
  artery occlusive disease
Endoscopic retrograde
  cholangiopancreatography
  (ERCP) 257, 258f, 258,
  259, 266
Endovascular
  intervention 164
Epididymis 302f
Escherichia coli 254, 259
Esophagogastric variceal
  bleeding 242–244
Esophagus
  anatomy and
    physiology 81, 81f
  manometry 89
  pneumatic dilatation 89
Esophagus, Barrett's 85–86
Esophageal cancer 87–88
Esophageal perforation 89–91
Esophageal sphincters 81, 81f
Esophagitis 85
Estrogen receptors 124
External inguinal ring 290f, 291, 291f

F

Falciform ligament 237f

Familial adenomatous
  polyposis 215
Fever 32t
Fibroadenomas 117, 118, 119
Fine needle aspiration (FNA)
  thyroid 48, 49, 54
Fine needle aspiration biopsy
  (FNAB), breast 118
Fluids and electrolytes 11–16
  concentration in body
    fluids 13t
  hypocalcemia,
    hypercalcemia 14
  hypokalemia,
    hyperkalemia 14
  hypomagnesemia,
    hypermagnesemia 14
  hyponatremia,
    hypernatremia 14
  losses 13, 13t
  water compartments 12f
Focal nodular hyperplasia,
  liver 244
Fournier's gangrene 133–135

G

Gallbladder carcinoma 259–260
Gallstone ileus 255
Gardner's syndrome 215
Gastrectomy 189, 191
Gastric cancer 189–191
Gastric hormones 183t
Gastric ulcer types 184, 186f
Gastrin 188, 189
Gastrinoma 73, 187, 188, 271, 272t
Gastroesophageal reflux
  disease (GERD) 82–84, 90
  barium swallow 83
  hiatal hernia types 82, 82f, 83f
Gastrojejunostomy 276
GI bleeding, algorithm 324–326
GIST tumors 200
Glucagonoma 272t

Grey-Turner's sign 267
Goiter 57–58, 59f
  toxic nodular 51
Granuloma 97, 115, 221
Graves' disease 51

H

Hamartoma 74, 97
Hartmann's pouch 251f
Heart, anatomy 139–140, 139f, 140f
Hemangioma, liver 244, 245
Hematochezia 211, 217
Hematuria 304, 307
Hemoptysis 99–100
Hemorrhoids 232–233
Hepatectomy 247
Hepatic abscess 259
Hepatic
  encephalopathy 241, 242
Hepatic venous pressure
  gradient 239
Hepatic wedge pressure 240
Hepatomegaly 246
Her2/neu receptors 124
Hereditary non-polyposis
  colorectal cancer (Lynch
  syndrome) 225
Hernia 292–295
  direct 291f, 292
  epigastric 294
  femoral 291f, 292
  hiatal. *See also*
    gastroesophageal reflux
    disease
  incarcerated 293, 294f
  indirect 291f, 292
  Littré 295
  pantaloon 292
  processus vaginalis 292
  recurrent 293
  Richter's 295
  sliding 295
  spigelian 295
  strangulated 293, 294f
  umbilical 294
Hesselbach's triangle 290f, 292
Hiatal hernia, types 82, 82f, 83f

HIDA (hepato-iminodiacetic acid) scanning 253
Hinchey stages of diverticulitis 209t
History and physical 3–4, 4t
Hollenhorst plaques 158
Homan's sign 171
Horner's syndrome 101
H. pylori 183, 185, 189
Hydrocele 312
Hypercalcemic crisis 60
Hyperparathyroidism 59–61, 60f
  causes and treatment 62t
  ultrasound 60
Hypersplenism 285
Hyperthermia, malignant 9
Hyperthyroidism 51–53

I

IgG antiplatelet 282
Ileus 196
Immune thrombocytopenic purpura 282–284
Immunoglobulin 284
Incidentaloma, adrenal 70–71
Inferior epigastric vessels 291f, 292
Inferior mesenteric artery (IMA) 204f
Inflammatory bowel disease
  Crohn's disease 220–222
  ulcerative colitis 217–220, 218t
Infliximab 222
Inguinal hernia. See hernia
Insulinoma 271, 272t
Internal fistulas 222
Internal inguinal ring 290f, 291f, 292
Intraductal papillary mucinous tumors (IPMTs) 270
Intraductal papilloma of breast 118
Intraoperative cholangiogram 257
Intravenous pyelography

(IVP) 304
Ischemic colitis 222–223
IVC (inferior vena cava) filter 174

J

Jaundice 257, 258, 261, 269
  algorithm 316–319
Jejunum 193
Juvenile polyp 214t

K

Kallikrein 200
Keratoses, actinic 129
Klatskin tumor 261
Klebsiella pneumonia 254, 259, 303
Kultchitsky cells 200

L

Lactulose 242
LaPlace law 230, 343
Large bowel obstruction 227–230, 229f
Leriche syndrome 162
LeVeen shunt 242
Levothyroxine 55, 57
Limb ischemia, algorithm 327–330
Linea alba 289f
Linea semilunaris 295
Lipase 267
Liver and portal system, anatomy 237, 237f
Liver tumors
  benign 244–246
  malignant 246–247
Lobular carcinoma in situ (LCIS) 119, 122
Lumpectomy 124
Lung
  anatomy 95–96, 95f, 96f
  granuloma 97
Lung cancer 100–104
  common lung cancers 101t

paraneoplastic syndromes 102t
pleural effusion, malignant 122
Lynch syndrome 225

M

Magnetic resonance imaging (MRI) 245
Mackler's triad 90, 339
Magnetic resonance imaging, cardiac 141, 143
Magnetic resonance pancreatography (MRCP) 267
Mallory-Weiss syndrome 186–187, 341
Mammogram 118, 124
Marginal artery of Drummond 204f
Manometry, esophageal 89
Meckel's diverticulum, diverticulitis 198–199, rule of 2s 198, 341
Melanoma 130–133, 132t, 133f
  ABCDs 130
  biopsy 131
  Breslow's thickness 131, 133t
  lymphoscintigraphy 132
Menin, MEN1 gene 73
Mesenteric ischemia 211, 222, 223
  algorithm 331–335
Metronidazole 242
Mohs micrographic surgery 128, 130
Multiple endocrine neoplasia, (MEN) I and II 72–75, 188
  marfanoid habitus 74
  medullary thyroid cancer 73, 74
  MIBG scan 75
  multifocal tumors 73
  types 72
Murphy's sign 254, 255, 344
Mycetoma 97, 102

Myocardial infarction 35

N

Nasogastric suction 198
Necrotizing fasciitis 133–135
Necrotizing infections 32t
Needle thoracostomy 107
Nephrectomy 306
Nephrolithiasis 303–305, 305f
Neuroendocrine tumors 271–274, 272t, 273f
Nipple discharge 118
Nocturia 308
Nutrition, in wound healing 22–23

O

Obstruction
 biliary 276
 large bowel 227–230
 small bowel 195–198
Obturator sign 205, 342
Octreotide 201, 244
Ogilvie's syndrome (pseudoobstruction) 228, 230
Oral contraceptives 244
Orchiectomy 311
Orchyopexy 310
Orphan Annie eye nuclei 54
Osmolality 12
Overwhelming postsplenectomy infection 286–287

P

Paget's disease, breast 123
Pancoast tumor 101
Pancreas, anatomy 265, 265f
Pancreatic
 adenocarcinoma 274–277, 275f, 276f, 277f
 chemotherapy 276
 Courvoisier's sign 274
 mortality 274
 radiation therapy 276
Pancreatic lymphoma 275
Pancreatic neuroendocrine tumors 271–274, 272t, 273f
Pancreatitis, acute 266–269, 266f, 268t
Pancreatic pseudocyst 269–271, 270f
Pancytopenia 285
Papilloma of breast, intraductal 118
Paracentesis 242
Paraneoplastic syndrome 102t
Parathyroid glands 47, 47f
Peptic ulcer disease 183–186, 186f
 H. pylori 183, 185
 upper GI endoscopy 184, 185
Percutaneous transhepatic cholangiography (PTC) 259, 261
Perforation, esophageal 89–91
Pericardial effusion 172
Pericardiocentesis 154
Pericarditis 152–154
Perioperative physiologic monitoring 9–10
Peripheral vascular disease 160–165, 161f, 163t, 164t, 165f
 claudication 162
 rest pain 162
Pernicious anemia 188
Peutz-Jeghers syndrome 214t, 215
Pheochromocytoma 68–70, 74
 rule of 10s 69, 339
Pleural effusion, malignant 103
Pleurodesis 103, 107
Pneumococcal vaccine 286, 287
Pneumonia 33–34
Pneumothorax
 classification and causes 105t
 recurrent 107
 primary 105
 secondary 123
 spontaneous 104–107
 tension 106f, 107
Polyps, colonic 213–216
Porcelain gallbladder 259
Portal hypertension 238–242
Postoperative care 11–16
 acid-base abnormalities 15t
Postoperative complications See complications 31
Postsplenectomy infection, overwhelming 286–287
Prehn's sign 309, 345
Preoperative care 3–7
 intraoperative care 8–10
 preoperative questionnaire 4
 preoperative testing 6
Progesterone receptors 124
Prolactin level 72
Prolactinoma 71–72
Prostate cancer 307–308
Prostate-specific antigen (PSA) 308
Proton pump inhibitors (PPIs) 85, 185, 189
Psammoma bodies 54
Pseudomembranous enterocolitis 219
Pseudopolyps 219
Psoas sign 205, 342
Pulmonary bleb 104
Pulmonary contusion 102
Pulmonary embolism 40–41, 105–106, 172–175
Pulmonary nodule, solitary 97–99, 98f

R

Radial scar 123
Radioactive iodine (RAI) 52, 55
Ranson's criteria 267, 268t

Rectal cancer 224–227
Recurrent laryngeal
 nerve 47f
Renal cell carcinoma
 (RCC) 305–306
Renal stones. *See*
 nephrolithiasis
RET gene 73, 74
Reynold's pentad 258, 344
Rib fractures 106
Riedel's struma 56
Risk
 anesthesia 6
 ASA class 7t
 cardiac 5, 3t
 Goldman criteria 5
 perioperative 5–6
 specific factors 5–6
Rovsing's sign 205, 342
Rubber banding of
 esophageal varices 244

S

Sclerotherapy 244
Segmental mastectomy
 (lumpectomy) 124
Sentinel node
 breast 125
 melanoma 132
Signs and syndromes 339–345
Sister Mary Joseph's
 node 190, 274
Skin, anatomy 127, 127f
 melanocytes 127f, 130
Small bowel capsule
 endoscopy 201
Small bowel
 obstruction 195–198
 air fluid levels 197, 197f
 fluid resuscitation 198
Small intestine,
 anatomy 193–194, 193f, 194f
Solitary pulmonary
 nodule 97–99
Somatostatinoma 272t
Spectrin 284
Spermatic cord 290f, 291f, 292, 294f

Spermatocele 312
Spherocytosis,
 hereditary 284–285
Sphincter of Oddi 251f
Sphincterotomy,
 endoscopic 257
Spironolactone 242
Splenectomy 284
 and sepsis 286–287
 indications 283t
Splenomegaly 285–286
Spleen, anatomy 281, 281f
Squamous cell
 carcinoma 129–130
Staghorn calculus 303
Stomach and duodenum
 anatomy 181–183, 181f
 gastric cells 182t
 gastric hormones 183t
String sign 222
Struvite stones 303
Stroke 158, 159
Superior mesenteric artery
 (SMA) 204f
Syndrome of apparent
 mineralocorticoid
 excess 66

T

Technetium scan 212
Testicular cancer 311
Testicular torsion 309–310, 310f
Thumbprinting 223
Thyroid anatomy 47, 47f
Thyroid cancer 53–55
 familial medullary 73, 74
Thyroid cytopathology 50t
Thyroidectomy 50, 54
Thyroid disease,
 inflammatory 55–57
Thyroiditis 55–57
 Hashimoto's 55
 de Quervain 55
 acute suppurative 55–56
 invasive fibrous (Riedel's struma) 56
 chronic lymphocytic (Hashimoto's) 55
Thyroid lobectomy 50

Thyroid nodule 48–50
 ultrasound 49f
Thyroid storm 52–53
Thyroxine (T_4) 47
TIA (transient ischemic
 attack) 158
TNM staging
 definitions 104t
Toxic megacolon 220
Transesophageal
 echocardiography
 (TEE) 141
Transitional cell carcinoma
 (TCC) 307
Transjugular intrahepatic
 portosystemic shunt
 (TIPS) 244
Transthoracic
 echocardiography
 (TTE) 141
Transurethral resection
 (TUR) 307
Triangle of Calot 251f
Trousseau's sign 14
Tuberculosis 97, 99, 102
Tube thoracostomy 107

U

Ulcerative colitis 217–220, 218t
Ultrasound
 abdominal aortic 169
 breast 119
 carotid 159
 endoscopic 87
 hepatic 240
 peripheral vascular 162
 parathyroid 60
 scrotal 311
 thyroid 48, 49, 49f, 54, 49f
 transrectal 308
Urea breath test 185
Urease assay 184
Urease producing
 organisms 303
Uric acid stones 303
Urinary complications
 infection 37–38
 retention 37

Urologic problems,
  anatomy 301–302, 301f, 302f

V

Vagotomy, types 186
Valvular disease
  aortic and mitral 144–149
  etiology 145, 146f
  murmurs 147
  treatment 148–149
Variceal bleeding 241, 242, 242–244
Variceal rubber band ligation 244
Varicocele 312
Vascular anatomy 157, 157f
Vas deferens 302, 302f
Venous thromboembolism (VTE) 170–175
  Homan's sign 171
  incidence 171
VIPoma 272t
Virchow's node(s) 190, 274
Volvulus 230–232, 231f
Von Hippel-Lindau syndrome 74, 271, 305

W

Water, total body 11, 12t
Wells score 172, 173t
Westermark's sign 172
Whipple procedure 274, 276, 277f
Whipple triad 344
Wilms' tumor 305
Wound care 23
  classification of surgical wounds 24–25, 25t
  closure techniques 27, 28f
  timing of closure 26
  types of wounds 23, 24t
Wound healing 17
  phases 17–20, 21f,
  cellular activity of wound healing 20t
  factors affecting healing 21–23
  types of wounds 23–25, 24t, 25t
  types of wound healing 25–26
Wound infection 41–42
Wound management 26–28, 28f

Z

Zollinger-Ellison syndrome (ZES) 187–189, 341
  gastrin levels 188
  gastrinoma 73, 187
  gastrinoma triangle 188

CPSIA information can be obtained at www.ICGtesting.com
Printed in the USA
LVOW05s0356180915

454422LV00002B/4/P

9 780991 316908